Principles of Pediatric Neurosurgery

Series Editor: Anthony J. Raimondi

Principles of Pediatric Neurosurgery

Head Injuries in the Newborn and Infant

The Pediatric Spine I: Development and Dysraphic State
The Pediatric Spine II: Developmental Anomalies
The Pediatric Spine III: Cysts, Tumors, and Infections

Cerebrovascular Diseases in Children

Intracranial Cyst Lesions

Posterior Fossa Tumors

Edited by Anthony J. Raimondi, Maurice Choux,
and Concezio Di Rocco

Posterior Fossa Tumors

Edited by Anthony J. Raimondi,
Maurice Choux, and Concezio Di Rocco

With 86 Figures

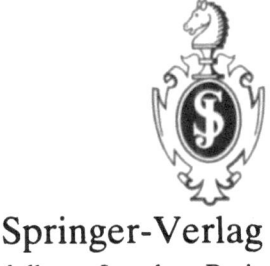

Springer-Verlag
New York Berlin Heidelberg London Paris
Tokyo Hong Kong Barcelona Budapest

ANTHONY J. RAIMONDI, M.D. University of Rome, "La Sapienza,"
30 Viale dell'Università, Rome, Italy

MAURICE CHOUX, M.D., Hôpital des Enfantes de la Timone, Rue Sainte
Pierre, 13005 Marseille, France

CONCEZIO DI ROCCO, M.D., Istituto di Neurochirurgia, Università Cattolica
del Sacre Cuore, Largo Gemelli 8, 00168 Rome, Italy

Library of Congress Cataloging-in-Publication Data
Posterior fossa tumors / [edited by] Anthony J. Raimondi, Maurice Choux, Concezio
  Di Rocco.
      p.   cm.—(Principles of pediatric neurosurgery)
    Includes bibliographical references and index.
    ISBN 0-387-97915-8.—ISBN 3-540-97915-8
    1. Cranial fossa, Posterior—Tumors—Surgery. 2. Cranial fossa,
  Posterior—Tumors. 3. Intracranial tumors in children.
  I. Raimondi, Anthony J., 1928– . II. Choux, M. (Maurice) III. Di
  Rocco, C. (Concezio) IV. Series.
      [DNLM: 1. Brain Neoplasms—in infancy & childhood. 2. Cranial
  Fossa, Posterior.]
  RD663.P68 1993
  618.92'9948059—dc20
DNLM/DLC
for Library of Congress   92-49986

Printed on acid-free paper.

Production managed by Terry Kornak; manufacturing supervised by Vincent Scelta.
Typeset by Asco Trade Typesetting Ltd, North Point, Hong Kong.
Printed and bound by Edwards Brothers, Inc., Ann Arbor, Michigan.

9 8 7 6 5 4 3 2 1

ISBN-13: 978-1-4613-9301-6   e-ISBN-13: 978-1-4613-9299-6
DOI: 10.1007/978-1-4613-9299-6

Series Preface

It is estimated that the functionally significant body of knowledge for a given medical specialty changes radically every 8 years. New specialties and "sub-specialization" are occurring at approximately an equal rate. Historically, established journals have not been able either to absorb this increase in publishable material or to extend their readership to the new specialists. International and national meetings, symposia and seminars, workshops, and newsletters successfully bring to the attention of physicians within developing specialties what is occurring, but generally only in demonstration form without providing historical perspective, pathoanatomical correlates, or extensive discussion. Page and time limitations oblige the authors to present only the essence of their material.

Pediatric neurosurgery is an example of a specialty that has developed during the past 15 years. Over this period neurosurgeons have obtained special training in pediatric neurosurgery and then dedicated themselves primarily to its practice. Centers, Chairs, and educational programs have been established as groups of neurosurgeons in different countries throughout the world organized themselves respectively into national and international societies for pediatric neurosurgery. These events were both preceded and followed by specialized courses, national and international journals, and ever-increasing clinical and investigative studies into all aspects of surgically treatable diseases of the child's nervous system.

Principles of Pediatric Neurosurgery is an ongoing series of publications, each dedicated exclusively to a particular subject, a subject which is currently timely either because of an extensive amount of work occurring in it, or because it has been neglected. The two first subjects, "Head Injuries in the Newborn and Infant" and "The Pediatric Spine," are expressive of those extremes.

Volumes will be published continuously, as the subjects are dealt with, rather than on an annual basis, since our goal is to make this information available to the specialist when it is new and informative. If a volume becomes obsolete because of newer methods of treatment and concepts, we shall publish a new edition.

The chapters are selected and arranged to provide the reader, in each instance, with embryological, developmental, epidemiological, clinical, therapeutic, and psychosocial aspects of each subject, thus permitting each specialist to learn what is most current in his field and to familiarize himself with sister fields of the same subject. Each chapter is organized along classical lines, progressing from introduction through symptoms and treatment, to prognosis for clinical material; and introduction through history and data, to results and discussion for experimental material.

Contents

Contributors

PETER W. ASCHER, M.D.
University of Graz, 8036 Graz, Austria

OLIVIER BERTRAND
INSERM, Brain Signals and Processing Laboratory, Lyon, France

ERICA CIRO, R.N., BSN
Department of Pediatric Neurosurgery, Loyola University of Chicago Medical Center, Maywood, IL 60153, U.S.A.

CATHERINE FISCHER, M.D.
Hôpital Neurologique, Lyon, France

FLEMMING GJERRIS, M.D.
Department of Neurosurgery NK, Rigshosptalet, 2100 Copenhagen, Denmark

FILIPPO GULLOTTA, M.D.
Institut für Neuropathologie der Universität Münster, 4400 Münster, Federal Republic of Germany

JENS HAASE, M.D.
Department of Neurosurgery, Aalborg Sygehus Syd, 9100 Aalborg, Denmark

YOON SUN HAHN, M.D.
Loyola University Medical Center, Maywood, IL 60153, USA

ELIZABETH HOPPE-HIRSCH, M.D.
Servica de Neurochirurgie Pédiatrique, 75730 Paris, France

JEAN-FRANCOIS HIRSCH, M.D.
19, Avenue des Sycomores, 75016 Paris, France

ALESSANDRO MAURO, M.D.
Clinica Neurologica II, Università di Torino, 10126 Torino, Italy

PH. MEYER, M.D.
Hôpital Necker-Enfants Malades, Service de Neurochirurgie Pédiatrique, Paris, France

H. STACY NICHOLSON, M.D.
Department of Hematology-Oncology, Children's National Medical Center, Washington, D.C. 20010-2970, USA

ROGER J. PACKER, M.D.
Department of Neurology, Children's National Medical Center, Washington, D.C. 20010-2970, USA

IGNACIO PASCUAL-CASTROVIEJO, M.D.
Servicio de Neurologia, Hospital Infantil "La Paz," 28046 Madrid, Spain

ANTHONY J. RAIMONDI, M.D.
University of Rome, "La Sapienza," 30 Viale dell'Università, Rome, Italy

JOHN R. RUGE, M.D.
619 N. Oak Park Avenue, Oak Park, IL 60302, USA; and Department of Pediatric Neurosurgery, Lutheran General Children's Medical Center, Children's Memorial Hospital, Chicago, IL, USA

JANIS RYAN, MSN
Department of Oncology and Neurology, Children's National Medical Center, Washington, D.C. 20010-2970, USA

PROF. DAVIDE SCHIFFER
Istituto di Clinica delle Malattie del Sistema Nervoso, Clinica Neurologica II, 10126 Torino, Italy

D. SUHR, M.D.
Neurochirurgische Klinik, Krankenhaus Nordstadt, 3000 Hannover 1, Federal Republic of Germany

H. VON GÖSSELN, M.D.
Neurochirurgische Klinik, Krankenhaus Nordstadt, 3000 Hannover 1, Federal Republic of Germany

ROBERT A. ZIMMERMAN, M.D.
Children's Hospital of Philadelphia, Philadelphia, PA 19104, USA

CHAPTER 1

Epidemiology and Classification of Posterior Fossa Tumors in Children

Flemming Gjerris

Treatment of malignant brain tumors in children is a challenge for neurosurgeons, pediatricians, and neuro-oncologists. Important to this treatment is a thorough knowledge of the frequency and taxonomy of brain tumors. The classification has changed during the last five decades from a pure cellular description to a clinical and prognostic neuropathological division.[1-4] During the last 20 years the prognosis of brain tumors in children has not improved very much, only in certain subgroups, in contrast to the general improvement in cancer in childhood (Table 1.1).

Intracranial tumors in children are the second most common type of tumor after leukemia; their rate of occurrence is about 25%.[5-7] In adults, brain tumors only constitute 3% of all malignancies.[8] Figures from cancer registry studies are dependent on the rate of notification, which is high in many European countries. It is also influenced by different coding practices[6,9,10] or, in larger countries, by differences in neuropathological judgment.[2,11] In addition, lack of clarity on the criteria of tumor definitions, considerable variation in range of ages accepted as representing childhood, and variation in the selection of materials make the comparison of incidence, classification, and survival in the various series difficult.[6]

After definitions and a survey of the general epidemiology and classification of brain tumors in children, it is my intention to describe these relations in the posterior fossa tumors in children, especially the location and histological patterns.

Table 1.1. Five-year survival rates in children with different tumors.

	Years of diagnosis		
	1970–1974	1975–1979	1980–1984
Wilms' tumor	70	75	81
Brain	45	55	55
Acute lymphatic leukemia	45	56	63

General Epidemiology of Brain Tumors in Children

Many articles dealing with brain tumors in children have problems in misclassification and selection biases. The rate of histological verification in most publications is as high as 85% to 90%.[6,9,12] In specific locations, i.e., the basal nuclei and the brain stem, it is still acceptable to have only a radiological verification, especially after the application of such imaging methods as contrast roentgen computer tomography (CT) and magnetic resonance imaging (MRI).

Epidemiology of brain tumors in children is a study of the variations in frequency among population groups and the possible etiological factors that influence these variations.[13,14] The principal goal is to find the causes of brain tumors so that preventive measures may be implemented.

Epidemiologic (demographic) studies also concern the frequency of tumors in population areas in order to uncover peculiarities in the distribution of brain tumors in children.[7-10,13,15-18] Correlational (ecological) studies explore the rate of brain tumors in a population area and compare it with a geographic distribution of suspected risk factors. The knowledge about risk factors in brain tumors in children is sparse. Some congenital or genetic factors are known, i.e., the well-known influence of heredity in Recklinghausen's neurofibromatosis and in von Hippel-Lindau disease.

Epidemiology in brain tumors in children is studied by a cohort or a case-control study. The cohort study is a follow-up (retrospective) investigation or a prospective analysis in which groups of individuals are identified and followed over time. The case-control study identifies children with brain tumors, uses a group of similar children without brain tumors as controls, and evaluates survival, disability rate, and social events. The tools used to measure frequency are

1. the number of individuals influenced by disease,
2. the length of the study period, and
3. the population under investigation.

Definitions

Brain tumors are intracranial neoplasms verified either by histology, by operation, by subsequent autopsy, or by radiological examinations. They arise from the brain itself, from the meninges, or from the inside of the skull. Tumors that are located exclusively in the skull, i.e., dermoids or eosinophilic granulomas and vascular arteriovenous malformations, are not included.

Age limits used for childhood are the 15 annual groups from 0 to 14 years of age.

Posterior fossa location is defined as the posterior fossa space in its entirety, including cerebellum, brain stem, and the adjacent parts of the base of the skull.

Radiological verification in the posterior fossa is accepted for those brain stem tumors that have been imaged by methods such as CT and MRI, or in older materials by pneumoence-

Table 1.2. Age-specific (5 years) incidence rates per 100,000 children in 1985 in leukemia and brain tumors.

	Boys			Girls		
	0–4	5–9	10–14	0–4	5–9	10–14
Leukemia	6.8	11.7	11.8	17.4	9.6	10.7
Brain	3.8	2.8	2.2	2.9	2.6	1.7

Modified after SEER program, 1985.

phalography (PEG) or angiography, only if the tumor is later verified by autopsy.

Incidence rate is the probability of developing brain tumors in children. It is defined as the number of children developing a brain tumor in a part of time (generally 1 year) divided by the population at risk within that time. The incidence rate is usually expressed per 100,000 persons (Table 1.2).

Mortality (death) rate is the number of children dying of brain tumor in a period of time divided by the population at risk during that period.

Prevalence rate is the total number of children with brain tumors at a given point in time divided by the total population at risk at that time.

Incidence Rates

In the literature, the frequency of brain tumors in childhood is mostly based on materials from single departments, i.e., pediatric and neurosurgical clinics, neuropathological institutes, or on reports referring to selected histological tumor types.[11,19-24] These studies give only a limited view of the epidemiological pattern of brain tumors in children. Brain tumor materials based on cancer registry studies or population materials have shown an annual incidence of between 2.2 to 3.5 per 100,000 brain tumors in children below 15 years of age (Table 1.3).[6,7,9,18,25,26] Other reports show differences both in location and histological typing,[23,27] mostly caused by varying age range for childhood, as emphasized by Gjerris.[6]

Table 1.3. Incidence in different series of intracranial tumors in children.

Year of publication	Authors	Region	Period	Number of cases	Pathoana-tomical diagnosis review	Incidence (100,000)
1958	Bergstrand	Stockholm	1947–56	55	–	3.6
1975	Teppo	Finland	1953–70	561	–	2.5
1976	Gjerris	Denmark	1945–59	183	+	2.5
1978	Gjerris et al.	Denmark	1935–59	533	+	2.1
1978	Ericsson	Sweden	1958–74	923	–	3.3[a]
1986	Young	United States	1973–81	1,014	–	2.6[a]
1988	Birch	England	1971–83	399	+	2.6[a]
1989	Lannering	Sweden	1970–84	186	+	3.5
1992	Gjerris et al.	Denmark	1960–84	912	+	3.7

Modified from Lannering, ref. 7.
[a] Spinal tumors included.

Table 1.4. Incidence of brain and spinal tumors in children in some European countries and parts of the United States.

Country	Sex	Years	Rates/million (age groups) <1	1–4	5–9	10–14	Adj.	HV%
Denmark	Males	1978–82	40.0	33.0	33.5	33.6	33.9	87.8
	Females	1978–82	27.9	37.7	21.5	23.9	27.7	88.6
Finland	Males	1970–79	40.9	42.5	30.1	26.2	33.7	87.8
	Females	1970–79	23.1	38.1	24.9	24.1	28.6	90.1
East Germany	Males	1976–80	26.7	30.8	30.8	21.8	27.9	74.4
	Females	1976–80	15.0	26.1	26.0	20.8	23.5	78.3
West Germany	Males	1982–84	17.2	18.5	13.4	9.8	14.2	21.0
	Females	1982–84	17.0	17.1	11.5	7.3	12.5	15.5(?)
Hungary	Males	1975–84	17.2	24.9	23.6	12.7	20.3	73.0
	Females	1975–84	14.2	17.4	19.5	12.6	16.4	81.3
Norway	Males	1970–79	34.0	33.3	31.8	24.0	30.2	87.5
	Females	1970–79	25.0	19.1	25.3	22.7	22.6	88.6
Sweden	Males	1970–82	33.8	47.3	31.9	32.7	37.0	91.8
	Females	1970–82	27.9	35.7	27.1	28.6	30.3	94.0
Canada	Males	1970–79	21.6	31.2	26.0	24.0	26.9	77.4
	Females	1970–79	12.4	31.7	20.4	19.4	23.0	68.6
United States (SEER)	Males	1973–82	—	27.3	28.2	23.3	26.4	89.5
	Females	1973–82	—	25.1	22.8	21.6	23.3	89.3

Modified from Parkin et al., ref. 9.

Table 1.4 displays the incidence of brain tumors in children in different European countries and parts of North America, and includes years of interest, sex, and 15 annual groups. Incidence, correlated to adjusted rate (age), i.e., calculated from the World Standard Population for age groups below 15 years and rate of histological verification (HV%) are also shown. The annual incidence differs between 1.3 and 3.7 per 100,000 with an average incidence of 3.0 per 100,000 for boys and 2.5 per 100,000 for girls.[9]

The location and histology of brain tumors in children were estimated in two Danish series from the years 1935–59 and 1960–84.[6,28] The first study was retrospective and the second retrospective/prospective. The social system in Denmark ensures that children with symptoms of a brain tumor will sooner or later be admitted to a hospital and reported to the Cancer Registry. The average annual population of children in Denmark during the 50 years of study was taken from the Statistical Yearbooks of Denmark (about one million individuals below 15 years of age). The population was stable and all the children were subject to follow-up. We found 533 children in the first period and 912 children in the second period who had brain tumors, which gives an average annual incidence in the first period of 2.1 per 100,000 and in the second period of 3.6 per 100,000. In both periods the incidence was a little higher in boys.

The annual incidence rates in the first period studied are a little lower than in some other countries (Canada, Israel, New Zealand) but close to the rates for the other Scandinavian countries, England, Holland, Scotland, and the United States. Studies using the usual pediatric upper limit for childhood of 15 years of age also show varying age rates of incidence. Hendrick et al.[21] saw a sharp fall in incidence after the age of 10 years and Schoenberg et al.[27] found a peak incidence rate at 6.4 years. Teppo et al.[26] and Gjerris et al.[28] demonstrated no significant difference in age distribution from the child populations in Finland and in Denmark. Moreover, other studies[27,29] took the age of 20 to be the upper age limit for childhood. Acceptance of this high upper age limit will cause inclusion of supratentorial tumors, typically found in adults, and comparison between individual studies in some countries is difficult, as most population statistics take the end of the 14th year to be the upper age limit of childhood.[6]

Taxonomy of Brain Tumors in Children

Location

Brain tumors can be classified according to localization. The intracranial space is by convenience divided into the supratentorial and the infratentorial compartments. The infratentorial area is divided into cerebellar (including fourth ventricle), brain stem, and cerebellopontine angle partitions.

Thirty years ago intracranial tumors in children were described as being far more frequent in the infratentorial than in the supratentorial compartment; in particular, tumors of the cerebral hemispheres were reported as being less frequent. Later it was reported from Sweden, Southern England, and Denmark that supratentorial tumors constituted about 40% to 45% of all intracranial tumors in childhood.[20,24,25,28,30,31] Koos and Miller[23] found identical rates of supratentorial and infratentorial tumors, but the upper age limit for childhood was 16 to 17 years, which implies a relative rise in the number of supratentorial tumors. Other authors also include further space-occupying disorders, such as aneurysms, arteriovenous malformations, arachnoid cysts, osteomas, and cranial dermoid cysts,[23] which in my opinion should *not* be included in tumor series.

Histological Types

At present, histology more than the anatomical location defines brain tumors in children. Previous studies have often been based on site rather than histology. The World Health Organization (WHO) Classification of brain tumors has been used for many years and has been revised two times during the last 10 years, and again in a new version in Japan in 1990.[1,2,4,9,11,12] In children, the International Classification of Diseases for Oncology (ICD-O) has been used.[32] The pathological classification is based on the tissue of origin, and the morphological criteria of malignancy are anaplasia, invasiveness, recurrence, and metastatic growth.[1,4,32] All the different histological types of brain tumors are shown in Tables 1.5 and 1.6. Tumors are graded in degree of malignancy according to the histological features in four malignancy groups I to IV. Grade I includes juvenile astrocytomas and ependymomas, grade IV includes glioblastomas and medulloblastomas. These grading system are most useful in neuroepithelial tumors, especially in regard to survival rates.[7,12,25,28,31]

In children the majority of the tumors (80%)

Table 1.5. Classification of brain tumors in children.

I.	Tumors of neuroepithelial tissue	A.	Glial tumors
			1. Astrocytic tumors (astrocytoma, anaplastic astrocytoma)
			2. Oligodendroglial tumors
			3. Ependymal tumors (ependymoma/anaplastic/ myxopapillary)
			4. Choroid plexus tumors (plexus papilloma/anaplastic)
			5. Mixed gliomas (new category)
			6. Glioblastomatous tumors (glioblastoma)
			7. Gliomatosis
		B.	Neuronal tumors
			1. Gangliocytoma/anaplastic
			2. Ganglioglioma/anaplastic
		C.	"Primitive" neuroepithelial tumors (new category)
			1. "Primitive" neuroectodermal tumors
			2. Medulloepithelioma
		D.	Pineal cell tumors
			1. Pineoblastoma
			2. Pineocytoma
II.	Tumors of meningeal and related tissues	A.	Meningiomas
		B.	Meningeal sarcomatous tumors
III.	Tumors of nerve sheath cells	A.	Neurilemoma/anaplastic
		B.	Neurofibroma/anaplastic
IV.	Primary malignant lymphomas		
V.	Tumors of blood vessels	A.	Hemangioblastoma
VI.	Germ cell tumors	A.	Germinoma
		B.	Embryonal carcinoma
		C.	Choriocarcinoma
		D.	Endodermal sinus tumor
		E.	Teratomatous tumors
VII.	Malformative tumors	A.	Craniopharyngioma (Rathke's cleft cyst)
		B.	Epidermal cyst/dermoid cyst
		C.	Colloid cyst of third ventricle
		D.	Lipoma
		E.	Hamartoma
VIII.	Tumors of neuroendocrine origin	A.	Adenoma/carcinoma
		B.	Paraganglioma
IX.	Local extensions from regional tumors		
X.	Metastatic tumors		
XI.	Unclassified tumors		

Modified from Rorke et al., ref. 32.

originate in neuroepithelial tissue. Astrocytomas are the most common, followed by medulloblastomas, ependymomas, and oligodendrogliomas (Tables 1.5 and 1.6). Two epidemiological studies in Denmark have shown that there are fewer tumor types in the posterior fossa than in the supratentorial space.[19,28] Pituitary adenomas, acoustic neurinomas, and meningiomas are uncommon in childhood. Primitive neuroectodermal tumors (PNET) are highly malignant tumors commonly seen in infants.

Posterior Fossa Tumors in Children

The only well known primary cause for posterior fossa tumors in children is heredity in families suffering from Recklinghausen's disease (i.e., meningiomas and acoustic neurinomas) and from von Hippel-Lindau disease (i.e., cerebellar angioblastomas). Neurofibromatosis is also linked to many cerebral disorders, i.e., genetic types of hydrocephalus and congenital defects in the skull.[12] The most distinct differences of intracranial tumor types

Table 1.6. Histology and grading in brain tumors in children.

Tumor type	Grade I, benign	Grade II, semibenign	Grade III, semimalignant	Grade IV, malignant
Angioblastoma	+++			
Choroid plexus papilloma	+++		+	
Craniopharyngioma	+++			
Epidermoid	+++		+	
Gangliocytoma (-glioma)	+++	++	+	
Meningioma	+++			
Pineocytoma	+++	++	+	
Subependymoma	+++		+	
Pilocytic astrocytoma	+++		+	
Anaplastic astrocytoma		++	+	
Oligodendroglioma		++	+	
Ependymoma	++	+++	+	+
Germinoma				+++
Medulloblastoma + PNET				+++
Pinealoblastoma				+++
Sarcoma				+++

Reprinted from Zülch, ref. 4.
Explanation: +++ = usual; ++ = less frequent; + = rare.

Table 1.7. Location and most prominent tumor types in the posterior fossa in children and adults.

Location	Histological tumor types	
	Adults	Children
Cerebellum	Angioblastoma	Medulloblastoma
	Astrocytoma, pilocytic	Astrocytoma, pilocytic
	Metastases	Angioblastoma
		Dermoid cyst
Fourth ventricle	Meningioma	Medulloblastoma
	Ependymoma	Ependymoma
	Subependymoma	Papilloma
Cerebellopontine angle	Schwannoma	Ependymoma
	Meningioma	Papilloma
	Epidermoid cyst	
	Glomus tumor	
Brain stem	Astrocytoma, anaplastic	Astrocytoma, anaplastic
	Astrocytoma, pilocytic	Astrocytoma, pilocytic

between children and adults are shown in Table 1.7.

Incidence Rates

The above-mentioned figures give a manifest annual incidence of 15 to 20 per million brain tumors in children in European and white North American populations. The incidence values of location and histological types in 489 Danish children during 25 years are shown in Tables 1.8 and 1.9. When the population figures of boys and girls are known in the different European countries the expected number of new posterior tumors are easily calculated. If the discovered annual number is much higher over a period of time (i.e., 10 to 20 years), suspicion of other causes than the "usual" (i.e., Chernobyl or a similar disaster) could be entertained.

Table 1.8. Frequency and histological types in 489 posterior fossa tumors in children in Denmark from the years 1960–84.

Tumor type	Number	Percent	Incidence (million/year)
Juvenile astrocytoma	89	18.2	3.5
Diffuse astrocytoma	58	11.9	2.3
Polymorphous astrocytoma	32	6.5	1.3
Ependymoma	55	11.2	2.2
Medulloblastoma	180	36.8	7.2
Gangliocytoma	4	0.8	
Spongioblastoma	1	0.2	
Glioblastoma	5	1.0	
Glioma nonclassificatum	5	1.0	
Plexus papilloma	5	1.0	
Teratoma	1	0.2	1.4
Neurinoma	3	0.6	
Sarcoma	1	0.2	
Meningioma	2	0.4	
Hemangioblastoma	7	1.4	
Metastasis	1	0.2	
No histology	40	8.2	1.6
Total	489	100.0	20.0

Modified from Gjerris et al., ref. 19.

Table 1.9. Annual incidence of the most common posterior fossa tumors in 489 children (per 100.000) in Denmark 1960–84.

Year	Medulloblastoma	Juvenile astrocytoma	Diffuse astrocytoma	Ependymoma
1960–64	0.73	0.21	0.32	0.28
1965–69	0.72	0.28	0.16	0.24
1970–74	0.61	0.33	0.21	0.20
1975–79	0.62	0.36	0.21	0.18
1980–84	0.53	0.44	0.14	0.06

Modified from Gjerris et al., ref. 19.

The frequency of posterior fossa tumors during 50 years in Denmark and the distribution between location and histological types during the years 1960–84 are shown in Tables 1.8, 1.10, and 1.11.

Location

The posterior fossa is small and holds the cerebellum, fourth ventricle, brain stem, vessels, and CSF. In children the majority of the posterior fossa tumors are localized in the cerebellum or the fourth ventricle. The grouping of brain tumors in the posterior fossa in children in Denmark during 50 years is shown in Table 1.10; 77% of the tumors were placed in the cerebellum or the fourth ventricle, 21% in the brain stem, and less than 2% in the cerebellopontine angle. Nearly the same distribution is found in Cancer Registry materials in Europe and North America.[12,14]

Histology

Cerebellar Tumors

The most common types are astrocytomas, medulloblastomas, and ependymomas (Tables

Table 1.10. The location and histology in infratentorial tumors in children in the years 1935–59 ($n = 314$) and 1960–84 ($n = 489$) in Denmark.

Histology	1935–59			1960–84		
	Cerebellum	Brain stem	Angle	Cerebellum	Brain stem	Angle
Astrocytoma, juvenile	91	—	—	89	—	—
Astrocytoma d-p.	—	29	—	33	57	—
Ependymoma	43	1	—	52	3	—
Medulloblastoma	86	1	1	178	2	—
Plexus papilloma	5	—	—	5	—	—
Acoustic neurinoma	—	—	3	—	—	3
Hemangioblastoma	3	—	—	7	—	—
Others; no histology	24	23	4	12	44	4
Total	252	54	8	376	106	7

Modified from Gjerris et al., refs. 19 and 28.

Table 1.11. Frequency and years of diagnosis (5-year intervals) in 489 children with posterior fossa tumors.

Years	Number	Percent
1960–64	103	21.06
1965–69	102	20.86
1970–74	96	19.63
1975–79	105	21.47
1980–84	83	16.97
Total	489	100

Modified from Gjerris et al., ref. 19.

1.7, 1.8, 1.10). In children, the difference between benign and malignant tumors can be difficult to determine except in cases of ependymomas and juvenile astrocytomas. In malignant tumors the differentiation between medulloblastomas, ependymoblastomas, and sarcomas can be almost impossible. The histology of 489 posterior fossa tumors in children in Denmark, verified by histology, operation, radiology, and/or postmortem studies are shown in Tables 1.8, 1.9, and 1.10. In 93% of the children the diagnoses were primarily established on histological grounds. Medulloblastomas, juvenile or diffuse astrocytomas, and ependymomas (Tables 1.8 and 1.10) were most frequent. As in the period 1935–59[14] we found very few acoustic neurinomas. None of the

children, all in the age group 10 to 14 years, suffered from neurofibromatosis.

Astrocytomas are derived from the astrocytes. Most cerebellar astrocytomas are grade I (Tables 1.7, 1.8, and 1.9) of fibrillar or pilocytic type.[12,33,34] They are generally circumscribed, well demarcated, and noninvasive. Cysts are very common, containing albuminous fluid with a tumor nodule in the wall. Further subdivisions have been made on histological grounds,[6,35,36] (e.g., the categories of juvenile and diffuse astrocytomas) in an attempt to compare the microscopic picture to prognosis. The occurrence of anaplastic astrocytoma and glioblastoma in the cerebellum is uncommon.[37]

Medulloblastomas have a peak age incidence of about 5 to 9 years and are found twice as frequently in boys as in girls.[12,22,28,38–40] They originate from embryonal medulloblasts in the germinative zone of the anterior or posterior medullary velum; most of them are placed in the cerebellar vermis. They are soft, grayish, and often well demarcated, and in older children often placed in the cerebellar hemispheres. From the cerebellar vermis they extend into the fourth ventricle. The tumors are very cellular and highly malignant, and are composed of poorly differentiated small round cells with hyperchromatic nuclei. Pseudorosettes are typical. All medulloblastomas are grade IV. They are divided into a classical and

Table 1.12. Medulloblastoma staging system (T and M system).

I. Children above 3 years of age; stages T_1 and T_2
T_1 Tumor less than 3 cm; limit to mindline position
T_2 Tumor 3 cm or greater; partially filling fourth ventricle
II. Children above 3 years of age; stages T_3 and T_4
T_3 Invades adjacent structures; complete filling fourth ventricle; marked hydrocephalus
T_4 Tumor spreads to mesencephalon, pons, and medulla
III. Children below 3 years of age
IV. Additional risk factors (TNM-staging)
M_0 No evidence of gross CSF or systemic metastases
M_1 Microscopic tumor cells in CSF
M_2 Gross nodular seeding in cerebral/cerebellar subarachnoid space or ventricular system
M_3 Gross nodular seeding in spinal subarachnoid space
M_4 Metastases outside cerebrospinal axis

Modified from Chang et al., ref. 41, and Laurent and Cheek, ref. 42.

a desmoplastic type. Medulloblastomas seed in the cerebrospinal fluid (CSF) space, and extraneural metastases are common in up to 30% of cases.

An operative staging system has been described by Chang et al.[41] and further developed by Laurent and Cheek.[42] It is based on CSF estimation of tumor cells and on postoperative myelography or CT. It includes T (T_{1-4} = size, invasiveness, and location of the tumor) and M (M_{0-5} = CSF metastasis) and is shown in Table 1.12.

Ependymomas originate from ependymal cells and are generally localized in the fourth ventricle, but can be found in the cerebellar hemisphere or cerebellopontine angle. They are well defined, poorly encapsulated, and often grossly calcified. Benign ependymomas are cellular with a regular histologic pattern and perivascular pseudorosettes are common. They can be classified in many types, a staging system for infratentorial ependymomas has been described, and about 40% are malignant.[43] Both the benign and malignant ependymoma cells seed into the CSF compartment.

Hemangioblastomas are uncommon (Table 1.10) and often found together with von Hippel-Lindau disease. Most of them are benign and cystic. Twenty percent of the patients have multiple hemangioblastomas.

Brain Stem Tumors

These tumors are located in the mesencephalon, pons, and medulla oblongata. Most of the tumors are benign or anaplastic astrocytomas[12] (Table 1.10). Glioblastomas are also found (Tables 1.8 and 1.10). They are most common in the pons, where they infiltrate the cranial nerve nuclei and grow along the longitudinal tracts. The tumors can be purely intrinsic, but often exophytic masses are seen, either in the fourth ventricle, in the cisterna magna, or in the cerebellopontine angle.

Cerebellopontine Angle Tumors

Many are cerebellar tumors that grow into the angle or are pushed out of the foramen of Luschka, i.e., plexus papillomas, ependymomas, and astrocytomas. Angle tumors, which are common in adults, are seldom diagnosed in children. They are mainly acoustic neurinomas, epidermoids, dermoids, and lipomas, and are nearly always found in children aged 10 to 14 years. The epidermoids consist of a thin capsule containing keratin and cholesterol crystals with a white pearly appearance.

Final Remarks

An average annual number of 20 new diagnosed posterior fossa tumors per million children (Tables 1.8, 1.10, 1.11, and 1.13) is to be expected in a future European population. Of these, 16 will be located in the cerebellum and 3 to 4 in the brain stem or the cerebellopontine angle. Seven will be astrocytomas, 7 medulloblastomas, 2 to 3 ependymomas, and the remainder will be distributed among glioblastomas, papillomas, hemangioblastomas, gangliocytomas, acoustic neurinomas, and other very uncommon tumors. In less than 10%, no histology will be obtained.

The introduction of CT and MRI has opened

Table 1.13. Location of posterior fossa tumors in 489 children in the years 1960–84 in Denmark.

| | Number | | | Incidence |
	Total	Boys	Percent	(million/year)
Brain stem	106	46	21.7	4.3
Cerebellum	182	99	37.2	7.3
Fourth ventricle	194	120	39.7	7.8
Cerebellopontine angle	7	7	1.4	0.3
Total	489		100	20

Modified from Gjerris et al., ref. 19.

up new possibilities of early diagnosis of intracranial tumors in children, and of monitoring the effects of neurosurgery and other therapy (radiotherapy and chemotherapy). CT and MRI make it possible to establish the location as well as the size of a tumor and frequently allow one to get an impression of the tumor type as well.

Far and wide knowledge of epidemiology and a uniform standardized classification system in brain tumors in children are necessary tools both for the correct treatment of the single child, for the evaluation of the long-term prognosis in children with different tumor types, and for comparison of rates of tumors between different centers and countries. It also makes it possible to analyze difficult cases over a long time and to identify and treat high-risk groups. Epidemiological and cancer registry studies have shown a low incidence and a corresponding poor prognosis of many tumor types. We must therefore consider the possibility of joint European efforts in multicenter treatment and follow-up studies.

References

1. Jellinger K. Pathology of human intracranial neoplasia. In: Jellinger K, ed. *Therapy of Malignant Brain Tumors*. Wien-New York: Springer-Verlag; 1987:1–90.
2. Russell DS, Rubinstein LJ. *Pathology of Tumours of the Nervous System*. 4th ed. London: Edward Arnold; 1977.
3. Zülch KJ. *Atlas of the Histology of Brain Tumours*. Berlin-Heidelberg-New York: Springer-Verlag; 1971.
4. Zülch KJ. *Brain Tumours: Their Biology and Pathology*. 3rd ed. New York: Springer-Verlag; 1986.
5. Allen JC. Childhood brain tumors: Current status of clinical trials in newly diagnosed and recurrent disease. *Pediatr Clin North Am.* 1985;32:633–651.
6. Gjerris F. Intracranial tumours in childhood—incidence and long-term prognosis. *Dan Med Bull.* 1979;26:253–260.
7. Lannering B. *Brain Tumours in Children. A Population Based Study on Incidence, Survival and Late Effects*. Thesis, Gothenburg; 1989.
8. Bahemuka M. Worldwide incidence of primary nervous system neoplasms. *Brain.* 1988;111:737–755.
9. Parkin DM, Stiller CA, Draper GJ, et al., eds. *International Incidence of Childhood Cancer*. Lyon: Int Agency Res Cancer; 1988.
10. Schoenberg BS, ed. *Neurological Epidemiology: Principles and Clinical Applications. Advances in Neurology*, Vol. 19. New York: Raven Press; 1978.
11. Zülch KJ. Principles of the new World Health Organization (WHO) classification of brain tumours. *Neuroradiology* 1980;19:59–66.
12. Jacobi G, Kornhuber B. Malignant brain tumor in children. Pathology of human intracranial neoplasia. In: Jellinger K, ed. *Therapy of Malignant Brain Tumors*. Wien, New York: Springer-Verlag; 1987:396–493.
13. Cohen ME, Duffner PK. *Brain Tumors in Children. Principles in Diagnosis and Treatment*. New York: Raven Press; 1984.
14. Schoenberg BS. The epidemiology of central nervous system tumors. In: Walker MO, ed. *Oncology of the Nervous System*. Boston: Martinus Nijhoff; 1983.
15. Doll R, Muir C, Waterhouse J. *Cancer Incidence in Five Continents*. Vol. II. Berlin; Heidelberg, New York: Springer-Verlag: 1970.

16. Muir C, Waterhouse J, Mack T, et al. *Cancer Incidence in Five Continents*. Vol. V. Lyon: Int Agency Res Cancer; 1987.

17. Schottenfeld D, Fraumeni JF Jr. *Cancer Epidemiology and Prevention*. Philadelphia: WB Saunders; 1982.

18. Waterhouse JAH. *Cancer Handbook of Epidemiology and Prognosis*. London: Churchill Livingstone; 1974.

19. Gjerris F, Agerlin N, Børgesen SE, et al. Incidence of intracranial tumours in children in Denmark 1960–84. 1992; to be published.

20. Heiskanen O. Intracranial tumours of children. *Childs Brain*. 1977;3:69–78.

21. Hendrick EB, Hoffman HJ, Humpreys RP. Treatment of infratentorial gliomas in childhood. In: Hekmatpanah, ed. *Gliomas*. Berlin: Springer-Verlag; 1975.

22. Kasantikul V, Shuangshoti S. Cerebellar medulloblastomas: A study of 35 cases with particular reference to cellular differentiation. *Surg Neurol*. 1986;26:532–541.

23. Koos WT, Miller MH. *Intracranial Tumours of Infants and Children*. Stuttgart: Georg Thieme Verlag; 1971.

24. Naidich TP, Zimmerman RA. Primary brain tumors in children. *Semin Roentgenol*. 1984; 21(2):100–114.

25. Lannering B, Marky I, Nordborg C. Brain tumors in children in West Sweden— Epidemiology and survival. *Cancer*. 1990; 66:604–609.

26. Teppo L, Salonen T, Hakulinen T. Incidence of childhood cancer in Finland. *J Natl Cancer Inst*. 1975;55:1065–1067.

27. Schoenberg BS, Schoenberg DG, Christine BW, Gomez MR. The epidemiology of primary intracranial neoplasms in childhood. *Mayo Clin Proc* 1976;51:51–56.

28. Gjerris F, Harmsen A, Klinken L, Reske-Nielsen E. Incidence and long-term survival of children with intracranial tumours treated in Denmark 1935–1959. *Br J Cancer*. 1978; 38:442–451.

29. Farwell JR, Dohrmann GJ, Flannery JR. Central nervous system tumours in children. *Cancer*. 1977;40:3123–3132.

30. Ericsson JL, Karnström L, Mattson B. Childhood cancer in Sweden. *Acta Pædiatr Scand*. 1978;67:425–432.

31. Gjerris F. Clinical aspects and long-term prognosis of intracranial tumours in infancy and childhood. *Dev Med Child Neurol*. 1976; 18:145–159.

32. Rorke LB, Gilles F, Davis RL, Becker LE. Revision of the World Health Organization Classification of brain tumors for childhood brain tumors. *Cancer*. 1985;56:1869–1885.

33. Garcia DM, Lafiti HR, Simpson JR, Picker S. Astrocytomas of the cerebellum in children. *J Neurosurg*. 1989;71:661–664.

34. Laws ER, Bergstralh EJ, Taylor WF. Cerebellar astrocytoma in children. *Prog Exp Tumor Res*. 1987;30:122–127.

35. Gilles FH, Leviton A, Hedley-White ET, Jasnow M. Childhood brain tumor update. *Hum Pathol*. 1983;14:834–845.

36. Winston K, Gilles FH, Leviton A, et al. Cerebellar gliomas in children: Clinical considerations and a proposed classification. *J Natl Cancer Inst*. 1977;58:833–838.

37. Shinoda J, Yamada H, Sakai N, et al. Malignant cerebellar astrocytic tumours in children. *Acta Neurochir (Wien)*. 1989;98:1–8.

38. Choux M, Lena G. Le médulloblastome. *Neurochirurgie*. 1982;28 (suppl):1–299.

39. Raimondi AJ, Tomita T. The advantages of total resection of medulloblastoma and disadvantages of whole brain postoperative radiation therapy. *Childs Brain*. 1979;5:50–59.

40. Landberg TG, Lindgren ML, Cavallin-Ståhl EK, et al. Improvements in the radiotherapy of medulloblastoma, 1946–1975. *Cancer*. 1980; 45:607–678.

41. Chang CH, Housepian EM, Herbert C. An operative staging system and a megavoltage radiotherapeutic technique for cerebellar medulloblastoma. *Radiology*. 1969;93:1351–1359.

42. Laurent JP, Cheek WR. A new staging method versus TNM staging in children with posterior fossa primitive neuroectodermal tumor (medulloblastoma). *Childs Brain*. 1986;2: 238–241.

43. Dohrmann GJ, Farwell JR, Flannery JT. Ependymomas and ependymoblastomas in children. *J Neurosurg*. 1976;45:273–283.

CHAPTER 2

Functional Basis of Posterior Fossa Tumor Symptoms and Signs

Ignacio Pascual-Castroviejo

Tumors of the posterior fossa in children are usually located in the cerebellum (vermis and/or cerebellar hemispheres), brain stem, fourth ventricle, or more rarely in the clival-cerebellopontine angle regions.

Signs and symptoms observed in patients with tumors in the posterior fossa are caused not only by the direct action of the tumor but also and especially by the increased intracranial pressure that is mainly due to obstructive or secondary hydrocephalus. There are wide differences in the incidence of the signs and symptoms caused by these tumors depending on whether or not they are associated with hydrocephalus.[1] The most frequent symptoms are headache, nausea, vomiting, unsteady gait, ocular squint, lethargy, head tilt, increased head circumference, irritability, and muscle weakness with hypotonia. The main signs are papilledema; Parinaud sign, increased head circumference, and osteotendinous hyper-reflexia (which are only seen in hydrocephalic patients); cerebellar ataxia and dysmetria; oculomotor disorders (especially abducens palsy); other cranial nerve signs; motor disorders with hypotonia; pyramidal disease with Babinski sign or with increased osteotendinous reflexes; and nystagmus. Other rarer or more specific symptoms or signs include the Cushing response, hemifacial pain, hemifacial spasm, and breath-holding episodes.

Headache

Headaches are an unlikely symptom of intracranial tumor in childhood.[2] They are, however, observed in 69% of children with brain tumors,[3] 65% of whom have the tumor in the posterior fossa[1] if there is association with hydrocephalus. The incidence of headaches is less than 30% in patients without hydrocephalus.[1] The headaches caused by brain tumors are often similar in character to those associated with more benign causes. However, they show some features that may distinguish them from those of other origin such as migraine.[3] Among the types of headaches that are considered to be alarming symptoms of a brain tumor are the following: (a) recurrent morning headaches; (b) headaches that repeatedly awaken the child from sleep; (c) intense, prolonged, and incapacitating headaches; (d) headaches that change in quality, frequency, or pattern; and (e) headaches that occur in association with vomiting and/or progressive neurological symptoms or signs, due to the raised intracranial pressure.

Headaches may be due to the direct effect of the tumor and the vasogenic peritumoral edema on the surrounding zones capable of producing pain, or to the increased intracranial pressure that acts by stretching meninges and/or vessels (arteries, veins, and venous sinuses). All these structures contain a high number of pain-sensitive endings. Although the pathophysiological mechanism of the headache in posterior fossa tumors has not yet received a convincing explanation, it could have in part the same neurobiological origin as some types of vascular head pain do. It seems likely that substance P participates in the production of these headaches. This neurotransmitter peptide is contained in trigeminovascular neurons and their peripheral unmyelinated nerve fibers. Substance P is transported from ganglion cell bodies to afferent nerve fibers, where the neurotransmitter is released into the wall of the cerebral blood vessel because of an induced depolarization. The pathophysiological action of substance P is carried out by dilatation of pial arteries, increase of vascular permeability, activation of cells that participate in the inflammatory response, and perhaps other still unknown ways.

Papilledema

The incidence of papilledema in children with posterior fossa is 69%.[1-5] It is mainly caused by elevated intracranial pressure. The incidence and severity of papilledema is proportional to the incidence and severity of complicating hydrocephalus.

The papilledema may be incipient or early and fully developed in accordance with the appearance of the disk, its margins, the size of the physiologic cup, the degree of capillary and venous engorgement, and the position and number of hemorrhages and exudates. The spontaneous venous pulsation usually is missing at the beginning of the disease. Although it has not been unquestionably accepted as an explaination of the pathophysiology of the papillar edema, it is thought that it is produced by the transmission of the increased intracranial pressure to the optic nerve layer. Hyperemia or blurring of the disk, distention of the retinal veins, or forward protrusion of the disk margins are suggestive of incipient papilledema. Early papilledema begins with dilatation of the capillaries within the substance of the optic disk, which results in the disk tissue becoming red. This hyperemia increases as capillary dilation increases. Venous distention and absence of venous pulsation are suggestive of incipient papilledema, although moderate widening and tortuosity may occur in some healthy people or in cases of anomalies of the optic disk, including pseudopapilledema.

As the intracranial pressure increases, the venous blood has more difficulty in returning to the heart through the intracranial venous sinuses and is retained extracranially. This explains the extracranial congestive veins and the papilledema. After the hyperemic phase, the disk's semitranslucent appearance is lost at its borders and gray, glistening, radial striations appear, most prominently above and below the disk. The initial blurring at the upper and lower margins of the disk is related to the anatomic arrangement of the nerve fibers entering the disk. When edema occurs, the resulting gray opacification appears first and is most prominent where the layer of the nerve fibers is thickest and most richly supplied with capillaries.

Small hemorrhages in the nerve fiber layer at the border of the disk in the presence of disk hyperemia and disk blurring are a definite and reliable sign of early papilledema. Hemorrhages, usually appearing as radial linear red streaks in the nerve fiber layer, are caused by rupture of distended segments of the interneural capillary plexus overlying the disk margin. Several types of "exudative" phenomena may occur as papilledema progresses. These soft white exudates reflect local concentrations of edema that have opacified part of the nerve fiber layer. Some of the exudates represent focal ischemic areas in the nerve fibers similar to the "cotton wool" patches of hypertensive retinopathy. Although the retinal arterioles maintain their normal caliber, they seem narrow when compared with the veins. A prolonged maintenance of high intracranial pressure may lead to an irreversible optic atrophy caused by degeneration of the nerve fibers. Successful decompression by shunt and/or by craniotomy with removal of the tumor is usually followed by the disappearance of the intracranial hyperpressure and the papilledema within a relatively short period of time.

Vomiting

Vomiting is seen as a symptom in patients with brain tumors, but it rarely leads to diagnosis in the absence of a recognized neurological deficit. Gastroesophageal disorders may be clinical manifestations of the tumors of the posterior fossa. The vomiting, including the physiologic correlates of nausea, gag reflex, and retching, are controlled by the central nervous system. Although a so-called vomiting center has been traditionally located in the brain stem, recent evidence has refuted the existence of this center. The brain stem has been said to be the main structure involved not only in vomiting but also in gastroesophageal reflux. Children with brain stem glioma have been described who initially present with gastroesophageal reflux during atypically late timing of presentation for infantile reflux,[6] and the same type of tumor has been related to upper gut motility disorders.[7] In these cases, the tumor infiltrates between normal neural structures, separating them more than actually destroying them. The brain stem may therefore modulate esophageal motility through vagus nerve projections to the esophagus and also to the stomach.

Several specific zones of the medulla are involved in the control of vomiting and in the esophagus motility. A so-called vomiting center is situated in the medullary zone corresponding to the nucleus solitarius of the vagus and the lateral portion of the reticular formation,[8,9] which are near to other medullary centers related not only to important respiratory, secretory, and vasomotor functions, but also to other cranial nerve motor nuclei controlling jaw, mouth, and tongue movements. They are even related to pathways to the motor neurons that control respiratory muscles and the striated abdominal muscles that are of prime importance in the expulsive phase of vomiting. There are efferent fibers to the vestibular nuclei, but mainly in the lateral reticular formation, situated in the upper medulla and the lower pons.[10] The main afferents to the vomiting center come from the area postrema and from the gut via both vagus and sympathetic splanchnic nerves.[11] Experimentally, there have been found to be several other connections in the brain stem related to vomiting, such as ascending fibers from the lateral reticular formation of the medulla and from the area postrema to the dorsolateral pontine tegmentum where they end on, or ventral to, the parabrachial nuclei.[11–13]

After experimental studies,[14,15] the neurophysiological basis of esophageal motility was determined to have its origin in the dorsal motor nucleus of the vagus and in the nucleus ambiguus.

Recent studies, however, have cast doubt on the concept of a single anatomic zone that can be considered as a vomiting center,[16] although they have not invalidated the basic concept that the motor control of vomiting is situated in the medulla. In this way, an alternative mechanism has been suggested for the act of vomiting, consisting in the interaction of several effector nuclei involved in the motor output of vomiting instead of the classical concept of a single vomiting center as coordinator of outputs from several sources.

The medullary center or centers of vomiting may be stimulated by afferent impulses arising from several extracranial and intracranial structures. The extracranial zone involved in the origin of vomiting is the posterior pharynx; vomiting is stimulated by an unpleasant taste or smell, by visual or auditory sensations from the corresponding sense organs, and by the stomach. Intracranial impulses arising from the chemoreceptor trigger zone situated in the area postrema of the floor of the fourth ventricle may activate the medullary center of vomiting.[17,18] This area has been shown to be very sensitive to several chemical agents, although it is considered an afferent intermediary way for vomiting, which is activated directly by endogenous or exogenous agents. However, the connections of these centers with other structures such as the cerebellum, vestibular system, and other sensory nuclei of the brain stem and spinal cord may also be involved in the genesis of vomiting. In any case, the chemoreceptor trigger zone incorporates receptors for dopamine and opiate neurotransmitters that can also be found peripherally. Hence, agents affecting these receptors may have either a central or peripheral effect.

Increased intracranial pressure, posterior fossa or brain stem mass lesions, and vestibular or cerebellar disorders probably affect the vomiting center through poorly defined neurotransmitter pathways.[19] The phenomenon of a mechanoreceptor being stimulated directly by the presence of a tumor has not yet been demonstrated.[18] Absence of neurologic findings in a patient having history of cyclic vomiting for longer than 3 months, especially with documented weight loss, should prompt a more detailed investigation of the central nervous system.[20]

Gait Disturbances and Equilibrium

Tumors located anywhere in the posterior fossa may affect the sense of equilibrium and the ability to walk. Although these disorders are usually seen in lesions situated in the midline or vermis and paravermis of the cerebellum, they can also be found in the brain stem and in fourth ventricle tumors. From experimental studies as well as from human observations, disturbance of equilibrium has been ascribed to lesions of the posterior vermis, including the flocculonodular lobe or archicerebellum. It is reciprocally connected with the vestibular nuclei of the brain stem through the inferior cerebellar peduncle.

The vestibulospinal system helps to maintain upright posture and head stability. The semicircular canals and their short latency connections to the neck motoneurons, largely via the medial vestibulospinal tract, respond to angular accelerations so as to stabilize the head in space. The paired otolith organs, the utricles, placed approximately horizontally, and the saccules, placed vertically, respond to linear acceleration, including gravity. Their influence leads, via the lateral vestibulospinal tract, to excitation of ipsilateral extensor motoneurons of the limbs and trunk, and to inhibition of reciprocal flexor motoneurons.[21] Many neck motoneurons are influenced by all six semicircular canals, with a highly specific excitatory or inhibitory drive from canal pairs.[22] Lesions of Deiters' nucleus or the lateral vestibulospinal tract produce very similar effects on the trunk and extremities. In patients with this lesion, the body curves to the ipsilateral side and the ipsilateral limbs are flexed.

The importance of the anterior vermis and paravermis zones in the control of locomotion is supported by experimental studies that demonstrate that lesions of the anterior lobe of the cerebellum result in increased muscle tone, especially in the antigravity muscles having influence in the tone, posture, and locomotion of the entire body. This occurs mainly through the direct or indirect connections of the vermis with the lateral vestibulospinal tract and with the reticular formation of the brain stem. The fastigial nucleus may act as an intermediary via. These brain stem structures, in turn, send motor control signals to spinal and motoneurons through vestibulospinal and reticulospinal tracts. Any destructive or compressive lesion in the anterior vermis, in the lateral zones of the brain stem, or in the otolith organs may provoke disorders of gait and of equilibrium. It is very rare to have lesions restricted to only one of the zones involved in the physiological mechanism of these functions. In any case, humans are more able to compensate for lesions of this area than are animals, according to experimental studies.

Equilibrium and locomotion cannot be regarded as independent functions. To have a normal gait, it is necessary to have a well-maintained equilibrium. On the other hand, in cerebellar diseases disturbance of gait may sometimes occur without any disturbance of equilibrium. Although gait ataxia is the only sign that can be ascribed with some degree of certainty to anterior lobe lesions in man,[23] posterior vermis lesions also cause difficulties in gait owing to disturbed equilibrium. Neocerebellar lesions may cause ataxia and hypotonia in the lower limbs, disturbing gait because of deviation and tendency of the patient to fall toward the side of the lesion.

Cerebellar Ataxia

Ataxia is the clinical expression of the incoordination of movements. It is caused by alterations of cerebellar function. From a simplistic point of view, the cerebellar hemispheres modulate limb movement of the ipsilateral side, whereas the midline vermis is primarily involved in station and gait.

The midline vermal structures project to the fastigial and vestibular nuclei and participate mainly in postural and locomotion functions. Large cells that originate in the red nucleus constitute the rubrospinal tract, which crosses the midline and descends to the spinal cord at all levels. Although the term *ataxia* is almost exclusively used to define limb or gait ataxia, speech disturbances such as dysarthria may also be considered a speech ataxia.

Ataxia occurring in neocerebellar diseases is usually restricted to the limbs. Superior phylogenetic species (man and primates) show a major development of the neocerebellum and the dentate nucleus that contribute to limb ataxia in case of injury. The symptoms are particularly severe and prolonged when the dentate nucleus and/or its efferent projection, the brachium conjunctivum, are involved. Clinical manifestation of cerebellar ataxia is also related to the activity of the cerebral motor cortex in connection with the spinal motor centers by means of various pathways (corticospinal, corticorubrospinal, corticoreticulospinal tracts, and possibly others). A disturbance in the force control and timing of movements in cerebellar ataxia is ultimately due to disorders in the cerebral control of voluntary movements.

The cerebral motor cortex is influenzed by the neocerebellum by means of the dentatorubrothalamocortical tract. The cerebellum receives input from the cerebral cortex via the inferior olive, pontine nuclei, lateral reticular nucleus, and possibly other reticular nuclei.[24] The Purkinje cells are able to depress the tonic discharge of the dentate nucleus by means of their inhibitory signals to dentate neurons.

The cerebellar cortex has a marked modulating effect on the signals from the dentate nucleus to the cerebral motor cortex.[25] The functional organization of the reciprocal cerebrocerebellar influence makes the dentate nucleus an important link in the corticopontothalamo cortical loop. The motor cortex sends command signals at the same time to the spinal motor centers (interneurons, α- and γ-motoneurons) and to the cerebellum. The central nervous system including the cerebellum receives a constant feedback of proprioceptive and exteroceptive signals during movement, via several pathways.[26] This information enables the cerebellum to correct errors of posture and movements. The cerebellum may in this way operate in relation to the motor cortex, influencing the number and frequency of descending motor control signals and determining the speed, range, and force of movement.[25]

When the cerebellum is affected, its error detector function is interfered with, resulting in disturbances in the temporospatial organization of movement, which are manifested clinically as cerebellar ataxia. This ataxia of cerebellar origin cannot be corrected to any great extent by visual guidance, in contrast to sensory ataxia in which the cerebellum is unaffected. The gamma system is markedly influenced by the cerebellum, which is considered essential to the normal execution of voluntary tracking movement.[27] The cerebellum increases the sensitivity of the muscle spindles to stretch. Cerebellar lesions cause depression of the γ-motoneuron activity, which probably decreases the sensitivity of spindles to measuring the correct muscle length and changes in muscle length during movement. Motoneurons α and γ are coactivated by descending motor control signals in order to operate in concert. These signals are conducted in several descending supraspinal pathways (corticospinal, rubrospinal, reticulospinal, vestibulospinal, and others), all of which can be influenced by the cerebellum. A disturbance in the coactivation of α- and γ-motoneurons by motor control signals occurs in cerebellar ataxia.

Speech Disturbances

Speech disturbances may be considered as incoordination or ataxia of speech and are occasionally the first signs of neocerebellar damage. It affects phonation more than articulation. Mainly bilateral or diffuse cerebellar lesions are associated with speech disturbances, although the midportion of the vermis and the adjacent paravermian regions—that is to say, the neocerebellum—seem to have more influence in the coordination of the motor part of the speech by disturbing the control of force and timing of the movement of phonation, articulation, and respiration.

Hypotonia

Decreased muscle tone is a common finding in cerebellar and brain stem tumors. Being affected unilaterally causes ipsilateral hypotonia with decreased resistance to passive stretching of muscle and a cerebellar hemiparesis consisting in deviation of gait and decreased muscle tone. Although it is possible that many factors participate in muscle tone, it primarily depends on the integrity of the γ-loop and the γ-motoneurons innervating the intrafusal fibers of the muscle spindles. The γ-system is influenced by the cerebellum. This influence is mainly exerted on the static γ-motoneurons. Cerebellar hypotonia may be caused by a depression of the activity of these neurons.[28] Decrease of γ-motoneuron activity causes a lowering of the tonic stretch response of the muscle spindle afferents, thereby explaining the tonic myotatic reflexes and its tendency to be pendular in the cerebellar lesions. However, in cerebellar disorders, hypotonia only occurs in lesions of the neocerebellum.

Nystagmus

Cerebellar nystagmus is physiologically related to damage of other structures of the posterior fossa such as the brain stem and the vestibular nuclei and/or their connections. It is unclear whether pure cerebellar lesions may cause nystagmus. However, two types of cerebellar nystagmus are described—spontaneous and positional. Spontaneous nystagmus may be caused by lesions in the cerebellar hemispheres, although there are authors who think it is more likely to be the result of a disturbance in the posterior vermis including the flocculonodular lobe[19] and possibly the fastigial nucleus. Nystagmus with the rapid component toward the side of the lesion has been provoked by unilateral destruction of the flocculonodular lobe. Cerebellar nystagmus in man is more irregular in its excursions than is labyrinthine nystagmus, and only appears in asymmetrical and unilateral disease of the posterior vermis, but not in bilateral lesions. A physiological explana-

tion for this may be the existence of a symmetrical inhibitory controlling influence on vestibular elicited eye movements at the vestibular nuclei level by the posterior vermis.

Cerebellar nystagmus may be regarded as a phenomenon in which the vestibular nuclei are released from the control of the posterior vermis. The positional nystagmus occurring in cerebellar disease is therefore most probably caused by lesion of the posterior vermis. It may be due to the symmetrical inhibitory controlling influence on vestibular elicited eye movements at the vestibular nuclei level by the posterior vermis. In this way, the cerebellar nystagmus may be regarded as a release phenomenon of the vestibular nuclei from the control of the posterior vermis. The existence of cerebellar nystagmus in man, however, may be questioned because of difficulties in deciding whether there is a concomitant involvement of the vestibular nuclei of the brain stem and their fiber connections.[23] In any case, nystagmus, slower and coarser on ipsilateral gaze, seems to represent either invasion or compression of the brain stem rather than a direct consequence of cerebellar dysfunction.

Increased Intracranial Pressure

Raised intracranial pressure in patients with tumors in the posterior fossa are mostly due to obstructive hydrocephalus from the compression of CSF pathways, by aqueductal stenosis, or by obstruction of the foramina of Luschka and Magendie. Tumors located in the clivus or basal zone are associated with communicating hydrocephalus that is caused by impairment of circulation of CSF from the basal cisterns through the subarachnoid space to the zone of absorption in the superior sagittal sinus. Many of the clinical symptoms and signs appearing in cases with tumors of the posterior fossa are due to increased intracranial pressure. Among these symptoms and signs, are headache; papilledema; altered mental state; vomiting; palsies of cranial nerves (mostly strabismus or setting-sun sign when the patient is an infant); altered vital signs such as elevated blood pressure, decreased pulse, and respiration counts; full fontanelle; macrocrania; irritability or lethargy; and even signs of herniation. Acute intra-cranial hypertension causes changes in the amplitude of auditory brain stem responses demonstrating the neuroelectrical alteration of some of the nuclei, centers, and projections of the brain stem.

Moreover, vomiting, headache, papilledema, hydrocephalus, and other symptoms and signs are also related to the increased intracranial pressure. One of the most significant is the abducens palsy, which can be either unilateral or bilateral and does not always cause diplopia. This palsy is due to the short *traject* and the early stretching of the abducens since the intracranial pressure begins to increase.

Enlargement of the Head

Enlargement of the head is observed in infants and young children with a long-standing increase of intracranial pressure. Cerebellar astrocytoma and ependymoma of the fourth ventricle are the tumors of the posterior fossa that are primarily implicated in obstructive hydrocephalus. This is usually associated with macrocephalus, although it does not inevitably occur. The pathophysiology of the enlarged head has a mechanical origin. The increased intracranial pressure causes a separation of the open sutures during the first years of life, which is carried out very easily due to the elasticity of the tissues at these ages.

Head Tilt

Head tilt or even torticollis and neck stiffness can be due to tonsillar herniation through the foramen magnum and to herniation of the cerebellar superior zone upward through the tentorial opening. Both may occur as the result of the presence of an expanding mass (tumoral, hemorrhagic, or fluid) in the posterior fossa, which is under much greater pressure as compared with the spinal canal or the middle fossa.

Downward herniation of the cerebellar tonsils into the foramen magnum will result in compression and stretching of the upper cervical nerve roots and edema followed by necrosis of the medulla and the upper cervical cord if unrelieved. Herniation may also be caused by a lumbar puncture by rapidly decompressing an already present inequality of pressure above and below the foramen magnum and the tentorium. Herniation of the cerebellar tonsils can lead to severe disorders in lower cranial nerves, respiratory irregularities, and cardiac rhythm alterations that can be followed by cardiorespiratory failure and even by death. Patients present with torticollis as an antialgic posture and any head movement may cause pain because of the stretching of the sensitive spinal roots, vessels, and meninges. However, a persistent head tilt may be adopted to avoid diplopia due to the disturbance of the sixth cranial nerve.

"Upward herniation" consists of antero-superior displacement of the cerebellum and brain stem through the tentorial notch. The result is the compression of the dorsal surface of the mesencephalon, the deformation of the posterior zone of the third ventricle and the compression and distortion of the deep venous system (veins of Rosenthal and Galen), raising the supratentorial pressure. It usually occurs after a rapid evacuation of a large supratentorial space-occupying lesion (e.g., releasing pressure through an ventriculoperitoneal shunt in cases of considerably unequal pressure above and below the tentorium). The incidence of upward herniation has been reported to be between 3%[1] and 6%,[30] occurring 24 to 38 hr after insertion of the precraniotomy shunt. Clinical symptoms of upward herniation are hyperventilation, progressive obtundation, conjugate downward gaze or loss of upward gaze, and autonomic dysfunction.

The Cushing Response

A marked increase in intracranial pressure produces a concomitant increase in systemic blood pressure (the Cushing response) and a fall in heart rate. It is observed with a frequency of 3% in children with brain tumors.[3] Although the phenomenon had been known for many years, Cushing[31] was the first to demonstrate the quantitative nature of this response, showing that it was graded and occurred when the pressure within the head exceeded that of the systolic blood pressure. Cushing suggested that ischemia of the brain stem was the stimulus for the response and that it was mediated by the medulla. Other stimuli that have been suggested are hypoxia, pain, pressure, stretch, or axial distortion of the brain stem.[32,33] Some of these, however, require such specific conditions to cause the Cushing response that they are very seldom produced.

Experimentally, it has been observed that the Cushing response is due to stimulation of structures highly localized in the medulla and spinal cord. The adequate stimulus appears to be pressure and/or stretch of neural tissue.[34,35] However, when the pressure is sustained, vasomotor reflexes elicited by tissue hypoxia may serve a secondary role in maintaining elevated blood pressure. The identity of the brain stem nuclei beneath the fourth ventricular surface that are involved in the response is unknown. However, it is of some interest that the area sensitive to pressure and stretch along the floor of the fourth ventricle overlies the so-called vasomotor region of the brain stem, the integrity of which is necessary to maintain blood pressure at normal levels.[36] Increased intracranial pressure may act by producing ischemia and/or hypoxia in some critical areas of the brain.[37] The local distortion or pressure may cause focal ischemia in areas of the brain stem. The existence of intracranial baroreceptors[38] has, however, not been accepted.[37] Children with brain tumors rarely have abnormal (slow) pulse rate, although it may be observed in cases with masses in the posterior fossa during herniation of the brain through the foramen magnum.

Hemifacial Spasm

Hemifacial spasm is characterized clinically by paroxysmal bursts of involuntary tonic or clonic activity occurring in muscles innervated by the facial nerve. It is mostly unilateral due to compression of the facial nerve at its root exit zone. The incidence of serious compressive lesions is very low[39] and descriptions in children and young people are rare. It occurs predominantly in middle-aged or elderly persons. In most patients, the underlying cause of hemifacial spasm is of vascular origin, such as an aberrant vessel, aneurism, or arteriovenous malformation. However, tumors of the cerebellopontine angle may also be found, with epidermoid tumor, acoustic neurinoma, meningioma, and lipoma being the most frequently reported.[40,41] In children, it has only been reported in one case with ganglioneuroma of the fourth ventricle in which diagnosis was performed more than 5 years following the onset of symptoms.[42] However, paroxysmal segmental rhythmic myoclonus has also presented in children with tumors in the cerebellum.[43]

Typically, the spasm begins in the orbicularis oculi and over months or years may spread to involve the lower part of the face, including the platysma. The presence of other clinical symptoms is usually observed. Headache, cerebellar dysfunction, facial pain or numbness, and involvement of other cranial nerves are the most common symptoms. Synkinetic movements involving one side of the face can be explained by one or more of the following mechanisms:[39] (a) aberrant regeneration after nerve injury; (b) abnormal nuclear firing owing to a hyperexcitable facial nerve nucleus; and (c) transaxonal or ephaptic spread of the nerve impulse, resulting from an artificial synapse after nerve injury. The last two mechanisms may cause hemifacial spasm in cases of tumors in the posterior fossa. Facial pain may be caused by tumors of the posterior fossa that compress the sensory roots of the cranial nerves. The disease is very infrequent in adults and extremely rare in children. Trigeminal neuralgia has been reported in a child 5 years of age with fifth nerve schwannoma in the middle and posterior fossae.[44] Duration of pain before the diagnosis of the tumor may be long.

Breath-Holding Episodes

Breath-holding episodes occur very frequently in childhood, especially in the first year, although they may present up to the age of 5 or 6 years. They are mostly of unknown origin. Occasionally, they have been related in cases with invasive tumor involving the medulla and fourth ventricle.[45] The pathophysiology of these episodes is identified as prolonged expiratory apnea. The hallmarks of prolonged expiratory apnea are rapidity of onset, progression, and severity of arterial hypoxemia.[46] The onset follows noxious stimuli and is associated with crying or an attempt to cry, an opisthotonic posture, and convulsions. The electroencephalogram (EEG) shows changes due to cerebral hypoxemia, a gasp on recovery, and subsequent drowsiness. Progressive increase in frequency and severity of cyanotic episodes and/or other clinical evidence of brain stem dysfunction may indicate a mass in the brain stem.

References

1. Raimondi AJ, Tomita T. Hydrocephalus and infratentorial tumors. Incidence, clinical picture, and treatment. *J Neurosurg.* 1981;55:174–182.
2. Gordon J. Recurrent headaches in 100 children. *Childs Brain.* 1978;4:95–105.
3. Honing PJ, Charney EB. Children with brain tumor headaches: Distinguishing features. *Am J Dis Child.* 1982;136:121–124.
4. Rossi LN, Vassella F. Headache in children with brain tumors. *Childs Nerv Syst.* 1989; 5:307–309.
5. Tomita T. Statistical analysis of symptoms and signs in cerebellar astrocytoma and medulloblastoma. In: Amador L, ed. *Brain Tumors in the Young.* Springfield, IL; Charles C. Thomas; 1983:514–525.
6. Mahony MJ, Kennedy JD, Leaf A, et al. Brain stem glioma presenting as gastro-oesophageal reflux. *Arch Dis Child.* 1987;62:731–733.
7. Wood JR, Camilleri M, Low PA, et al. Brain stem tumor presenting as upper gut motility disorder. *Gastroenterology.* 1985;89:1411–1414.
8. Borison HL, Wang SC. Functional localization of central coordinating mechanism for emesis in cat. *J Neurophysiol.* 1949;12:305–313.
9. Borison HL, Wang SC. Physiology and pharmacology of vomiting. *Pharmacol Rev.* 1953; 5:193–230.
10. Ito J, Takahashi H, Matsuoka I, et al. Vestibular efferent fibres to ampulla of anterior, lateral and posterior semicircular canals in cats. *Brain Res.* 1983;259:293–297.
11. Mehler WR. Observations on the connectivity of the parvicellular reticular formation with respect to a vomiting center. *Brain Behav Evol.* 1983;23:63–80.
12. King GW. Topology of ascending brainstem projections to nucleus parabrachialis in cat. *J Comp Neurol.* 1980;191:615–638.
13. Shapiro RE, Miselis RR. An efferent projection from the area postrema and the caudal medial nucleus of the solitary tract to the parabrachial nucleus in rat (abstract). *Neuroscience.* 1982; 8:269.
14. Eliasson S. Activation of gastric motility from the brain stem of the cat. *Acta Physiol Scand.* 1953;30:199–214.
15. Paganini FD, Norman WP, Kasbekar DK, et al. Effects of stimulation of nucleus ambiguus complex on gastro-duodenal function. *Am J Physiol.* 1984;246:253–262.
16. Miller AD, Wilson VJ. Vomiting centre reanalyzed: an electrical stimulation study. *Brain Res.* 1983;270:154–158.
17. Borison HL. Area postrema: chemoreceptor trigger tone of the vomiting—is that all? *Life Sci.* 1975;14:1807–1817.
18. Borison HL, Borison R, McCarthy LE. Role of the area postrema in vomiting and related functions. *Fed Proc.* 1984;43:2955–2958.
19. Malagelada JR, Camilleri M. Unexplained vomiting: a diagnostic challenge. *Ann Intern Med.* 1984;101:211–218.
20. Squires RH. Intracranial tumors. Vomiting as a presenting sign. A gastroenterologist's perspective. *Clin Pediatr.* 1989;28:351–354.
21. Markham CH. Vestibular control of muscular tone and posture. *Can J Neurol Sci.* 1987; 14:493–496.
22. Wilson VJ, Maeda M. Connections between semicircular canals and neck motoneurons in the cat. *J Neurophysiol.* 1974;37:346–357.
23. Nyberg-Hansen R, Horn J. Functional aspects of cerebellar signs in clinical neurology. *Acta Neurol Scand.* 1972;48(suppl 51):219–240.
24. Brodal A. Cerebrocerebellar pathways. Anatomical data and some functional implications. *Acta Neurol Scand.* 1972;48(suppl 51):153–181.
25. Evarts EV, Thach WT. Motor mechanisms of the CNS: cerebrocerebellar interrelations. *Annu Rev Physiol.* 1968;31:451–498.
26. Oscarson O. Recent development on internal feedback. In: Evarts EV, ed. *Central control of movement. Neurosci Res Progr Bull.* 1971;9:98–103.
27. Phillips CG. Motor apparatus of the baboon's hand. *Proc R Soc Med.* 1969;173:141–174.
28. Gilman S, McDonald WI. Cerebellar facilita-

tion of muscle spindle activity. *J Neurophysiol.* 1967;30:1494–1512.

29. Down RS. Cerebellar syndromes. In: Vinken PJ, Bruyn GW, eds. *Handbook of Clinical Neurology.* Amsterdam: North-Holland; 1969: 392–431.

30. Hoffman HJ, Hendrick EB, Humphreys RP. Metastasis ·via ventriculoperitoneal shunt in patients with medulloblastoma. *J Neurosurg.* 1976;44:562–566.

31. Cushing H. Some experimental and clinical observations concerning states of increased intracranial tension. *Am J Med Sci.* 1902;124:375–400.

32. Thompson RK, Malina S. Dynamic axial brain stem distortion as a mechanism explaining the cardiorespiratory changes in increased intracranial pressure. *J Neurosurg.* 1959;16:664–675.

33. Weinstein JD, Langfitt TW, Bruno L, et al. Experimental study of patterns of brain distortion and ischemia produced by an intracranial mass. *J Neurosurg.* 1968;28:513–521.

34. Hoff JT, Reis DJ. The Cushing reflex: Localization of pressure-sensitive areas in brainstem and spinal cord of cat. *Neurology.* 1969;19:308.

35. Hoff JT, Reis DJ. Localization of regions mediating the Cushing response in CNS of cat. *Arch Neurol.* 1970;23:228–240.

36. Alexander RS. Tonic and reflex functions of medullary sympathetic cardiovascular centers. *J Neurophysiol.* 1946;9:205–217.

37. McGillicuddy JE, Kindt GW, Raisis JE, et al. The relation of cerebral ischemia, hypoxia, and hypercarbia to the Cushing response. *J Neuro-*

surg. 1978;48:730–740.

38. Rodbard S, Saiki H. Mechanism of the pressor response to increased intracranial pressure. *Am J Physiol.* 1952;168:234–244.

39. Auger RG. Hemifacial spasm: clinical and electrophysiologic observations. *Neurology.* 1979; 29:1261–1272.

40. Auger RG, Piepgras DG. Hemifacial spasm associated with epidermoid tumors of the cerebellopontine angle. *Neurology.* 1989;39:577–580.

41. Jannetta PJ, Abbasy M, Maroon JC, et al. Etiology and definitive microsurgical treatment of hemifacial spasm: operative techniques and results in 47 patients. *J Neurosurg.* 1977;44:321–328.

42. Lanstron JW, Tharp BR. Infantile hemifacial spasm. *Arch Neurol.* 1974;31:63.

43. Jayakar PB, Seshia SS. Involuntary movements with cerebellar tumour. *Can J Neurol Sci.* 1987;14:306–308.

44. Bullit E, Tew JM, Boyd J. Intracranial tumors in patients with facial pain. *J Neurosurg.* 1986;64;865–871.

45. Southall DP, Lewis GM, Buchanan R, et al. Prolonged expiratory apnoea (cyanotic 'breath-holding') in association with a medullary tumour. *Dev Med Child Neurol.* 1987;29:789–793.

46. Southall DP, Talbert GD, Johnson P, et al. Prolonged expiratory apnoea—a disorder resulting in episodes of severe arterial hypoxaemia in infants and young children. *Lancet.* 1985;2:571–577.

CHAPTER 3

Biology and Microscopic Morphology of Posterior Fossa Tumors

Filippo Gullotta

Introduction

Brain tumors are among the most frequent neoplastic diseases of childhood, being surpassed in frequency only by leukemia and, in early infancy, by renal neoplasms. Whereas in early infancy supratentorial tumors predominate, starting with the fourth or fifth year the number of infratentorial tumors exceeds that of cerebral neoplasms, the rates being 60% to 40%, respectively, in the statistics of Koos and Miller[1] or 55% to 45% according to Brett.[2] After adolescence, the figures fall rapidly down to about 20%, and supratentorial tumors are again predominant. A satisfying explanation of this and of many other biological aspects of childhood central nervous system (CNS) tumors is at present not available. These points have been recently discussed *in extenso* by Giuffré.[3]

The midline location of the greatest number of infratentorial tumors and/or the direct involvement of the brain stem and the fourth ventricle explains the early impairment of cerebrospinal fluid (CSF) circulation, the raising of intracranial pressure; and the problems related to prognosis. Given the limited size of the posterior fossa, even slowly growing and histologically benign tumors have to be regarded as potentially malignant because of the impairment produced by pressure on the vital centers of the brain stem. It is a well-known fact that prognosis of brain tumor bearers depends not only on the histology of the neoplasm, but also and primarily on its location and extension; this very important point has been recently emphasized by Raimondi and Taomoto.[4] However, in some cases, infratentorial tumors, surprisingly, do not produce neurologic signs for a long time. Clinicians and neuropathologists are frequently astonished by the presence of huge tumors or cysts involving the cerebellum or brain stem—without an equivalent clinical syndrome. This is often seen in histologically benign tumors.

Glial Tumors

Pilocytic Astrocytoma

This glioma, also called "spongioblastoma" or "juvenile astrocytoma" is, together with the medulloblastoma, one of the most frequent tumors of the posterior fossa and specifically the cerebellum (20–25%). Both sexes are equally affected. This slowly growing tumor is related to paleoencephalic structures, i.e., to the subependymal regions, and therefore usually arises in the midline. In its cerebellar localization it often extends into the hemispheres.

Macroscopically these astrocytomas appear usually well circumscribed, of firm or elastic consistency, and are frequently cystic. In some cases, a more or less strong mucoid degeneration is present, as well as small hemorrhages. These gliomas grow mainly by expansion, but histologically an infiltration of surrounding tissue is evident in the margin of the tumor. Tumor cells can also invade the leptomeninges.

Microscopically, pilocytic astrocytomas ap-

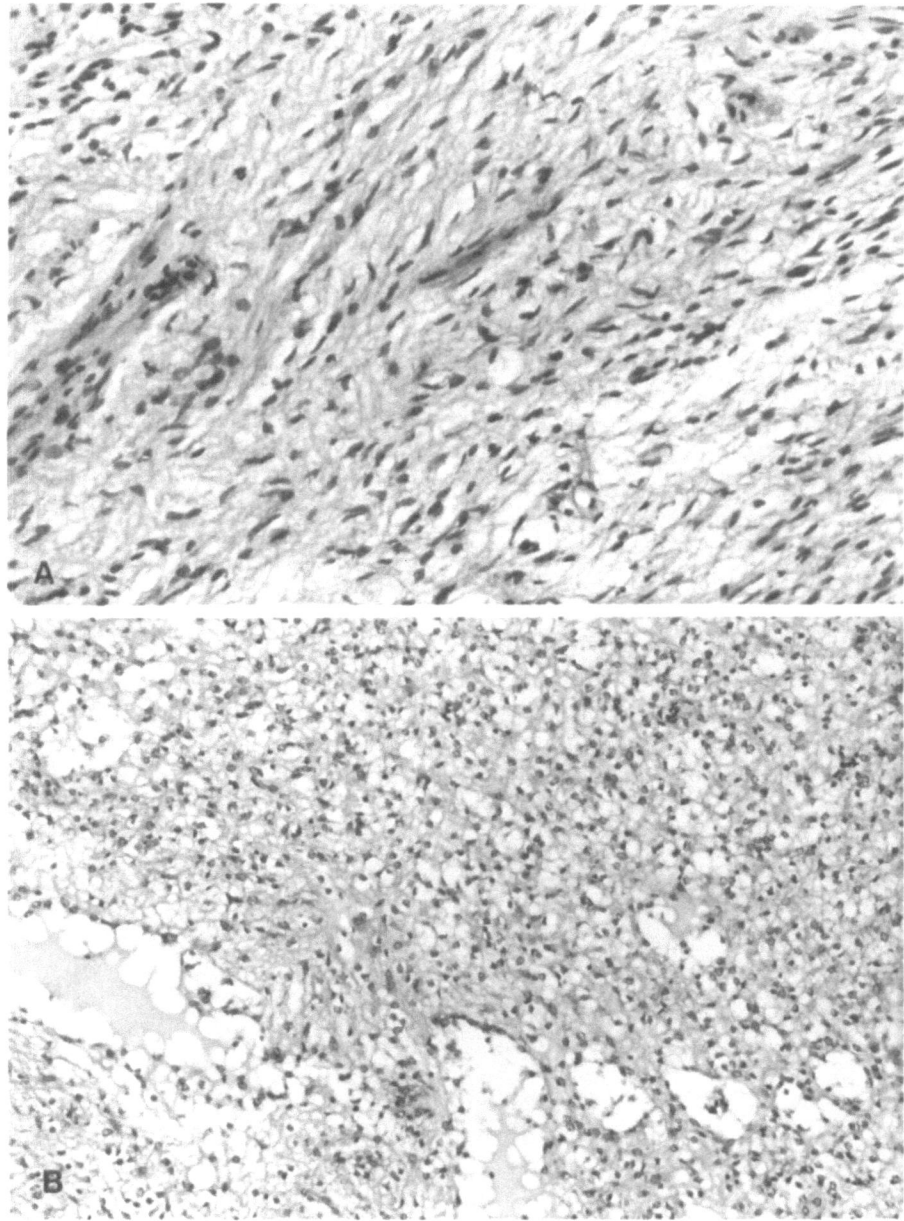

Figure 3.1. Pilocytic astrocytoma of cerebellum. (A) This compact area is composed of fibrillated fusiform and bipolar cells. Other tumor areas show (B) a reticular pattern, due to microcystic and mucoid degeneration of the spindle-shaped cells, which here appear as stellate astrocytes or oligodendrocytes. (H&E; A ×64; B ×40.)

pear as highly fibrillary tumors, the cells of which are slim, elongated, spindle shaped, bipolar ("spongioblasts"; "tanicytes") (Fig. 3.1.A). The morphology and biological behavior of these tumors are quite different from

that of supratentorial astrocytomas of adults. The controversial point concerning the pilocytic shape of tumor cells—whether this shape is a primary or secondary phenomenon—has been clearly resolved by in vitro investigations (see below). Tumor cells are frequently oriented in streams and whorls, and their nuclei are elongated. These cells usually demonstrate a strong positivity for the glial marker GFAP (glial fibrillary acidic protein), expecially if they invade the leptomeninges. Areas with moderate cellularity can alternate with strong fibrillary areas; in some tumors, areas characteristic of subependymomas are present.

The tumor cells have a high tendency to undergo mucoid and fibrillary degeneration; for this reason large tumor areas very frequently present a microcystic reticular appearance (Fig. 3.1B) Mucoid degeneration leads to cell swelling, producing aspects very similar to the honeycomb pattern of oligodendrogliomas: tumor cells appear rounded, the cytoplasm is swollen, and the hyperchromatic nucleus is centrally located. This tendency to microcystic degeneration explains the frequent, almost regular appearance of large cystic cavities within or beside the tumor. In some cases, only a small tumor nodule in the wall of a large fluid-filled cavity is found. A similar finding is frequently seen in cerebellar hemangioblastomas (Lindau's tumor).

A peculiar kind of fibrillary degeneration (Fig. 3.2), very typical for these astrocytes, is represented by the so-called Rosenthal fibers (or cytoid bodies). This name is applied to degenerated cells and cell remnants, which appear as eosinophilic rounded, ovoid, or corkscrew-shaped bodies, partially positive for GFAP. Investigations with the electron microscope and tissue cultures have confirmed that we are dealing here with a peculiar degenerative process of the cells that probably represents the end result of a defect of the metabolism of glial filaments, either an anabolic alteration (overproduction of glial filaments) or a catabolic defect (incomplete degradation) with intracellular overloading.[5,6] This peculiar kind of degeneration is very rare in other astrocytic cell populations; Rosenthal fibers are practically never seen in supratentorial protoplasmic and fibrillary astrocytomas. They are seldom found in glial scars, except for old scars in infantile brains, and mainly in the periventricular regions. Investigations with the electron microscope lead us to suppose that this kind of cellular degeneration could be a disorder akin to a storage dystrophy. This type of cellular degeneration confirms that pilocytic astrocytes are related to but not identical with the usual astrocytic cell population of the cerebrum.

Another peculiar type of degeneration detectable in these tumors is the presence of "granular bodies,"

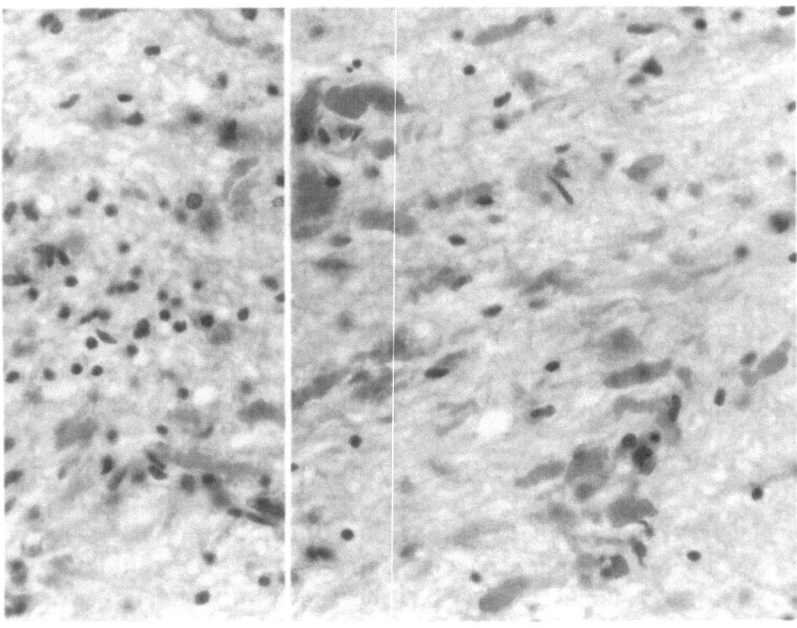

Figure 3.2. In the fibrillated area of this pilocytic astrocytoma, many round-ovoid eosinophilic bodies are evident; Rosenthal fibers. (H&E; ×100.)

first described by Zülch,[7] and related to Rosenthal fibers. Further signs of degeneration, i.e., of slow growth, are represented by less specific findings such as the presence of some small calcospherites irregularly distributed within the tumor, particularly in the highly fibrillary areas, and of some calcified and iron-positive neurons.

The cellular density of these tumors is usually low, and mitoses are scanty or absent. Frequently, atypical cells with large, hyperchromatic, and atypical nuclei, as well as multinucleated cells, can be found. This must not be regarded as a criterion of malignancy, however; rather, it is due to degenerative phenomena. A malignant transformation ("glioblastomatous" astrocytoma) of these tumors is a rare event. According to Garcia and Escalona Zapata,[8] true malignant histological features in these tumors are high cellular density, nuclear pleomorphism, frequent mitoses, and areas of coagulative necroses. It should be stressed, however, that with the exception of high cellular density all the features mentioned above can appear, as a single finding, on the basis of degenerative phenomena and can be depicted in almost every pilocytic astrocytoma. It is therefore very important to examine as much tumor tissue as possible; only a synoptical examination of different tumor areas allows one to get data that permit the evaluation of the biological behavior of the tumor as a whole. In cases of small stereotactic biopsies, the examiner should therefore be very careful in the biological grading of the samples, especially if endothelial proliferations are seen.

Pilocytic astrocytomas are generally poorly vascularized; in some cases, however, vessels with angiomatoid patterns can be present, particularly in young children. Such tumors are usually dysontogenetic in origin and in the past have been termed "angiogliomas." A similar pattern can also be detected in pilocytic astrocytomas invading the leptomeninges; in these cases, a kind of organoid pattern is evident, because large islands of astrocytoma are separated by arachnoid trabeculae and leptomeningeal vessels (Fig. 3.3). These are obviously secondary structures, as is the oligodendroglioma-like appearance frequently seen in some pilocytic astrocytomas, especially if they grow into the leptomeninges (Fig. 3.3).

Vascular proliferations similar to those detectable in malignant astrocytomas of the cerebrum and in glioblastomas are rarely seen. Endothelial buds and vascular coils are found at times in the margin of degenerated areas and cysts. The correct biological interpretation of these findings is very important; they are reactive and should therefore not be mistaken for the afinalistic endothelial proliferations that characterize a glioblastoma.

In some tumor areas, among the elongated tumor cells of piloid appearance, stellate astrocytes can also be seen. These cells can be actual stellate astrocytes, but more frequently they are pilocytic elements that develop this shape because of degenerative phenomena. This finding is in fact very frequent in microcystic and mucoid degenerated areas. The transformation (evolution) of pilocytic astrocytes into stellate astrocytes (and vice versa), as had been hypothesized on the basis of investigations in the past with metallic impregnations or, more recently with immunohistochemical markers, in fact does not occur; this has been confirmed by tissue culture investigations. A description of these results is therefore appropriate.

Tissue Cultures

In vitro studies of pilocytic astrocytomas of the cerebellum, spinal cord, and optic nerves have clearly demonstrated that these tumor cells are completely different from astrocytes of normal brain tissue and from cerebral astrocytomas.[9] Colonies of pilocytic astrocytomas are built up by elongated, slim, spindle-shaped cells with two or three short cytoplasmic processes (Fig. 3.4). A predictable or constant transformation of these elements in typical stellate astrocytes does not appear. Also, after a very long period of cultivation (many months), apart from degenerating signs with shortening and thickening of some cells and their cytoplasmic processes, no evidence of a change in to another glial form can be detected. In other words, pilocytic astrocytes are and remain "pilocytic" from the beginning until the last stage of cultivation, i.e., until degeneration. The morphological and biological differences from the usual "stellate" astrocytes are also demonstrated by the peculiar cellular degeneration leading to the formation of Rosenthal fibers,[6] as demonstrated by Fig. 3.5. Rosenthal fibers have never been seen

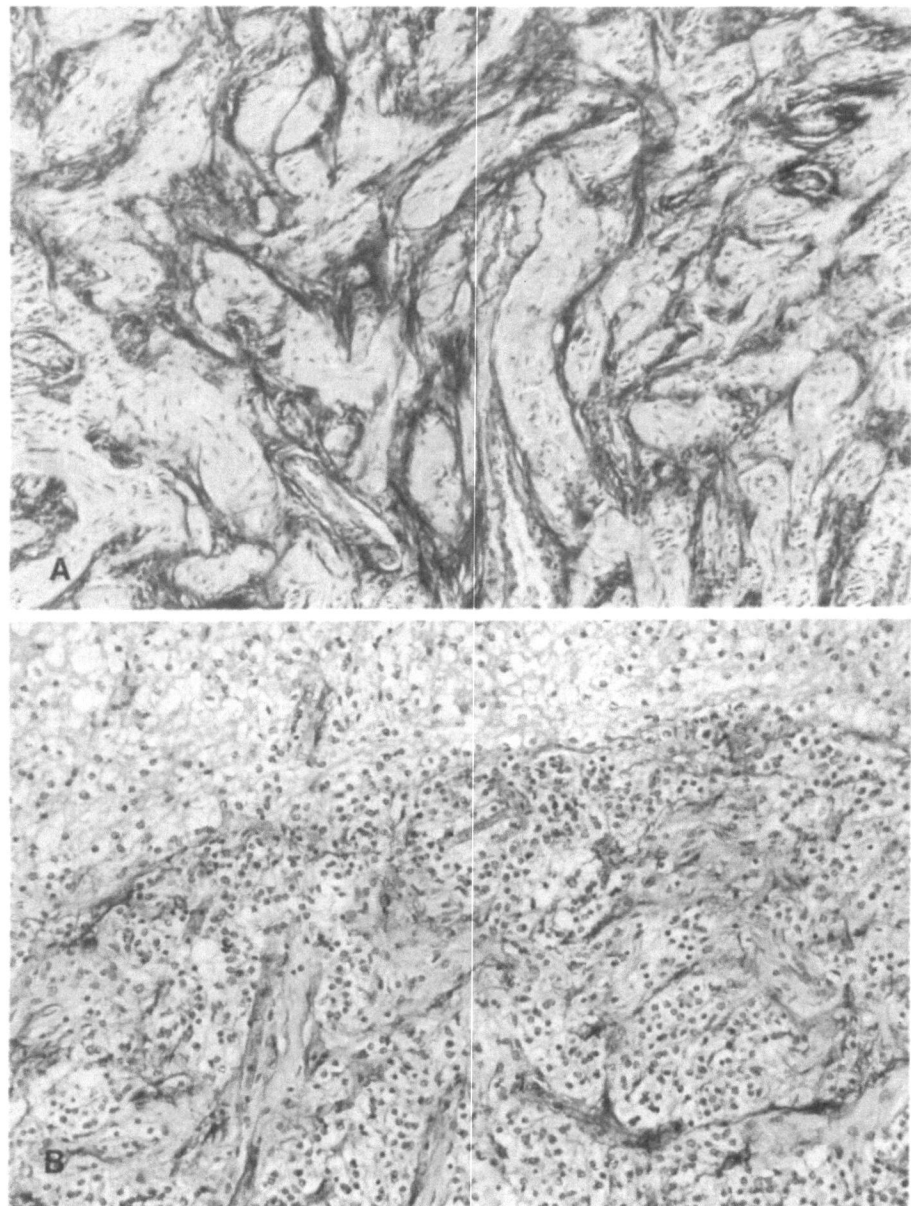

Figure 3.3. Invasion of leptomeninges by pilocytic astrocytoma. Large tumor cell areas are separated by meningeal vessels and fibrotic arachnoid trabeculae. Cells may undergo microcystic changes. A picture similar to "angioglioma" (A) or oligodendroglioma (B) can eventually appear. (Van Gieson; A ×40; B ×60.)

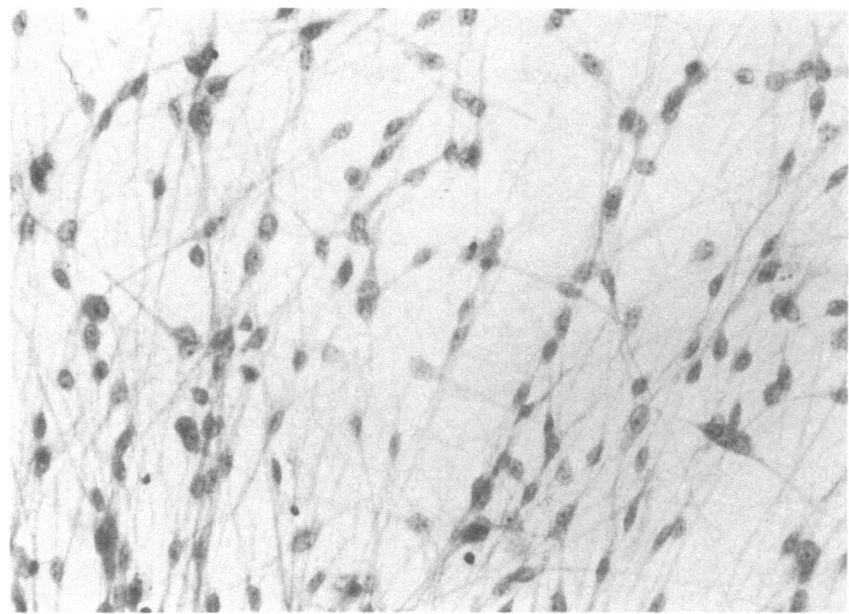

Figure 3.4. Tissue culture of a cerebellar astrocytoma. The pilocytic shape of the proliferating tumor cells is clearly evident. Cells are elongated, mostly bipolar. Stellate astrocytes are missing and will not appear, even in the late stage of cultivation. (H&E; ×60.) (From Gullotta,[57] reproduced with permission of the editor.)

in cultures of cerebral fibrillary or protoplasmic (gemistocytic) astrocytomas.

Biological Behavior

Pilocytic astrocytomas of the cerebellum are benign (grade I). They can however recur, especially if the excision was subtotal. Unfortunately, many of these tumors are located in unfavorable sites, often involving the brain stem as well.

Postoperative radiation of these tumors has been recently proposed. However, this treatment has probably no effect at all, the biological behavior of the tumors being primarily benign. This has been known since the 1931 report of Cushing,[10] and has been confirmed by the author of this chapter in a retrograde study[11] of 105 patients who had been operated on for cerebellar astrocytomas between 1950 and 1972. Thirteen years later, 32 patients were still alive, 14 had been operated on 20 to 30 years before, and 18 patients had been operated on 10 to 19 years previously. In two patients, the tumor had also infiltrated the brain

stem; both of them were still alive 25 and 10 years later. These results confirm the good prognosis of these tumors provided a total resection has been possible. This also demonstrates that patients with a pilocytic astrocytoma do not need postoperative radiotherapy or chemotherapy. These treatments can be applied in cases with certain anaplastic transformation, or in cases of small-celled and fast-growing astrocytomas.

Variants

Small Cell Astrocytoma

A rare cancer that occurs in particular in young children, small-celled astrocytic gliomas, can appear in the cerebellum, brain stem, or cerebrum. These tumors are highly cellular; their biological behavior is different from that of a pilocytic astrocytoma. They are highly malignant and correspond biologically to a medulloblastoma. Tumor cells are not pilocytic astrocytes but small astrocytoma- or oligoglia-like elements with small, round hyperchromatic

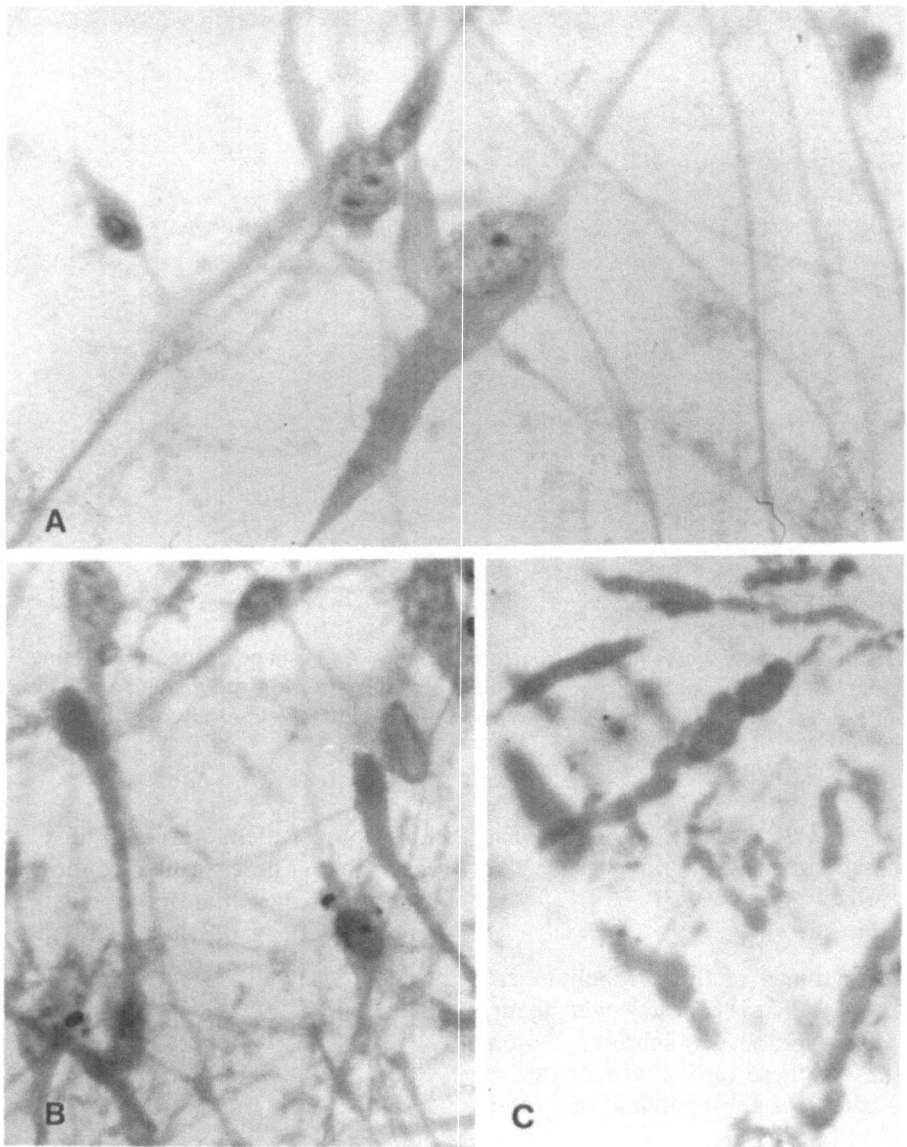

Figure 3.5. Tissue culture of a pilocytic astrocytoma. In the latest stage of cultivation, cells degenerate; they become thicker and strongly eosinophilic, the nucleus eventually disappears (A). Dead cells and cell remnants present the typical aspect of Rosenthal fibers (B, C). (H&E; ×100.) (From Gullotta,[57] reproduced with permission of the editor).

nucleus, and present a high number of mitoses. The tumor cells infiltrate diffusely the cerebellum and the brain stem; they can also invade the leptomeninges, spreading via the CSF to other regions of the brain. The prognosis is very poor.

Polar Spongioblastoma

According to Russell and Rubinstein,[12] this is a rare malignant tumor located in the walls of the fourth or the third ventricle, and histologically characterized by a rhythmic palisade-like dis-

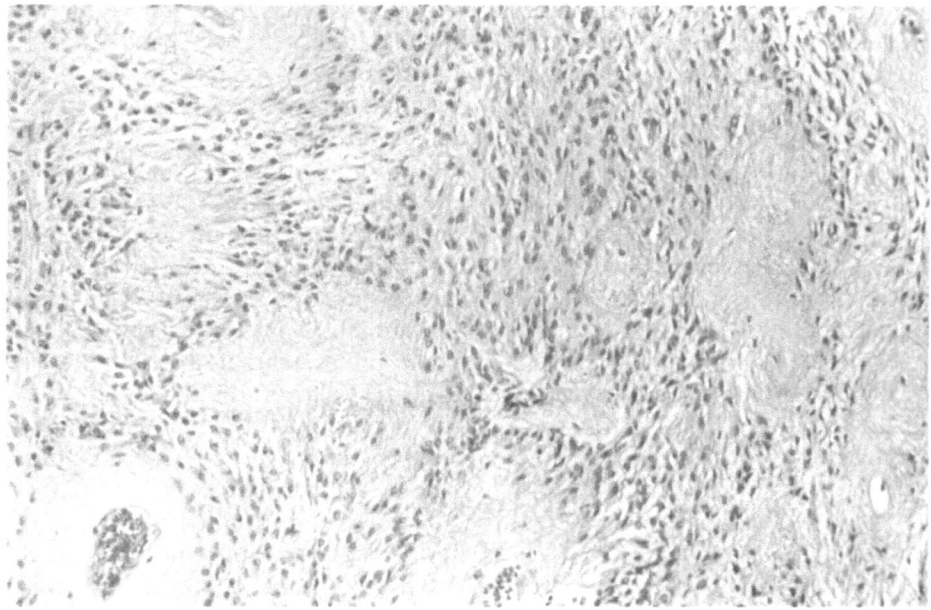

Figure 3.6. Subependymoma of the fourth ventricle. The overall view of the tumor shows highly fibrillated areas intermingled with small cell clusters (subependymal glomerulate astrocytoma). (HE; ×40.)

position of the spindle-shaped tumor cells. The existence of this evidently very rare neoplasm is still debated, however. Rhythmic structures such as those presented in the pictures of Russell and Rubinstein are in fact a frequent non-specific pattern detectable in many astrocytomas, especially in oligodendrogliomas (see Fig. 7 in ref. 13).

Oligodendroglioma

True oligodendrogliomas of the cerebellum are very rare, and benign. The oligoglia-like areas frequently seen in pilocytic astrocytomas are due to regressive cell changes.

Subependymoma

This term is usually applied to small glial nodules localized in the walls of the fourth ventricle or, more rarely, in the walls of cerebral ventricles. They are usually incidental autoptic findings. Histologically they are characterized by small or large clusters of ependymal cells intermingled with bundles of glial fibrils (Fig. 3.6). In some cases however, these nodules can be very large and become true

neoplasms ("subependymal glomerulate astrocytomas").

These tumors are built up by high fibrillary areas (bearing morphological similarities with pilocytic astrocytomas) and by areas with moderate or high cellularity (resembling an ependymoma). Both areas are often strictly intermingled; this explains why many neuropathologists do consider this tumor to be a mixed ependymoastrocytoma. The mixed structure of these tumors has in fact been clearly demonstrated by in vitro investigations.[14]

Subependymomas can also appear in the spinal cord, i.e., they are not restricted to the ventricular walls; "subependymoma areas" can also be easily found in many pilocytic astrocytomas of the cerebellum or spinal cord. This is an important point that may explain possible discrepancies between an initial and a subsequent histological diagnosis in recurring tumors. These divergent findings must not be interpreted as a sign of consecutive cell differentiation, but rather as a reflection of the mixed structure of the tumor, with either ependymal or astrocytic parts prevailing. It is very important for the clinicians to know that these tumors are histologically absolutely benign (grade I); their biological behavior corresponds more to that of a pilocytic astrocytoma than to an ependymoma. They do not need any postoperative treatment. Recurrence is of course possible, especially by tumors located in the spinal cord, and by tumors that were only partially excised.

In some cases, the histological investigation of small tumor specimens composed of ependymal cell clusters may present some differential diagnostic problems with regard to distinguishing ependymoma from medulloblastoma, especially if the tumor is located in the roof of the fourth ventricle.

Brain Stem Gliomas

Astrocytic tumors of the brain stem are composed of a mixed, pleomorphic cell population. They are basically pilocytic in type, but among pilocytic cells typical stellate and/or protoplasmic astrocytes, oligoglia-like elements and pleomorphic glia cells can also be found. In some cases, besides small calcospherites, foci of necrosis or of small ("anaplastic") cells can also be present, with or without proliferations of vascular endothelia (Fig. 3.7). Many of these tumors are therefore named *tout court* glioblastomas, but they differ fundamentally in morphology, behavior, age of incidence, etc. from the "classical" glioblastomas of the cerebral hemispheres. In my opinion, the definition "anaplastic astrocytomas" would be more appropriate here. Absolutely incorrect is the use of the term *primitive neuroectodermal tumor* (PNET) with astrocytic differentiation" (see below). Gliomas located in the lower portion of the brain stem (medulla) are usually histologically benign, whereas those appearing in the midbrain and pons are predominantly anaplastic (malignant).

According to their modality of growth, these gliomas can be divided in to two groups: focal and diffuse. Focal gliomas are mainly pilocytic in type, or subependymomas; they may also be cystic. Surgical treatment of these tumors is frequently successful.[15-18] Diffuse gliomas have a tendency to infiltrate the local structures, mainly respecting and engulfing nerve

cells and growing along and within fiber tracts. In these cases, the whole brain stem appears macroscopically enlarged; a tumor "nodule" is not detectable. Histologically, such a "neoplastic" brain stem shows a very pleomorphic picture, with different cell types, neurons, calcospherites, necrosis, etc. In some cases, tumor cells can also invade the leptomeninges, growing outside the brain stem (exophytic or extrinsic growth); this can be relevant for treatment and prognosis. In some unfavorable cases, the whole brain stem, from the midbrain to cervical medulla, is diffusely infiltrated by neoplastic glia cells. A brain stem glioma can in fact represent the first local manifestation of a diffuse gliomastosis.

The above-mentioned modalities of growth have prognostic relevance, because surgical therapy in focal gliomas, in cystic tumors, and in extrinsic growths can be successful. The statement of Matson[19] that these tumors, regardless of their specific histology, must all be classified as malignant, since their location itself renders them inoperable, can be only partially accepted today. The positive results presented by many authors[15-18,20,21] confirm that in many cases of brain stem gliomas, surgical excision was successful in prolonging the survival time of these patients.

Brain stem gliomas usually grow slowly, frequently with relapses and rarely regress.[11] Their clinical course generally does not correlate with their histology. In fact, as in some tumors that present a pleomorphic histologic picture ("glioblastoma"), an unexpected long survival time for patients can be seen, regardless of whether or not they underwent radio- or chemotherapy. This point must not be forgotten in the evaluation of nonsurgical treatments. "Recognition that certain patients with brainstem gliomas may have prolonged survival even in the absence of definitive treatment must be taken into consideration when new treatment regimens are being formulated."[21] There is in fact no actual evidence that modern therapies have significantly increased the survival time of these patients.[22] A brain stem glioma follows its own biological laws; its clinical course therefore remains unpredictable from a histologic point of view. Glioblastomas

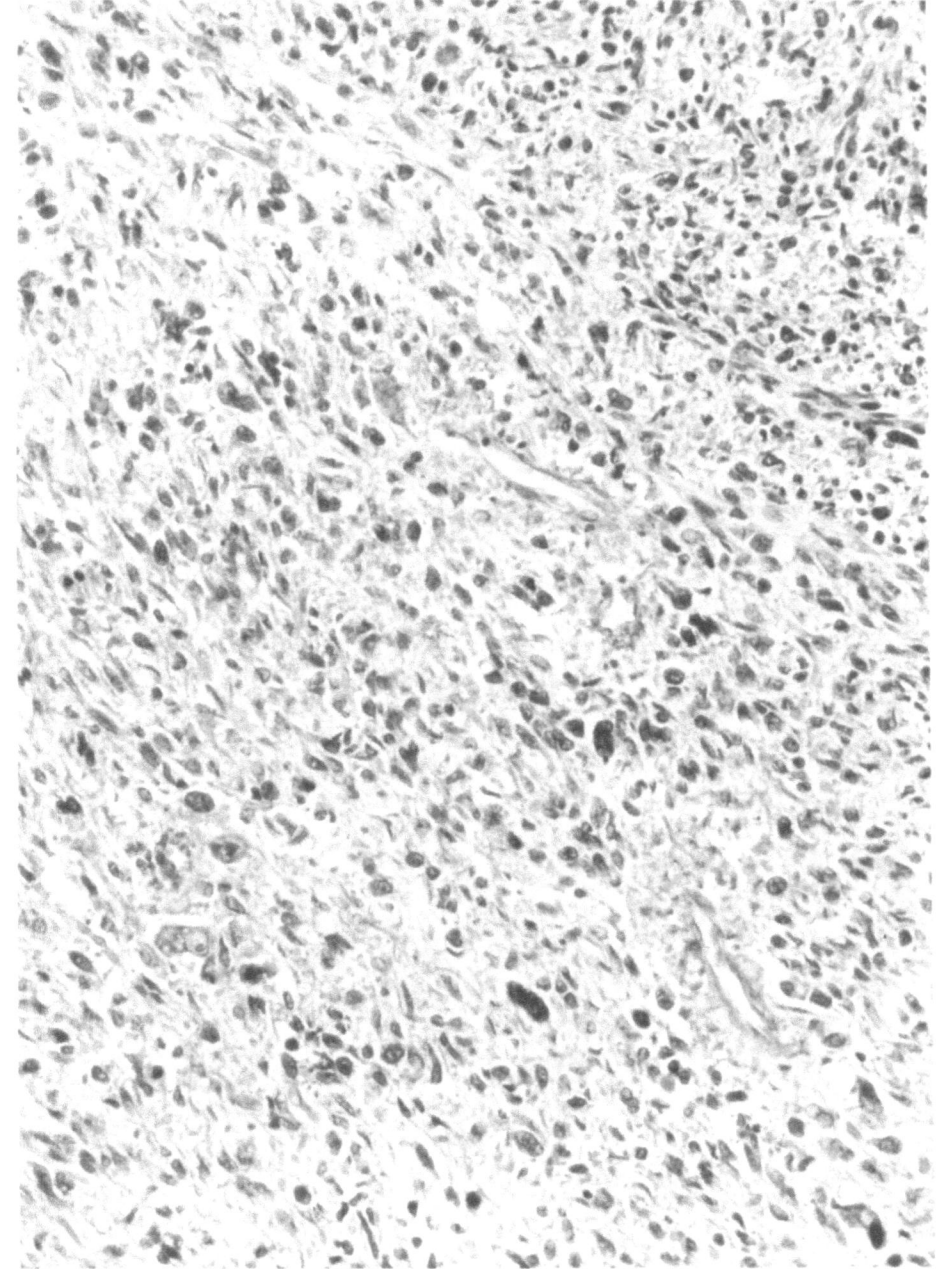

Figure 3.7. Brain stem glioma. This pons glioma, showing a basic pilocytic pattern, is characterized by a pleomorphic glial cell population. Micronecroses and vascular proliferations are missing, however. (HE; ×60.)

of the brain stem with a long survival time (e.g., 18 years[23]) are obviously incorrect histologic diagnoses.

Medulloblastoma and Primitive Neuroectodermal Tumor

Medulloblastoma

The medulloblastoma is the most malignant brain tumor of childhood; its frequency peak lies between 5 and 10 years of age, twice as many boys being affected than girls. These tumors account for about 20% of cerebral neoplasms of children. They can also appear in adolescents and adults, especially as the variant known as "desmoplastic medulloblastoma."

Medulloblastomas usually arise in the midline (vermis cerebelli; velum medullary inferior); they grow very quickly, infiltrating and destroying the local structures, spreading into the cerebellar hemispheres and the leptomeninges, and sometimes filling up the cavity of the fourth ventricle. This explains the high frequency of liquoral metastases. In adolescents and adults, but rarely in children, medulloblastomas are laterally localized in the cerebellar hemispheres; in these cases they are usually circumscribed and of firm consistency as they are rich in reticulin fibers ("desmoplastic medulloblastomas").

Macroscopically, the grayish-white tumor masses are soft and friable; their cut surface has a granular appearance. In rare instances calcospherites or cysts are seen. In some cases the tumor can appear well demarcated, but usually it infiltrates diffusely the surrounding structures, which in turn appear enlarged and whitish. The leptomeninges involved have a milky appearance.

Microscopically, medulloblastomas are high cellular tumors, composed of small undifferentiated cells with poorly defined cytoplasm and round–oval nuclei (Fig. 3.8). Cells can also appear beet- and carrot-shaped, without any peculiar architectural arrangement; in some areas they are vaguely disposed in concentric patterns, building what it is usually called

a pseudorosette, devoid of a lumen (Homer-Wright rosette). Cellular and/or nuclear pleomorphism is rarely seen and vascular stroma and reticulin fibers are usually scanty. Only in the variant known as *desmoplastic medulloblastoma* a high number of reticulin fibers is present, in the meningeal growths and in the intracerebellar tumor areas as well (Fig. 3.9A). This tumor variant presents histologically a lobulated pattern due to the fact that reticulin-free tumor islands are separated by strands of reticulin, meningeal cells, capillaries, and fibroblasts. This tumor is also known as "arachnoidal sarcoma." Reticulin fibers can also be found within small cell groups, surrounding single tumor cells. Rarely, in some medulloblastomas, striated or nonstriated muscle fibers and large, eosinophilic myoblastic-like elements are present ("medullomyoblastoma").

The prognosis of medulloblastomas is poor (grade IV), although in recent years good progress has been made with radiotherapy; survival times of 5 to 8 years can be observed, particularly in desmoplastic medulloblastomas. However, it must be stressed that desmoplastic medulloblastomas generally do present a longer survival time, independent of radiotherapy.[24]

Histogenesis

Since the first description of this tumor by Bailey and Cushing[25] 65 years ago, its histogenetic problem is still the object of discussion and scientific controversies. "Despite numerous cytologic, histochemical, and electron microscopic studies, evidence for the real existence of a common neural stem cell, the hypothetical medulloblast, is still lacking."[26]

Given the fact that in some tumors, some signs of a neuronal or glial differentiation can be found, the current histogenetic theories consider the medulloblastoma as a primitive neuroectodermal tumor with a glial, or a neuronal or a multipotential, differentiation capability. These theories are mainly based on these findings: (a) presence of Homer-Wright pseudorosettes in some tumors; (b) presence of mature glia and/or neurons among the undifferentiated tumor cells; (c) rhythmic palisading of tumor cells, suggestive of "spongioblastic" differentiation; (d) identification of astrocytoma- or oligodendroglioma-like areas within or at the periphery of the tumor; (e) evidence of neurofibrillary differentiation in

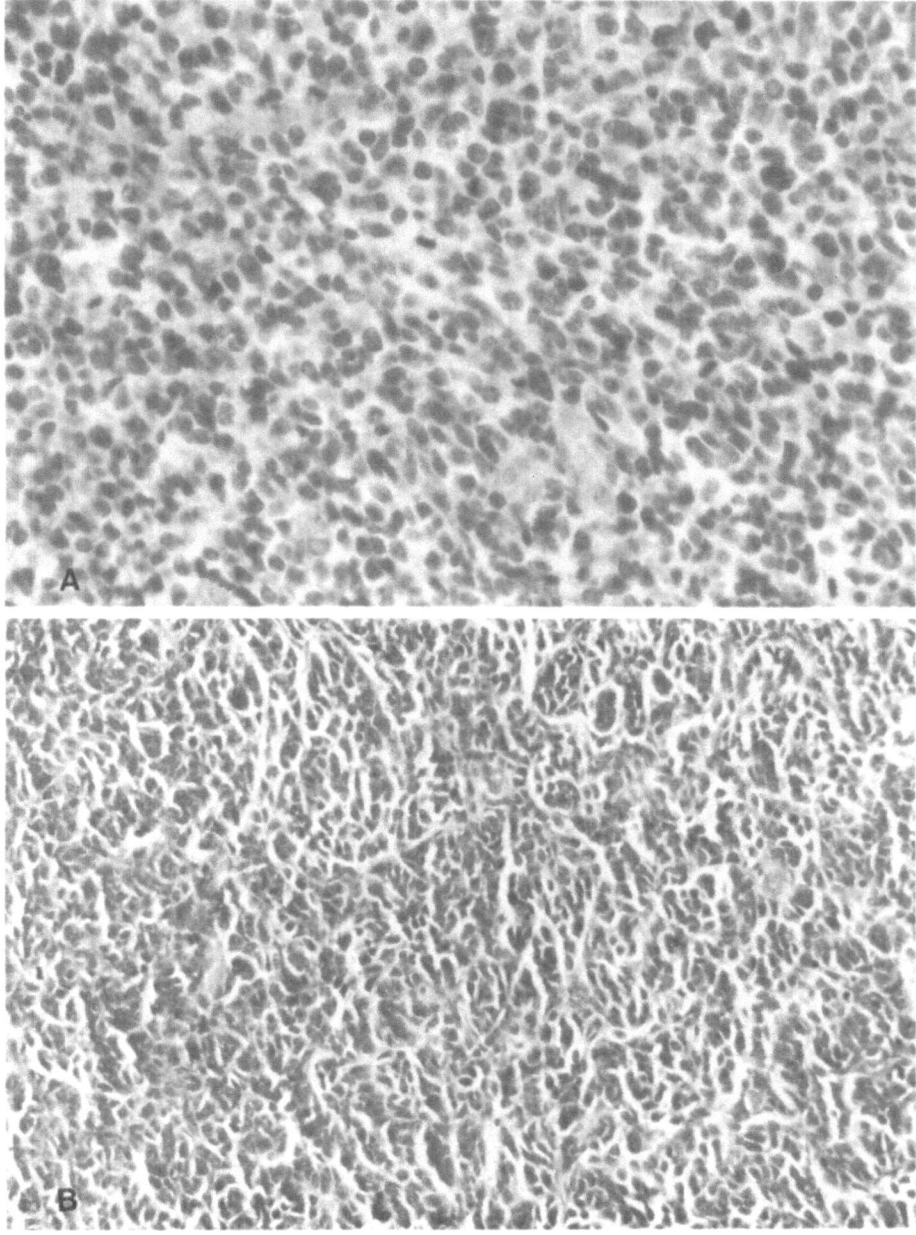

Figure 3.8. Medulloblastoma. (A) The highly cellular tumor is composed of small cells with hyperchromatic nuclei and many mitoses; no definite architectural pattern or any signs of cellular differentiation are detectable. (H&E; ×100.) (B) Desmoplastic medulloblastoma. The tumor cells are identical with those depicted in A, but they are arranged in small lobules or fields by strands of reticulin fibers (see also Fig. 3.9A). (H&E; ×64.)

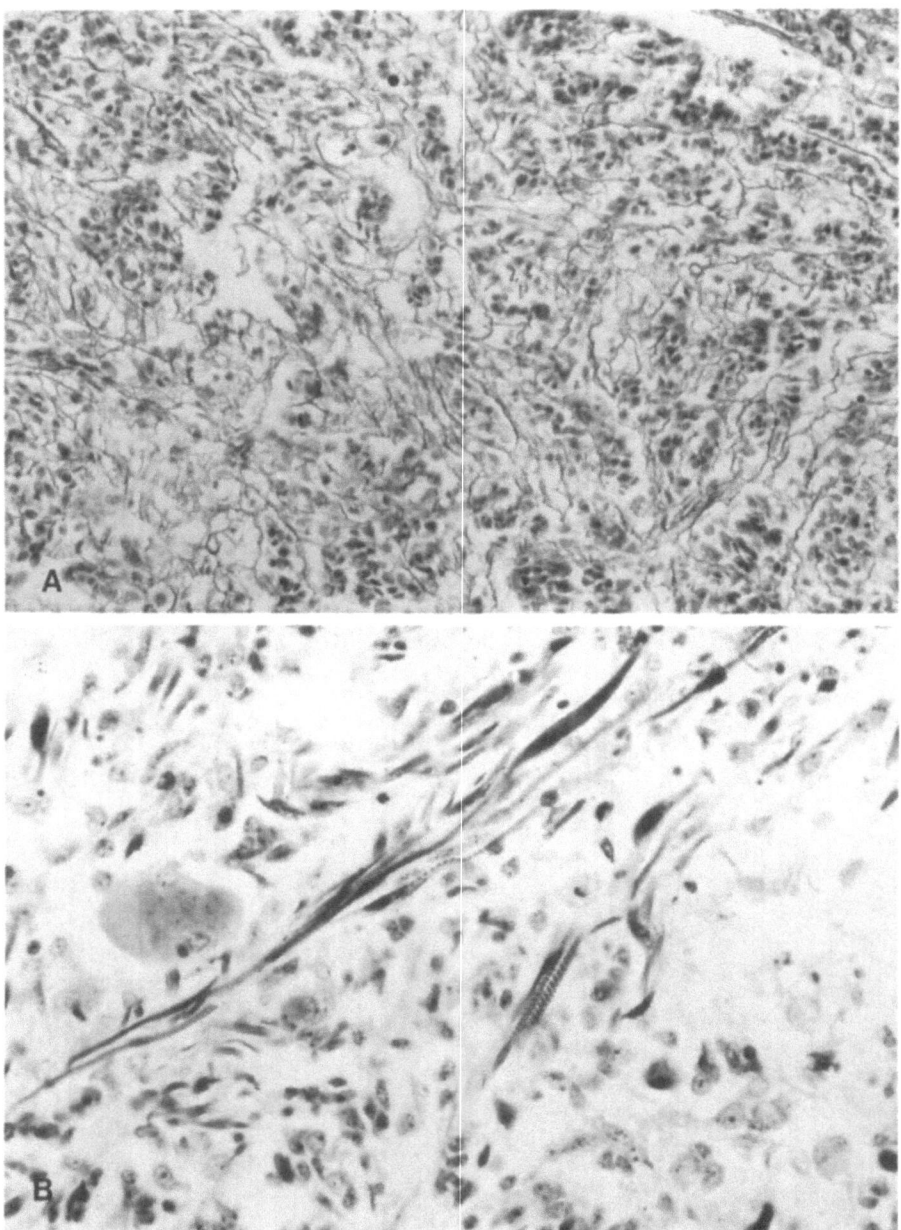

Figure 3.9. (A) Desmoplastic medulloblastoma. In this intracerebellar growth of the tumor, a dense meshwork of reticulin fibers separating cell groups or even single cells is clearly evident. This reticulin network is different from reactive fibrosis detectable in leptomeninges invaded by tumor cells (for comparison see Fig. 3.3). (Gomori; ×100.) (B) "Medullomyoblastoma." In this otherwise typical medulloblastoma, some striated muscle fibers and myoblast-like cells are evident. (Van Gieson; ×100.)

some tumor cells as revealed by metallic impregnations, electron microscopy, tissue cultures and histochemistry. However, the critical analysis of these points[27,28] has demonstrated that the above-mentioned cytological and histological features are not specific at all. In particular, the glial or neuronal elements occasionally found in medulloblastomas and intermingled with tumor cells are usually preexistent elements that have been entrapped by the proliferating tumor cells. This is already evident with conventional histological methods, and has been confirmed by immunohistochemistry.[29,30] Furthermore, the GFAP-positivity reported by some authors and regarded as the confirmation of the presumed glial differentiation of tumor cells, cannot be taken as a certain demonstration of this, because it is known that GFAP is not specific.[31,32]

The exact evaluation of the distribution of these cells within the tumor confirms that the greatest number of them are reactive and not neoplastic.[30,31] A certain neuronal differentiation has seldom been demonstrated.[8]

The neurofibrillary differentiation depicted in some tumor cells by metallic impregnations is not specific or at least very doubtful. The sporadic positivity for Synaptophysin occasionally detected in *some* cells demonstrates that these few cells show evidence of a neuronal differentiation. Immunocytochemical results obtained with neuron-specific enolase (NSE) and neurofilament protein (NP), and other "neuronal" markers as well, are worthless because all these markers (out of Synaptophysin) are *not* specific,[31] especially if they are employed on paraffin slides. It has to be stressed that the interpretation of immunohistochemical findings in medulloblastomas and in PNETs is usually subjective, problematic; and often controversial, especially since we know that different markers can be coexpressed by one and the same cell. However, even if we accept the "neuronal" results of immunohistochemistry, it remains to be explained why in these tumors only evidence of a molecular but not of a histomorphological neuroectodermal differentiation is seen.

The results of electron microscopical investigations also conflict with those of immunohistochemistry. This has been recently emphasized by Ishida.[33] The presence of filaments and dense-core vesicles in some tumor cells seems to demonstrate their neuronal origin or differentiation capability. If this were true, given the high frequency of medulloblastomas, we would expect to find a very large number of these tumors presenting light-microscopical evidence of a neuronal or a glial differentiation. This is not the case, however.

The results obtained by tissue culture investigations are controversial (see review[34]). A neuronal and/or glial differentiation of cultured tumor cells has been reported by Lumsden[35] and by Herman and Rubinstein[36] in single cases of medulloblastomas, whereas the systematic investigations of Kersting[9] and Gullotta and Kost,[37] on a large number of medulloblastomas, have failed to demonstrate any evidence of a constant glial or neuronal differentiation. Only in one of our 50 cultured tumors, a proliferation of neuroectodermal cells, similar to those detectable in sympathoblastoma was seen.[38] In the cell colonies of the other tumors a vigorous and incessant growth of short, fish-like cells, endothelial in type, was observed. In about 50% of these cultures, small clusters of granule-like cells or few, sporadic neuroectodermal elements were also present; these single cells or cell groups were permanently overgrown by the endothelia-like cells, however (for details see ref. 37). These results fit in with our histogenetic interpretation of medulloblastoma (see below).

A very important point should be stressed. The morphological investigation of small biopsy specimens is not adequate to comprehend the histogenetic problem of the medulloblastoma, because tumor cells usually infiltrate very deeply the cerebellar tissue, without destroying the underlying nervous substance, neurons, or glia cells (Fig. 3.10), which are thereby intermingled with neoplastic elements. Medulloblastomas are tumors of soft consistency and are therefore usually removed by suction; in most cases, the fragments employed for morphological investigations consist of infiltrated cerebellar tissue. This basic fact is usually neglected by many investigators; it easily explains the contradictory findings and the different histogenetic interpretations reported in the literature.

Conclusion

The origin of this tumor and the differentiation capability of its cells are still controversial. In my opinion, we are not dealing with a single oncotype, but with a *tumor group* that includes (a) rare, pure neuroectodermal tumors (neuroblastomas; small cell gliomas); (b) tumors with mixed cell populations, i.e., with intermingled neuroectodermal and mesenchymal cells; and (c) mesenchymal tumors, probably pial in origin (leptomeningeal sarcomas). All these cell populations derive from the neural crest (ectomesenchyme). In mixed tumors, there is

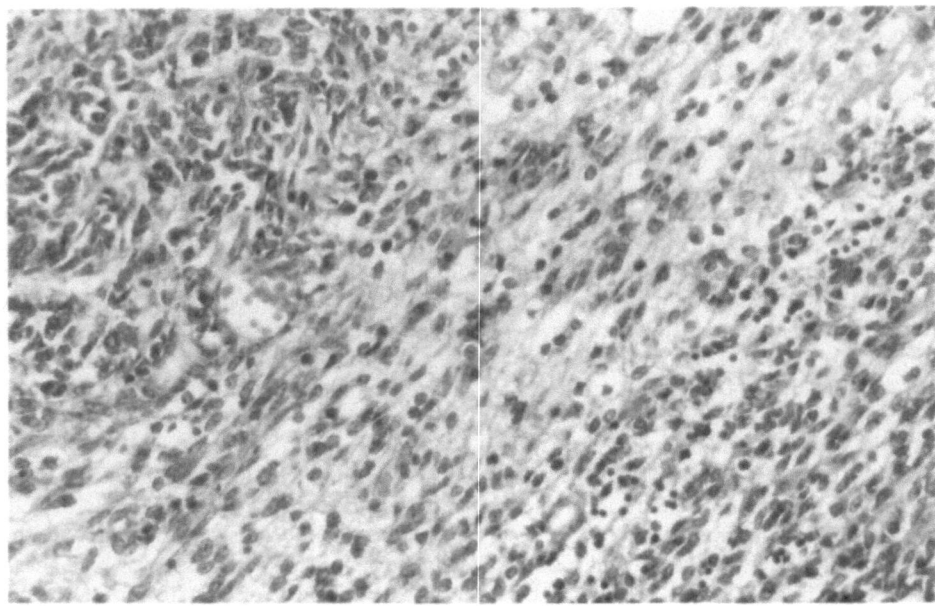

Figure 3.10. Medulloblastoma. The tumor cells have diffusely infiltrated the cerebellum and are intermingled with preexistent glia and nerve cells. The biopsy examination of such an area may give rise to misinterpretations about the hypothetical differentiation capability of "medulloblasts." (H&E; ×80.)

usually an overgrowth phenomenon of one of the two components (for details see refs. 13 and 27).

This hypothesis can help us to understand the pleomorphic appearance of the whole tumor group and of single cases as well. It also easily explains the presence of muscle fibers in some "medullomyoblastomas," the autochthonous production of reticulin fibers detectable in the intracerebellar growths of some desmoplastic medulloblastomas, and the presence of melanin granules in some "papillary" medulloblastomas (a finding that can be observed also in some meningiomas).

Many tumors reported in the literature as medulloblastoma with neuroblastomatous differentiation are true central neuroblastomas. In these cases, if the neuroblastoma-component prevails (and this is not infrequent), it would be correct to speak directly of central neuroblastoma (see below). For more discussion on medulloblastoma and PNETs, see the next chapter.

Primitive Neuroectodermal Tumors (PNET)

This definition was introduced by Hart and Earle[39] to describe small-celled, isomorphic, unclassifiable tumors of the CNS considered to be built up by undifferentiated or embryonic neuroectodermal elements. The name PNET was later extended by Rorke et al.[40] to any kind of CNS tumor consisting (or containing foci) of undifferentiated cells. This term is actually largely employed also in general pathology, to describe every kind of tumor devoid of sure signs of differentiation, and the cells of which react (or do not react) with "specific" neuroectodermal markers. The interpretation of these findings, however, varies from pathologist to pathologist; it is merely subjective, and the reliability of the employed markers is frequently questionable.[31]

The controversial points concerning the definition of cerebral PNET have been discussed by many authors and are reported in the monograph of Fields.[41] A very critical analysis of this term has been recently given by Schiffer et al.[30] As pointed out by these authors, if we apply the definition PNET in the classification of the CNS tumors, the only undifferentiated tumor deserving this name is the medulloblastoma. If we extend the definition PNET to all tumors of children and adults consisting (or containing foci) of small, "undifferentiated" (i.e., not classifiable) cells, we will have just a large heterogeneous group of different neoplasms. Taking into account, for instance, that in many brain stem gliomas foci of small unclassifiable cells are frequently present (anaplastic? dedifferentiated? undifferentiated? small astro- or oligocytes?), the consequent application of the PNET system would mean speaking not of mixed, pleomorphic, or anaplastic glioma or astrocytoma, but rather of PNET with glial/astrocytic/oligodendrocytic, etc. differentiation. The same applies for the supratentorial tumors.

The application of this nomenclature is clinically without any relevance. The biological behavior of a tumor will probably not change if instead of medulloblastoma we call it "PNET with medulloblastic or neuronal, or ependymal, or astrocytic differentiation." The PNET system will only oversimplify the histological categorization of different oncotypes, acting as a wastebasket category. This oversimplification represents an obstacle in comparing histological diagnoses among different pathologists, and creates disarray in the evaluation of the clinical course, *viz.* of the efficiency of the therapies employed.

There is no doubt that few single cases of supratentorial round-celled, unclassifiable, "medulloblastoma-like" tumors occur. In my opinion, the term *PNET* should be reserved only for these neoplasms and not employed in the broad sense, as it is.

Neuroblastoma and Gangliocytoma

Central *neuroblastomas* are rare malignant tumors that appear usually in childhood, mostly in the posterior fossa, but also in the supra-

tentorial regions. Their frequency cannot be exactly evaluated, because many of them are described actually as medulloblastomas or *tout court* PNETs. They are built up by small cells with round hyperchromatic nuclei, presenting features of neuroblastic differentiation in the form of slender, elongated cytoplasmic processes, many Homer-Wright pseudorosettes, nervous ground substance (very good evidence also in leptomeningeal spreading) and, rarely, ganglionic cells (ganglioneuroblastomas).

Macroscopically, these tumors can appear sharply demarcated, but histologically, characteristics of malignancy are evident: high mitotic rate, infiltration of surrounding tissue, and not infrequent leptomeningeal spreading, similar to that observed in medulloblastomas or in some cases of pineoblastomas. Synaptophysin and chromogranin markers are positive in many cells. The prognosis is poor (grade IV).

Microscopically, single tumor areas are practically indistinguishable from a medulloblastoma. It is therefore very important to examine many parts of the tumor, which facilitates the identification of the true neoplastic elements, primarily for the presence of the nervous ground substance and of slim, elongated, neuritic processes. The differences between neuroblastoma and medulloblastoma cells can be clearly detected by in vitro investigations (Fig. 3.11).

Rarely, *gangliocytomas* (gangliogliomas) can also be found in the cerebellum. As their supratentorial counterparts, these tumors are characterized by the presence of large ganglionic elements within a ground substance that clearly consists of glial tissue (Fig. 3.12). These tumors should not be identified with the gangliocytoma dysplasticum cerebelli (see below). Proliferating features of glial cells can usually be detected; the term *ganglioglioma* is therefore the most suitable one for these cases, especially if we consider that the slow progressive growth of these tumors is not so much due to the proliferation of neuronal elements as to that of glial cells. These cells are usually astrocytes but oligoglia can also be found.

In some cases, transitional forms between neuroblastoma and gangliocytoma can be present. But not every cluster of small rounded,

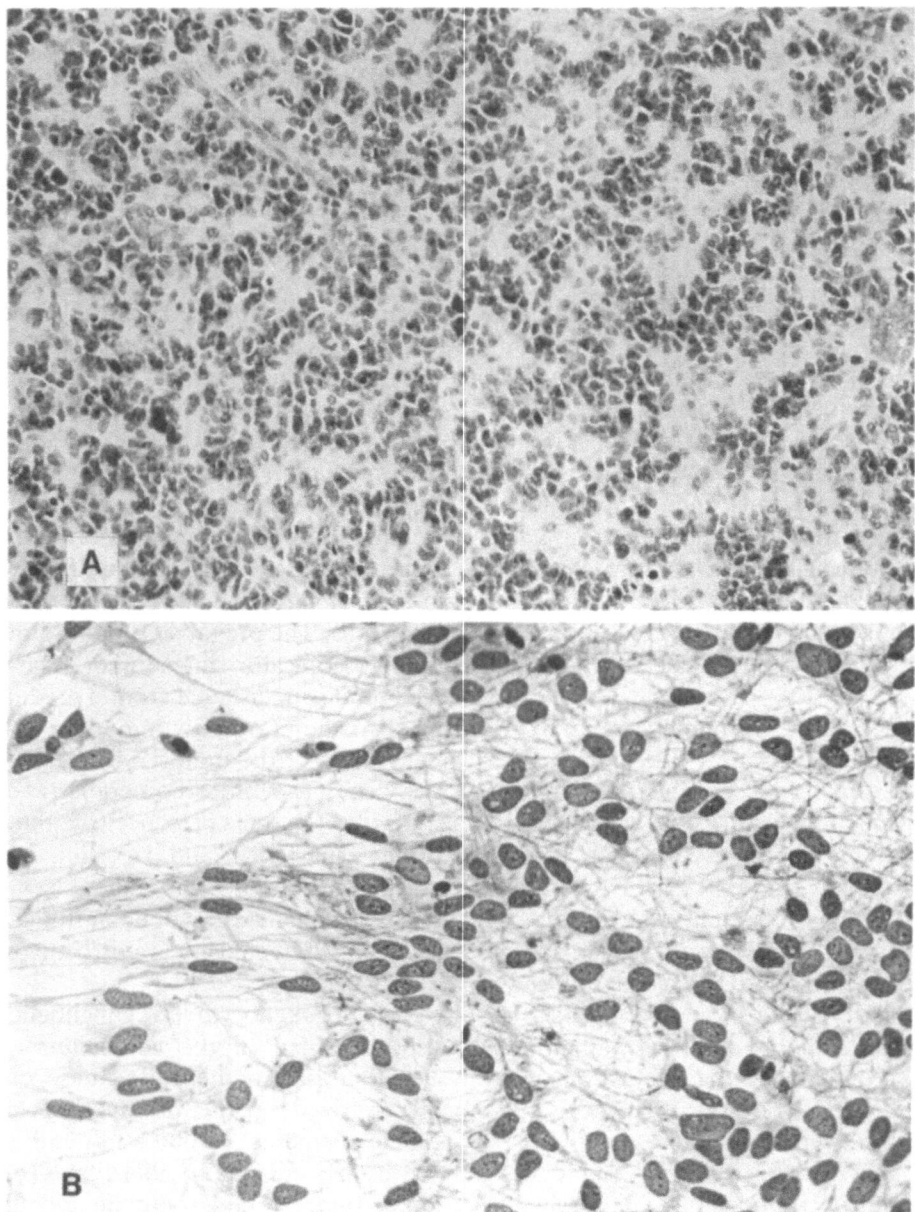

Figure 3.11. Cerebellar neuroblastoma. (A) Histology shows a tumor very similar to a medulloblastoma, with many rosette-like cell formations. These consist of delicate cell processes. The neuroblastic nature of the tumor is clearly demonstrated by tissue culture (B). The growing cells have very long and delicate cell processes, which build a network very similar to that detectable in cultures of embryonic nervous tissue or of sympathicoblastomas. This growth pattern in medulloblastoma cultures was missed.[37] (A, van Gieson, ×50; B, Bodian ×100.)

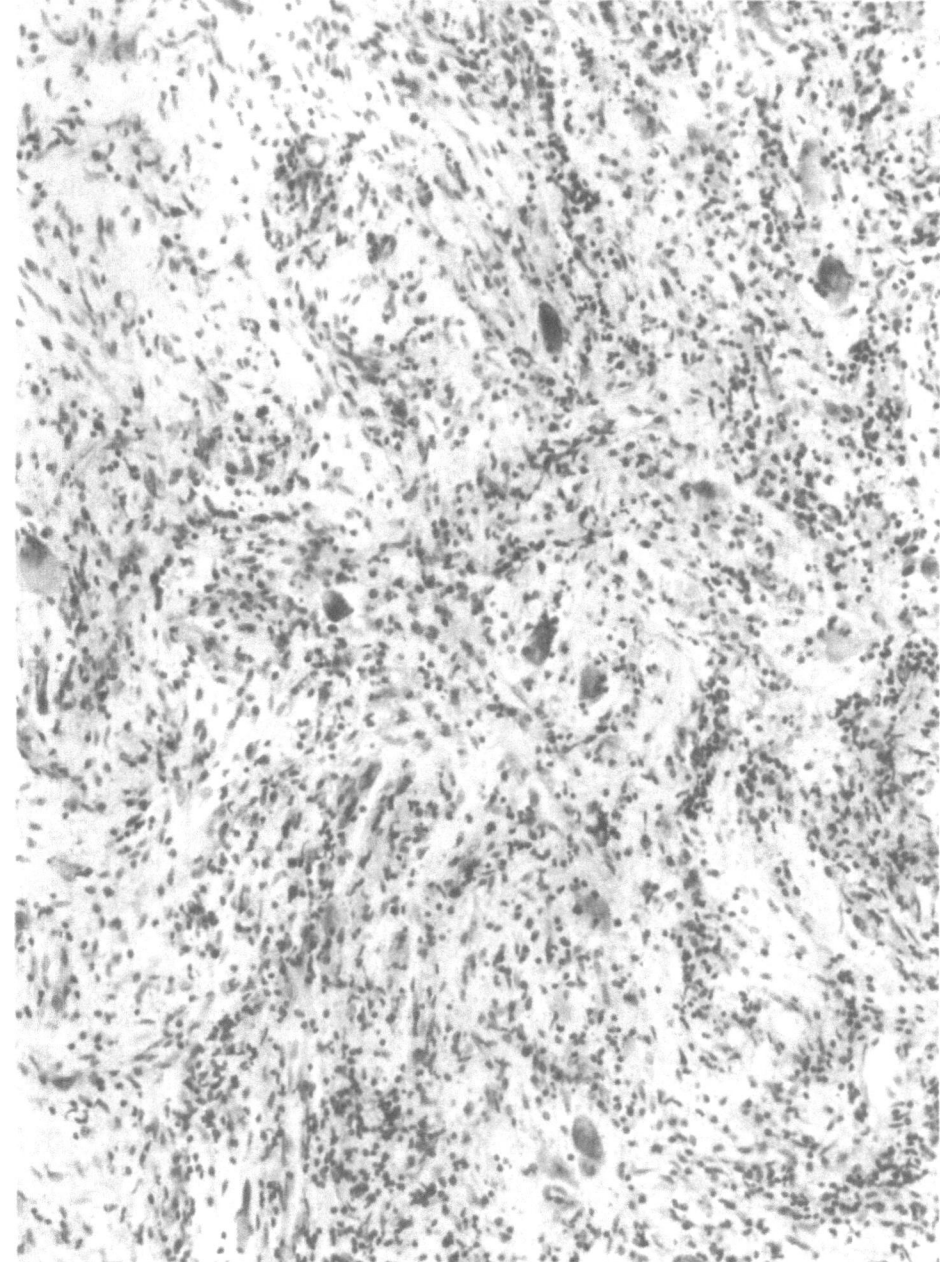

Figure 3.12. Ganglioglioma of the cerebellum. The tumor is built up by a gliomatous ground substance with many ganglionic cells of different size and shape. (Nissl; ×60.)

lymphocyte-like cells should be interpreted as "neuroblasts," for in slow-growing gliomas the presence of lymphocytic infiltrates is not infrequent. Gangliocytomas (gangliogliomas) are usually relatively well demarcated, their prog- nosis is therefore mainly dependent on their location and extension, not on their histology. The malignant transformation is rare and involves mainly the glial, not the neuronal, cell population.

Variant: Gangliocytoma Dysplasticum Cerebelli

The so-called Lhermitte-Duclos disease is a hamartomatous lesion of the cerebellar cortex, which can present itself as a tumor. The cortex appears macroscopically enlarged and of firm consistency. Histologically, the cortical layers are thickened, their architectural pattern is disorganized, and many large or medium-sized atypical nerve cells (Purkinje cells? granule cells? atypical neurons?) are seen (Fig. 3.13). Myelination of the molecular layer is a striking feature of this dysplastic lesion; it is associated with the hypertrophy of granule cells and the myelination of their axons. The neuritic patterns of ganglionic cells as demonstrated by the Golgi method, are different from those of normal cerebellar neurons; Ferrer et al.[42] therefore propose that dysplastic gangliocytoma cerebelli is an organized, self-regulated hamartoma. In some cases, other cerebral and extracerebral malformations (dysplasias) are present; this confirms the maldevelopmental origin of the Lhermitte-Duclos disease. Personal immunohistochemical investigations[43] have shown, that some dysplastic nerve cells share immunohistochemical features with Purkinje cells.[44] The prognosis is good.

Ependymal and Choroid Plexus Tumors

Ependymoma

Ependymomas are rarer than medulloblastomas and pilocytic astrocytomas, accounting—together with choroid plexus papillomas—for about 8% to 10% of infratentorial tumors in children. They arise from the ependymal lining of the fourth ventricle, rarely of the aqueduct, and may completely fill the ventricular cavity, projecting like a tongue into the cisterna cerebellomedullaris. In some rare cases they spread through the foramina of Luschka into the cerebellopontine angle. They are usually benign and grow mainly by expansion, compressing the adjacent structures but also adjusting themselves in form and size to their surroundings.[45] Also in benign ependymomas, histologically a slim layer of tumor cells is detectable on the floor of the fourth ventricle. In malignant forms, tumor cells clearly invade the surrounding structures, infiltrating more or less diffusely cerebellum and/or brain stem. No exact correlation between histology and biology of these tumors can be made, however (see below).

Macroscopically, ependymomas have been compared to placenta because of their reddish, cauliflower appearance. They are very well vascularized and are built up by small nodules and lobules. Microscopically they appear as highly cellular tumors; their cells are isomorphic with a large nucleus and scanty cytoplasm. The typical architectural pattern of ependymomas is the perivascular disposition of the neoplastic elements building up so-called vascular pseudorosettes or gliovascular systems (Fig. 3.14); these appear as nucleus-free perivascular cell cuffs, because the nuclei are displaced to the periphery of the cell. Another typical finding consists of small ependymal cysts (true rosettes, with lumen) or, rarely, ependymal tubules. In some cases, papillary structures can be present; this can create difficulties in differential diagnosis with a papilloma of plexus choroideus, especially in small biopsy specimens. Tumor vessels can undergo fibrohyalinotic and mucoid changes, a phenomenon that is frequently seen in myxopapillary ependymomas of the cauda equina, and in spinal ependymomas and in subependymomas. Mitoses, in benign ependymomas of the fourth ventricle, are rarely seen (they are frequent in supratentorial ependymomas). Mitoses are clearly present in the malignant tumors infiltrating the brain stem and cerebellum. The differential diagnosis with a medulloblastoma can be very difficult here, especially if only small tumor fragments are examined. The presence of gliovascular structures, ependymal cysts, true rosettes, and tubules can help in the diagnosis. Ependymal nuclei are usually larger than those of medulloblastomas. But in some cases a sure nosological identification of the oncotype is not possible. In malignant ependymomas, a metastatic dissemination through cerebrospinal fluid is rarely seen, although it can occur after surgery.

Electron microscopical investigation[46-48] have clearly demonstrated the ependymal nature of

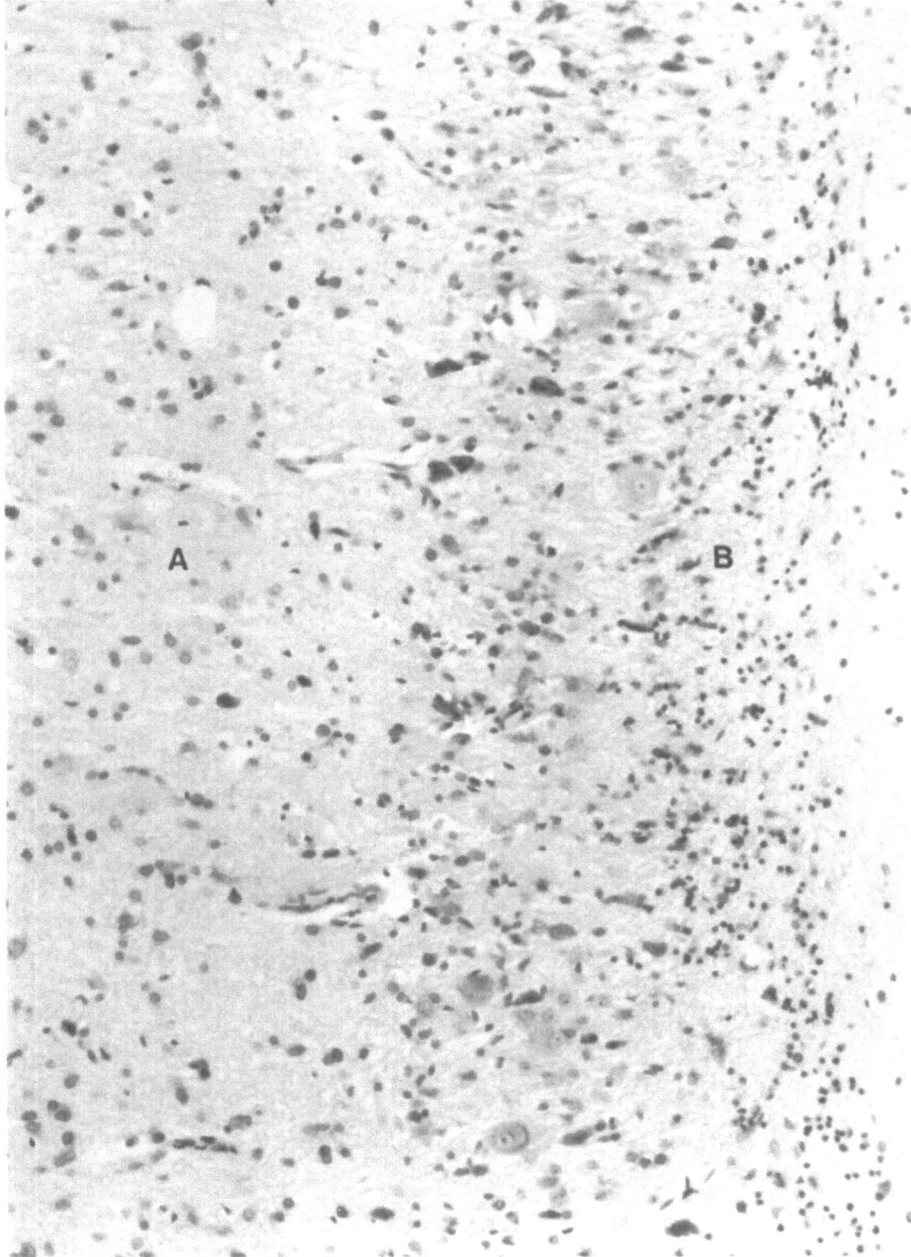

Figure 3.13. Lhermitte-Duclos disease. Dysplastic gangliocytoma is characterized by a diffuse or circumscribed hypertrophy of cerebellar cortex. The molecular layer (A) is greatly thickened and myelinated. The cell layers (B) consist of few remnants of granule cells and of many other neuronal elements of different size, some of which bear resemblance to Purkinje cells. (Nissl; ×60.)

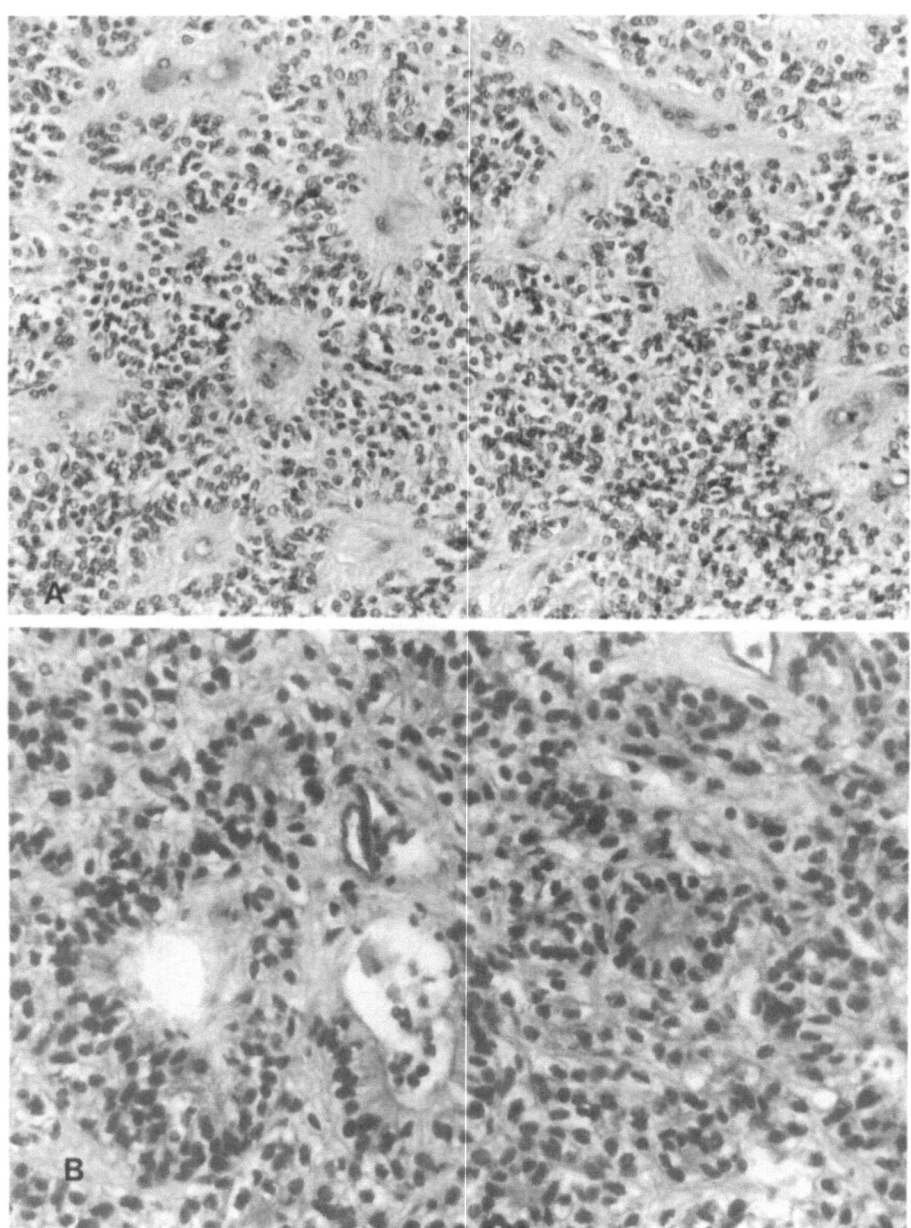

Figure 3.14. Ependymoma. The typical architectural pattern with many perivascular pseudorosettes in seen in A. In B, true ependymal rosettes with lumina are evident. (A, H&E; ×60; B, van Gieson; ×80.)

tumor cells and confirmed the presence of cilia, microvilli, glial filaments, and desmosomes (junctional complexes) between tumor cells. In some cases, cells with features similar to those present in pilocytic astrocytomas have been described.[48] Ependymoma cells express GFAP and S-100 protein, and in some cases also Vimentin.[32]

Tissue Cultures

Systematic investigations have shown that the in vitro proliferating cells are generally isomorphic and epithelial, with round nuclei and evident nucleoli.[9] Proliferating cells are flattened and lie tightly against one another, building up an epithelial carpet or organoid structures. Casentini et al.[14] confirmed these findings and demonstrated that in malignant or anaplastic ependymomas, the growing rates of cell colonies were very high; cell colonies were built up by atypical, multinucleated cells with many mitoses. In cultures of subependymomas, they observed a mixed cell population (pilocytic astrocytes and ependymal cells) growing up from the explanted tumor fragments. These findings confirmed the mixed structure of subependymomas.

Prognosis of infratentorial ependymomas depends primarily on their location and extension, not on their histological structure. Between the histology and biological behavior of ependymomas, no exact correlation can in fact be made.[49] In some cases histologically described as "anaplastic" or malignant, a very long survival time was seen. On the other hand, tumors devoid of histological features of malignancy can have a poor prognosis.

Ependymoblastoma and Medulloepithelioma

The term *ependymoblastoma* is often employed to describe a malignant (anaplastic) ependymoma, i.e., "an ependymoma containing areas of anaplasia, or a tumor resembling a glioblastoma or a medulloblastoma in which features indicative of ependymal differentiation can be recognized."[50] Rubinstein[51] stresses that this term should be reserved for a peculiar tumor, characterized by high cellularity, embryonal cell forms suggesting spongioblasts, ependymal rosettes, and tubules, but devoid of cellular pleomorphism and multinucleated and/or giant cells (as present in anaplastic ependymoma). Rubinstein's entity, however, is controversial and was not accepted by the World Health Organization (WHO) classification, which included it among anaplastic ependymomas. The application here of the PNET system would lead to the definition "PNET with ependymal differentiation."

Few cases of ependymoblastomas as described by Rubinstein have been reported in the literature, but their histological features correspond very well to another rare tumor of children called *medulloepithelioma*. This oncotype should be composed "of undifferentiated medium or tall columnar cells, with characteristic tubular or papillary pattern closely resembling that of primitive neural or medullary epithelium."[50] The picture presented in the few cases published show mainly ependymal rosettes and tubules. The same findings were detected in a personal case.[52] Hence, in my opinion, Rubinstein's

ependymoblastoma and medulloepithelioma represent very probably one and the same tumor. The discussion about the identity of these oncotypes is clinically meaningless, both of them being highly malignant (grade IV).

Subependymoma

A description of this tumor has been given in the chapter on pilocytic astrocytomas.

Choroid Plexus Papilloma and Carcinoma

Choroid plexus papillomas are rarer than ependymomas and occur, in children, mainly in the lateral ventricles and only occasionally in the fourth ventricle.[53] They appear as lobulated, papillary grayish-pink masses, similar to cauliflower. Histologically (Fig. 3.15) their structure closely recapitulates that of normal choroid plexus, with papillae covered by a single layer of cylindrical epithelium, whereas the supporting stroma of papillary ependymoma is built up by neuroglial tissue. Mitoses are scanty. If a high number of mitoses are seen, they should be regarded as a feature of potential malignancy. It has to be stressed, however, that in many plexus papillomas with some cellular atypias and mitoses, the tumors did not show (except in cases of recurrence) any further sign of aggressive growth. The term *carcinoma of the plexus* should therefore be reserved for those tumors presenting certain features of malignancy, e.g., high mitotic rate, cellular and nuclear pleomorphism, and multinucleated cells. Further features of malignancy (infiltration of surrounding structures) can be clearly seen only in autopsy specimens, not in biopsies. Carcinomas of plexus are rare and they generally appear as a malignant transformation of a primary benign papilloma, i.e., they are usually found in recurrences.[54]

Other Rare Space-Occupying Lesions

The *capillary hemangioblastoma* (Lindau's) is rare in children. It can appear as a solitary tumor of the cerebellum or together with a

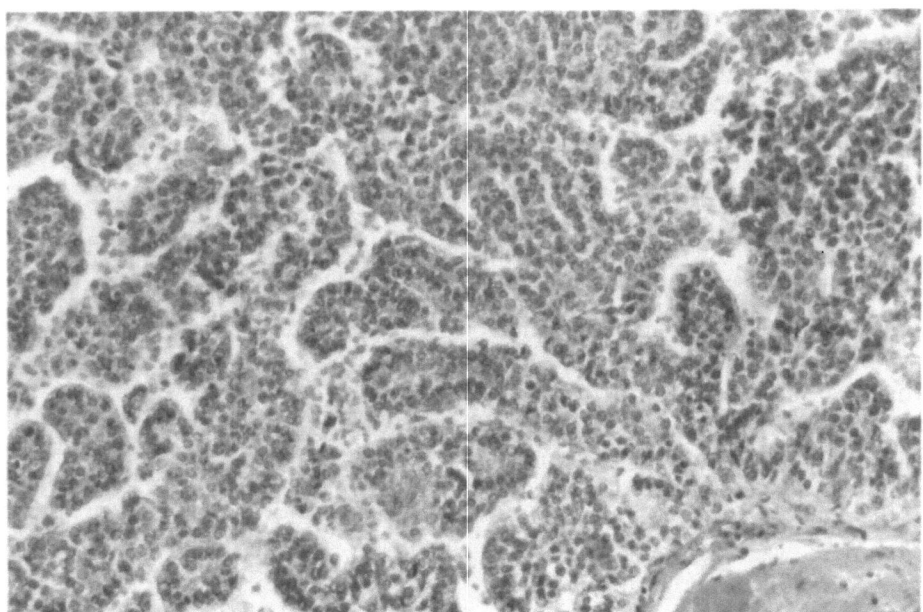

Figure 3.15. Plexus papilloma of the fourth ventricle. The typical papillary pattern of these neoplasias in shown. (H&E; ×60.)

retinal angiomatosis (von Hippel-Lindau disease). The cerebellar tumor macroscopically appears usually as a large fluid-filled cyst with a small reddish tumor nodule in its wall. This "solid" tumor is built up by a dense meshwork of capillaries with cavernous and angiomatoid vessels (Fig. 3.16). Tumor cells are endothelial in type. Among the newly built vessels, interstitial cells as well as glia elements are present. Interstitial cells are round or polygonal, their cytoplasm often presents a foamy appearance due to an overloading with lipid droplets; the round and hyperchromatic nuclei are centrally located. The exact nature of these cells is still debated; among the possibilities are endothelia, pericytes, glia cells, and pial cells. The tumor usually has contact with the leptomeningeal vessels, it is frequently superficially localized and can therefore be regarded as a kind of meningioma. It can also appear in the brain stem and the spinal cord, but rarely in supratentorial regions. This slowly growing tumor is benign, but has a tendency to infiltrate the cerebellar tissue; hence, recurrence is possible. Multiple haemangioblastomas, retinal angiomatosis, renal cysts and/or tumors,

and other lesions involving different internal organs can be found in patients with von Hippel-Lindau disease (see review[12]).

Meningiomas are rare in children, especially in the posterior fossa.[55] *Sarcomas*, vascular or meningeal in origin, are rare, too. They are clearly malignant, particularly the variant known as *diffuse meningeal sarcomatosis* (very difficult to differentiate from the leptomeningeal spreading of a medulloblastoma). In these cases, a diffuse proliferation of small- or medium-sized cells is found; these cells have the tendency to spread everywhere, infiltrating the underlying nervous structures. In many of these cases it is impossible to establish exactly the starting point of the neoplastic proliferation, because the basal meninges, the pineal region, and the cerebellar and spinal meninges are involved; there is also an involvement of the supratentorial regions. The macroscopical finding is characteristic; the leptomeninges present a milky appearance. Histologically, the differential diagnosis with a medulloblastoma is very difficult; easier is the diagnosis in cases of neuroblastomas or pineoblastomas, provided that characteristic differentiation fea-

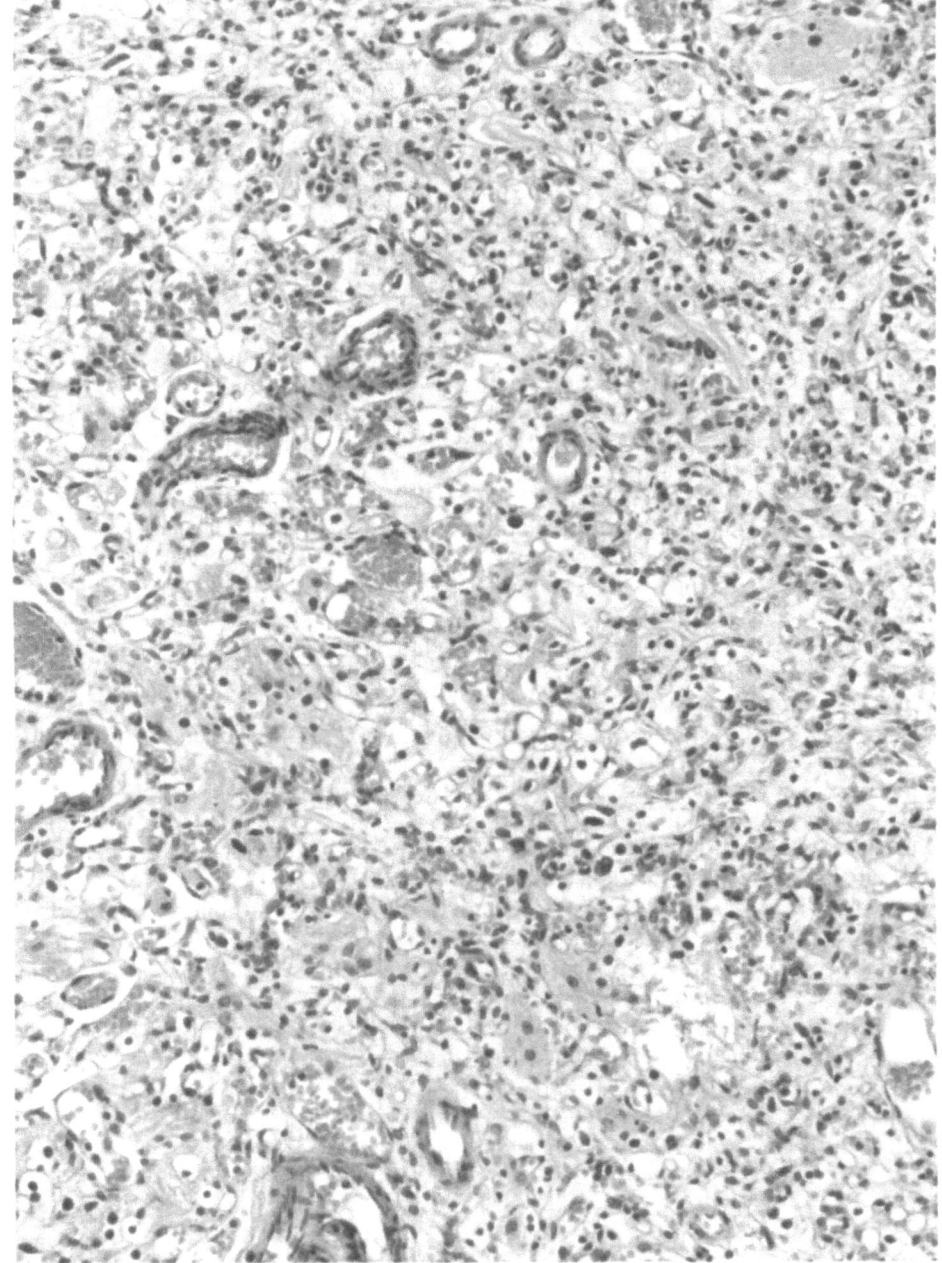

Figure 3.16. Hemangioblastoma of the cerebellum. The tumor is built up by a meshwork of capillaries and angiomatoid vessels, separated by large, pale stromal cells. (H&E; ×60.)

tures of these tumor cells are evident. The circumscribed arachnoidal sarcoma of cerebellum is identical with the desmoplastic medulloblastoma.

Acoustic schwannomas are infrequent in children. These benign, slowly growing tumors arise from the vestibular portion of the acoustic nerve, and are therefore located in the cerebellopontine angle. They grow compressing adjacent structures, mainly the brain stem. Their appearance in children, as a mono- or bilateral tumor, is suggestive of a diffuse neurofibromatosis (von Recklinghausen disease).

The *chordoma* is a relatively rare tumor that arises from remnants of the notochord and is therefore localized in the midline, usually at the superior or inferior end of vertebral column. In children, if located in the clivus or at the upper end of the column, it will compress the brain stem and cerebellum without infiltrating them. The large and vesicular tumor cells present frequently myxomatous changes; they infiltrate and destroy the bone structures. *Chondromas* and *chondrosarcomas* can also appear in the clivus region, but they are rare.

Dermoid and epidermoid cysts as well as *teratomas* can also appear in the posterior fossa, especially in young children (see review[56]). Epidermoid cysts are usually located in the cerebellopontine angle, frequently being slightly superior to dermoid cysts. Teratomas are mostly located in the pineal region. In some dermoid cysts, the malformation may be connected with the skin surface by way of a fistula (dermal sinus); this can lead to secondary inflammatory complications. *Arachnoidal cysts*, such as congenital malformations or as a result of leptomeningitis (adhesive arachnoiditis), can also be found in the cisterna cerebellomedullaris; they produce an impairment to CSF circulation and are therefore to be regarded clinically as a tumor. Histologically they consist of fibrotic leptomeningeal tissue and are benign.

References

1. Koos WTh, Miller M. *Intracranial Tumors of Infants and Children*. Stuttgart: Thieme Verlag; 1971.
2. Brett EM: *Pediatric Neurology*. Edinburgh-London-Melbourne-New York: Churchill Livingstone; 1983:430–471.
3. Giuffré R. Biological aspects of brain tumors in infancy and childhood. *Childs Nerv Syst*. 1989;5:55–59.
4. Raimondi AJ, Taomoto K. Pediatric brain tumors: a comparative analysis of histological classification, anatomical location, extent of resection, and age as indicators of extreme. *Childs Nerv Syst*. 1988;4:173–174.
5. Schlote W. Rosenthalsche Fasern und Spongioblasten im Zentralnervensystem. II. Elektronenmikroskopische Untersuchungen. *Beitr Pathol Anat*. 1966;133:461–480.
6. Gullotta F, Fliedner E. Spongioblastomas, astrocytomas and Rosenthal fibers. Ultrastructural, tissue culture and enzyme histochemical investigations. *Acta Neuropathol (Berl)*. 1972;22:68–78.
7. Zülch KJ. Über das sog. Kleinhirnastrocytom. *Virchows Arch [A]*. 1940;307:222–252.
8. Garcia JH, Escalona Zapata J. Tumors of the central nervous system (II). In: Garcia JH, Escalona Zapata J, Sandbank U, eds. *Diagnostic Neuropathology*. Vol. I. Philadelphia: Field A. Wood; 1988:127–312.
9. Kersting G. Tissue cultures of human gliomas. In: Krayenbühl H, Maspes PE, Sweet WH, eds. *Progress in Neurological Surgery*. Vol. 2. Basel: Karger; 1968:165–202.
10. Cushing H. Experiences with the cerebellar astrocytomas. *Surg Gynecol Obstet*. 1931;52:129–204.
11. Ferbert A, Gullotta F. Remarks on the follow-up of cerebellar astrocytomas. *J Neurol*. 1985;232:134–136.
12. Russell DS, Rubinstein LJ. *Pathology of Tumors of the Nervous System*. 5th ed. London: Arnold; 1989.
13. Gullotta F. Morphological and biological basis for the classification of brain tumors. In: Krayenbühl H, ed. *Advances and Technical Standards in Neurosurgery*. Vol. 8. Wien-New York: Springer-Verlag; 1981:123–165.
14. Casentini L, Möhrer U, Gullotta F. Clinical and morphological investigations on ependymomas and their tissue cultures. *Neurochirurgia (Stuttg)*. 1981;24:51–56.
15. Hoffman HJ, Becker L, Craven MA. A clinically and pathologically distinct group of benign brainstem gliomas. *Neurosurgery*. 1980;7:243–248.
16. Entzian W, Diaz L, Schumacher W. Spongioblastoma in childhood. Remarks on problems in diagnosis and treatment. In: Voth D, Gutjahr P, Langmaid C, eds. *Tumors of the Central Nervous System in Infancy and Childhood*. Berlin-Heidelberg-New York: Springer Verlag; 1982:399–403.

17. Soffer D, Sahar A. Cystic glioma of the brain stem with prolonged survival. *Neurosurgery*. 1982;10:499–502.
18. Epstein F, Wisoff JH. Intrinsic brainstem tumors in childhood: surgical indications. *J Neuroncol*. 1988;6:309–317.
19. Matson DD. *Neurosurgery of Infancy and Childhood*. 2nd ed. Springfield, IL: Charles C. Thomas; 1969.
20. Alvisi C, Cerisoli M, Maccheroni ME. Long-term results of surgically treated brainstem gliomas. *Acta Neurochir (Wien)*. 1985;76:12–17.
21. Cohen ME, Duffner PK, Heffner RR, et al. Prognostic factors in brainstem gliomas. *Neurology*. 1986;36:602–605.
22. Schmitt HP, Zeisner W. The diffuse brain stem astrocytoma in childhood. Morphology, course and prognosis. In: Voth D, Gutjahr P, Langmaid C, eds. *Tumors of the Central Nervous System in Infancy and Childhood*. Berlin-Heidelberg-New York: Springer Verlag; 1982: 149–153.
23. Hitchcock MH, Hollingshead AC, Chretien P, et al. Soluble membrane antigens of brain tumors. Controlled testing for cell-mediated immune responses in a long surviving glioblastoma multiforme patient. *Cancer*. 1977;40:660–666.
24. Gullotta F, Neumann J. Medulloblastome und cerebelläre Sarkome. Eine histologisch-katamnestische Untersuchung. *Neurochirurgia (Stuttg)*. 1980;23:35–40.
25. Bailey P, Cushing H. Medulloblastoma cerebelli. *Arch Neurol Psychiatr*. 1925;14:192–224.
26. Zeltzer PM, Bodey B, Marlin A et al. Immunophenotype profile of childhood medulloblastomas and supratentorial primitive neuroectodermal tumors using 16 monoclonal antibodies. *Cancer*. 1990;66:272–283.
27. Gullotta F. *Das sogenannte Medulloblastom*. Berlin-Heidelberg-New York: Springer Verlag; 1967.
28. Escalona Zapata J. *Atlas de Anatomia Patologica de los Tumores del Sistema Nervioso*. Madrid: Edit. de la Universidad Complutense; 1987.
29. Schindler E, Gullotta F. Glial fibrillary acidic protein in medulloblastomas and other embryonic CNS tumors of children. *Virchows Arch [A]*. 1983;398:263–275.
30. Schiffer D, Giordana MT, Vigliani MC. Brain tumors of childhood: nosological and diagnostic problems. *Childs Nerv Syst*. 1989;5:220–229.
31. Gullotta F. Immunohistochemistry in childhood brain tumors: what are the facts? *Childs Nerv Syst*. 1990;6:118–122.
32. Schwechheimer K. Spezielle Immunmorphologie neurogener Geschwülste. In: Doerr W, Seifert G, Schwechheimer K, eds. *Pathologie des Nervensystems*. Vol. IV. Berlin-Heidelberg-New York-London-Paris-Tokyo-Hong Kong: Springer-Verlag; 1990:1–305.
33. Ishida Y. Discussion on primitive neuroectodermal tumors and medulloblastomas. In: Fields WS, ed. *Primary Brain Tumors*. New York-Berlin-Heidelberg-London-Paris-Tokyo-Hong Kong: Springer-Verlag; 1989:79–81.
34. Escalona Zapata J. Tissue culture in the diagnosis of brain tumors. In: Garcia JH, Escalona Zapata J, Sandbank U, Cervós-Navarro J, eds. *Diagnostic Neuropathology*. Vol. II. Berlin-Heidelberg-New York-London-Paris-Tokyo-Hong Kong: Springer-Verlag; 1990:3–46.
35. Lumsden CE. The study by tissue culture of tumors of the nervous system. In: Russell D, Rubinstein LJ, eds. 3rd ed. London: Arnold; 1971:335–415.
36. Herman MM, Rubinstein LJ. Divergent glial and neuronal differentiation in a cerebellar medulloblastoma in an organ culture system: in vitro occurrence of synaptic ribbons. *Acta Neuropathol (Berl)*. 1984;65:10–24.
37. Gullotta F, Kost HG. In vitro studies of so-called medulloblastomas. *Pathologica*. 1980; 72:27–34.
38. Gullotta F, Fliedner E, Wüllenweber R, et al. Tissue culture, electron microscopic and enzyme histochemical investigations on a sympathetic ganglioneuroblastoma. *Acta neuropathol (Berl)*. 1973;24:107–116.
39. Hart MN, Earle KM. Primitive neuroectodermal tumors of the brain in children. *Cancer*. 1973;32:890–897.
40. Rorke LB, Gilles FH, Davis RL, et al. Revision of the WHO classification of brain tumors for childhood brain tumors. *Cancer*. 1985;56 (suppl):1869–1886.
41. Fields WS ed.: Primary Brain Tumors. *A Review of Histologic Classification*. New York-Berlin-Heidelberg-London-Paris-Tokyo-Hong Kong: Springer-Verlag; 1989.
42. Ferrer I, Marti E, Guionnet N, et al. Studies with the Golgi method in central gangliogliomas and dysplastic gangliocytoma of the cerebellum (Lhermitte-Duclos disease). *Histol Histopathol*. 1990;5:329–336.
43. Kuchelmeister K, Gullotta F. Das immunhistochemische Profil der Lhermitte-Duclosschen

Krankheit. *Verh Dtsch Ges Pathol.* 1990;74: 646.

44. Shiurba RA, Gessaga EC, Eng LF, et al. Lhermitte-Duclos disease. An immunohisto-chemical study of the cerebellar cortex. *Acta Neuropathol (Berl).* 1988;75:474–480.

45. Zülch KJ. *Brain Tumors. Their Biology and Pathology.* 3rd ed. Berlin-Heidelberg-New York-Tokyo: Springer Verlag; 1986.

46. Raimondi AJ. Ultrastructure and the biology of human brain tumors. In: Krayenbühl H, Maspes PE, Sweet WH, eds. *Progress in Neurological surgery.* vol. I. Basel: Karger; 1966:1–63.

47. Goebel HH, Cravioto H. Ultrastructure of human and experimental ependymomas. *J Neuropathol Exp Neurol.* 1972;31:54–71.

48. Friede RL, Pollak A. The cytogenetic basis for classifying ependymomas. *J Neuropathol Exp Neurol.* 1978;37:103–118.

49. Undjian S, Marinov M. Intracranial ependymomas in children. *Childs Nerv Syst.* 1990;6:131–134.

50. Zülch KJ, ed. *WHO Classification of Tumors of the Central Nervous System.* Geneva: World Health Organization; 1979.

51. Rubinstein LJ. The definition of ependymoblastoma. *Arch Pathol.* 1970;90:35–45.

52. Gullotta F, Entzian W. Klinische und morphologische Betrachtungen über das "Medulloepitheliom." *Neurochirurgia (Stuttg).* 1975; 18:193–198.

53. Spallone A, Pastore FS, Giuffré R, et al. Choroid plexus papillomas in infancy and childhood. *Childs Nerv Syst.* 1990;6:71–74.

54. Gullotta F, de Melo AS. Dar Karzinom des Plexus chorioideus. *Neurochirurgia (Stuttg).* 1979;22:1–9.

55. Kepes JJ. Meningiomas. *Biology, Pathology and Differential Diagnosis.* New York-Paris: Masson; 1982.

56. Fornari M, Solero CL, Lasio G, et al. Surgical treatment of intracranial dermoid and epidermoid cysts in children. *Childs Nerv Syst.* 1990;6:66–70.

57. Gullotta F. La genesi formale delle fibre di Rosenthal. *Acta Neurol (Napoli).* 1965;20:704–711.

CHAPTER 4

Experimental Pathology as a Basis for Understanding the Biology of Posterior Fossa Tumors

Alessandro Mauro and Davide Schiffer

The classification of childhood brain tumors mainly composed of undifferentiated cells with various degrees of recognizable differentiation has been a focus of great debate and can be quite confusing.[1-5] The term *primitive neuroectodermal tumor* (PNET) is increasingly used to classify these kinds of tumors that, according to other systems of classification, include medulloblastomas, pinealoblastomas, cerebral neuroblastomas, and ependymoblastomas. Medulloblastomas, the most common malignant pediatric brain tumors, are restricted to the cerebellum. They are composed of undifferentiated small cells of uncertain origin that in some cases may show neuronal and/or glial differentiation. The principal reason for uncertainties about medulloblastoma classification resides in the unknown origin of medulloblastoma cells; in the normal histogenesis of the central nervous system there are no embryonal cells that can be identified as "medulloblasts."

Three main sources of medulloblastomas have been proposed: the fetal external granular layer, primitive cells of the roof of the fourth ventricle (posterior medullary velum), and the internal granular layer. Nowadays, there is general agreement about the possibility that medulloblastomas originate from the external granular layer of the cerebellum.[4-6] The posterior medullary velum can be suggested as a source of some medulloblastomas, taking into account that embryonal cells migrate dorsally and laterally from that structure to form the external granular layer.[5-7] In contrast, the suggestion that the internal granular layer gives rise to medulloblastomas is supported primarily by data on chemical and viral neuro-oncogenesis in animals.[8-10]

This chapter focuses on experimental studies concerning embryonal posterior fossa tumors and, in particular, medulloblastomas.

Chemical Neuro-Oncogenesis

Medulloblastomas have been obtained only occasionally in chemical carcinogenesis experiments.

A single report concerns the result of oral administration of 2,7-acetylaminofluorene in a rat,[11] an approach that today can be considered to be of primarily historical interest.

In experiments using the technique of local implantation of pellets of polycyclic hydrocarbons such as methylcholanthrene, Zimmerman[8,12] succeeded in obtaining medulloblastomas in rodents. Implantation of carcinogen pellets in the cerebellum of adult mice (between 3 and 6 months of age) produced typical medulloblastomas. In this type of experimental neuro-oncogenesis the incidence and the type of tumors obtained are largely dependent on the site of implantation. Moreover, mixed tumors were frequently observed, probably because different cell types are transformed by the chemical due to the pellet size.[8] In fact, in one case a mixed medulloblastoma-astrocytoma tumor was observed.[12]

This experimental model of medulloblastoma is interesting from several points of view. The possibility of obtaining medulloblastomas from adult animals suggests that the cells that give origin to this tumor are not restricted to the fetal or neonatal brain, but are also present in the cerebellum in adult life. This cell population, which preserves immature features, must coexist with a more differentiated one of a glial nature representing the target of carcinogenesis in the previously mentioned mixed medulloblastoma-astrocytoma tumor. Moreover, in the original description[8,12] it seemed that the experimental medulloblastomas arose from the internal granular layer of cerebellum and were composed of cells resembling the small neurons of this layer.

These observations led Zimmerman[8] to identify the medulloblastoma with the neuroblastoma, suggesting its origin from the internal granular layer of the cerebellar cortex. Even though the origin of medulloblastoma from the internal granular layer is acceptable, at least for some of these tumors,[4] its identification with a pure neuroblastoma is hardly tenable in light of the general agreement on the possibility of glial differentiation in medulloblastomas. On the other hand, the existence of rare but *definite* cerebellar neuroblastomas has been repeatedly demonstrated.[13–17]

The most successful method of chemical neuro-oncogenesis, the transplacental induction with resorptive *N*-nitroso- compounds, is not useful in the production of medulloblastomas. It is well known that tumors obtained with this approach are almost always gliomas, characteristically mixed gliomas, and oligodendrogliomas.[18–20] Reports of neuronal tumors in rodents can be considered exceptional,[21,22] as well as those of medulloblastomas.[23,24] It is of particular interest that medulloblastomas have been obtained more easily in mice, that, in contrast to rats, show a relative resistance to the neuro-oncogenic action of *N*-nitroso-compounds. In the experiment of Jones et al.[23] only four brain tumors have been obtained with ENU in mice, and three of these neoplasms were medulloblastomas. These tumors showed continuity with subpial, densely packed islands of cells resembling remnants of the fetal external granular layer. Apart from these examples in mice, the extreme rarity of medulloblastomas

obtained in rats with nitrosoureas remains unexplained. This apparent lack of vulnerability cannot be attributed generically to the cerebellum, where, instead, in the neonatal period it seems that target cells for ENU-induced oligodendrogliomas are present.[25]

Viral Neuro-Oncogenesis

A wide variety of brain tumors has been obtained in viral carcinogenesis experiments.[26] In particular, different oncogenic DNA viruses can induce immature embryonal brain tumors when locally injected. Tumors of embryonal neuroectodermal origin have been obtained in different animals and with various locations using human adenovirus type 12.[27,28] Intracranial inoculation of this virus in different rodents (hamster, rats, and mice) induced embryonal tumors with limited differentiation, corresponding to medulloblastomas, neuroblastomas, primitive spongioblastomas, ependymoblastomas, and medulloepitheliomas.[28] Tumors identical with human medulloblastomas, sometimes showing typical Homer-Wright rosettes, have been described. In these experiments a relative species specificity was demonstrated, being the incidence of brain tumors obtained in mice and in hamsters (<37%) lower than that obtained in rats (>90%). Moreover, the incidence of infratentorial tumors was significantly higher in hamsters and in mice than in rats, and infratentorial tumors increased significantly if animals were inoculated during their intrauterine life. These observations suggest that the target of this DNA oncovirus may be a cell population in a definite differentiation stage. It is possible that the topographical and chronological distributions of target cells differ between animal species. Interestingly, infratentorial medulloblastomas in some cases seemed to originate from the posterior medullary velum, whereas no microtumors located in the external granular layer were described.[28] A surprising finding in experimental neuro-oncogenesis with adenovirus type 12, is the occurrence in some animals of supratentorial tumors resembling typical medulloblastomas.[28] This finding seems to be in agreement with the concept that undifferentiated tumors (PNETs) of similar cell composition may originate from primitive neuroepithelial cells at all levels of the CNS,[2] but in humans cerebral hemispheric tumors resembling medulloblastoma are at least rare.[7] A peculiar characteristic of adenovirus type 12–induced tumors is their markedly undifferentiated aspect with a scarce tendency to differentiate; in no cases neuronal or glial filaments were demonstrated. The absence of evident signs of differentiation may suggest that target cells after transformation do not retain a multipotential differentiation capability. The moderately divergent phenotypes described[28] may be the consequence of a different developmental stage at the time of transformation or, in some cases, of microenvironmental events. The histological features of differentiation are an unresolved matter of debate also in human medulloblastomas.[5]

Different strains of JC virus, the papovavirus that causes progressive multifocal leukoencephalopathy, have been shown to be highly neuro-oncogenic in hamster.[9,10,29–32] Cerebellar medulloblastoma was the predominant tumor induced in animals inoculated at birth (95% of brain tumors).[10] Histologically, medulloblastomas obtained in this way showed close resemblance to human medulloblastomas and in no cases expression of GFAP was demonstrated. However, Takakura and coworkers[33] described the establishment of a clonal cell line expressing GFAP from a 2-year in vitro culture of a JC virus–induced medulloblastoma. These clonal cells, when transplanted subcutaneously in hamster, originate a tumor similar to the human astrocytoma. This result, if a cultural artifact is excluded, may be in agreement with the suggested medulloblastoma capability of glial differentiation.[33]

Very important information about the origin of medulloblastomas can be derived from the JC virus experimental model. The tumors were located in the internal granular layer, where tumoral cells migrated from the external granular layer postnatally.[9,10] Virus is inoculated in the hamster brain when the external granular layer is present in the cerebellum. The presence of the viral T-antigen in cells of the external granular layer of the newborn

hamster seems to demonstrate that the cells of this structure are a target of the JC virus.[10]

A conclusive observation can be derived from these viral neuro-oncogenesis experiments. In the embryonal and perinatal cerebellum of rodents at least two cell populations exist that can give origin to tumors closely resembling human medulloblastomas: cells of the external granular layer and cells of the posterior medullary velum. Even though moderately differentiated phenotypes have been described, the lack of evident markers of differentiation cannot confirm a residual multipotent differentiation capability of the transformed cells.

Transgenic Mice Models

Few recent works have reported the induction of brain tumors in transgenic mice. Transgenic animals have integrated foreign DNA sequences in their genome, as a result of introduction of DNA fragments into the pronucleus of fertilized mouse eggs that subsequently are transferred to the oviducts of pseudopregnant females. Choroid plexus papillomas were generated in transgenic mice bearing a fragment of the simian virus 40 (SV 40).[34–37,59] The T-antigen of SV 40 seems to play a pivot role in the development of these tumors.[34,35,59] The SV 40 DNA fragment introduced into mouse genome in these experiments comprised regions encoding large T- and small t- (tumoral) antigens together with its own promoter and enhancer.[35,36] Other transgenic mice have been recently described, carrying the large T-antigen of SV 40 under the control of the Moloney murine sarcoma virus (MSV) enhancer and the promoter of the SV 40.[38] These transgenic mice developed heritable eye abnormalities of retina and lens and undifferentiated neuroectodermal brain tumors. Tumors histologically composed of small undifferentiated cells with hyperchromatic nuclei and occasionally forming rosettes occurred in adult mice. They were located in the midline of the brain and infiltrated the cerebellum and the occipital cortex. These tumors have been compared to human pineal cell tumors and certain medulloblastomas on the basis of their location and histology and of some immunohistochemical findings. In particular, these neoplasm have been shown to express S-antigen and rhodopsin,[39] two antigens that are considered indicative of photoreceptor-like differentiation. The two molecules have been found exclusively in retinal photoreceptors and a class of normal pinealocytes,[40] as well as in human pineocytomas and pinealoblastomas,[41,42] and in some medulloblastomas with photoreceptor-like features[43,44]; thus they are considered sensitive and specific markers for these tumors. The site of origin of tumors developed in these transgenic mice seems to be the pineal parenchyma, whereas the external granular layer of the cerebellum appears unaffected in young animals.[39]

This model of neuro-oncogenesis appears to be highly promising for the study of neuro-ectodermal undifferentiated tumors with photoreceptor-like differentiation and seems to confirm that some oncogenetic link may exist between pinealoblastomas and medulloblastomas.[7]

Tumors similar to medulloblastomas and PNETs have been obtained with a new experimental model of gene transfer into the nervous system.[60] Using a replication-defective retroviral vector, foreign potentially transforming genes are introduced into fetal rat brain cells that are grafted intracerebrally into syngenic host animals. These transplants will develop with formation of highly differentiated CNS tissue, providing a potent tool for study in vivo the expression of retrovirally transmitted genes in selected CNS cell populations. Fetal brain transplants exposed to a retroviral vector encoding the *large T* antigen of SV40 showed a high incidence of medulloblastoma-like tumors, after latency periods of 6–9 months.[60] In these neoplasms a potential for both neuronal and glial differentiation was demonstrated by the presence of neuroblastic rosettes and immunoreactivity for neuron-specific enolase, synaptophysin and GFAP.[60] A primitive neuroectodermal tumor has been obtained also in a neural graft exposed to a *v-gag/myc* retroviral vector.[61] However, the observation that only a single tumor was obtained introducing

this oncogene in 15 grafts suggests that a single *myc* oncogene probably have a very limited transforming potential in the brain. In contrast, results obtained with SV40 *large T* are extremely interesting. This gene encodes a nuclear phosphoprotein capable of complex with different cellular proteins including the tumor suppressors p53 and RB-1. Therefore, since a possible mechanism of transformation by SV40 *large T* is the interaction with and the inactivation of tumor suppressor proteins, this experimental model may provide a goog tool for the identification on neural suppressor genes.

Medulloblastoma Cell Lines and Transplantable Xenografts

Searching for models of human medulloblastoma, useful in the design of appropriate therapies, a small number of permanent medulloblastoma-derived cell lines and transplantable xenografts have been reported.[45–49] The phenotype of four medulloblastoma cell lines has been characterized in the last few years, yielding interesting results. Two of them, D-283 Med and D-341 Med, express neurofilament proteins, neuron specific enolase, and glutamine synthetase, but are negative for GFAP, S100 protein, and other antigenic markers collectively considered as glial.[48,50,51] In contrast, the pattern of antigenic expression of the other two lines, TE-671 and Daoy, has been considered of glial type in a recent study.[51] However, on the basis of a previous study,[52] TE-671 can be considered as having a limited potential for neuronal differentiation.[7] Different patterns of growth are associated with the aforementioned different patterns of antigenic expression: TE-671 and Daoy grow as adherent cell lines, whereas D-283 Med and D-341 Med lines grow in suspension. Moreover, TE-671 when injected intracerebrally in nude mice, produces a diffuse infiltration of the brain instead of a circumscribed proliferation. This different phenotype can be considered as reflecting the heterogeneity of medulloblastomas[48,51] and in particular the differentiation capabilities of these tumors. On the other hand, it is questionable that cell lines reflect perfectly the in vivo behavior of a tumor, and culture artifacts cannot be completely excluded. Tumoral cell populations that proliferate in vivo are not necessarily the same that have a selective advantage in vitro; moreover, genomic abnormalities may occur in culture giving a selective advantage to the mutated cells.

Some recent findings are extremely important in this regard. Few studies found oncogene amplifications in medulloblastoma specimens: N-myc amplification was found in 2 of 20 cerebellar PNETs[53] and an isolate medulloblastoma[54]; erb B1 was found in 1 of 20 cases.[55] On the other hand, oncogene amplification seems to be a relatively common feature of medulloblastoma cell lines. Two recent studies, from the same group, reported amplification in five out of six medulloblastoma cell lines tested[49,55]: c-myc was amplified in three cell lines, N-myc and erb B1 in one. Moreover, in two cases showing c-myc amplification, a cell line, and a xenograft, there was no evidence of amplification in the original biopsy tissue.[49] These findings suggest a positive selection, in vitro or in xenografts, for medulloblastoma cells presenting oncogene amplification.[56]

Moreover, a recent report showed that medulloblastoma cell line TE-671 produces a platelet-derived growth factor (PDGF)-like growth factor and that the biological activity of this growth factor can be blocked by antibodies against PDGF.[57] However, previous study in a single medulloblastoma[58] and our analysis of two medulloblastomas (unpublished data) failed to demonstrate sis mRNA expression.

Collectively, these findings suggest that results obtained with permanent medulloblastoma-derived cell lines must be extended very cautiously to human medulloblastomas in vivo.

References

1. Rorke LB. The cerebellar medulloblastoma and its relationship to primitive neuroectodermal tumors. *J Neuropathol Exp Neurol*. 1983;42:1–15.
2. Rorke LB, Gilles FH, Davis RL, et al. Revision of the World Health Organization Classification. *Cancer*. 1985;56:1869–1886.
3. Rubinstein LJ. Embryonal central neuroepithelial tumors and their differentiating potential. A cytogenetic view of a complex neuro-oncological problem. *J Neurosurg*. 1985;62:795–805.
4. Rubinstein LJ. Primitive neuroectodermal tumors. *Arch Pathol Lab Med*. 1987;111:310–312.
5. Schiffer D, Giordana MT, Vigliani MC. Brain tumors of childhood: nosological and diagnostic problems. *Childs Nerv Syst*. 1989;5:220–229.
6. Kadin ME, Rubinstein LJ, Nelson JS. Neonatal cerebellar medulloblastoma originating from the fetal external granular layer. *J Neuropathol Exp Neurol*. 1970;29:583–600.
7. Russel DS, Rubinstein LJ. *Pathology of Tumors of the Nervous System*. 5th ed. London: Arnold; 1989.
8. Zimmerman HM. Brain tumors. Their incidence and classification in man and their experimental production. *Ann NY Acad Sci*. 1969;159:337–359.
9. Zu Rhein GM, Varakis JN. Perinatal induction of medulloblastomas in Syrian golden hamster by a human polyoma virus (JC). *Natl Cancer Inst Monogr*. 1979;51:205–208.
10. Nagashima K, Yasui K, Kimura J, et al. Induction of brain tumors by a newly isolated JC virus (Tokyo-1 strain). *Am J Pathol*. 1984;116:455–463.
11. Snell KC, Stewart HL, Morris HP, et al. Intracranial neurilemmoma and medulloblastoma induced in rats by the dietary administration of N,N'-2,7-fluorenylene-bisacetamide. *Natl Cancer Inst Monogr*. 1961;5:85–91.
12. Zimmerman HM. The histopathology of experimental "medulloblastoma." *Acta Neuropathol (Berl)*. 1967;8:69–75.
13. Ermel AE, Brucher JM. Arguments ultrastructuraux en faveur de l'appartenence du medulloblastome à la ligne neuronale. *Acta Neurol Belg*. 1974;74:208–220.
14. Shin WY, Laufer H, Lee YC, et al. Fine structure of a cerebellar neuroblastoma. *Acta Neuropathol (Berl)*. 1978;50:139–142.
15. Hirano A, Shin WY. Unattached presynaptic terminals in a cerebellar neuroblastoma in the human. *Neuropathol Appl Neurobiol*. 1979;5:63–70.
16. Yagashita S, Itah Y, Chiba Y, et al. Cerebellar neuroblastoma: a light and ultrastructural

study. *Acta Neuropathol (Berl)*. 1980;50:139–142.

17. Pearl GS, Takei Y. Cerebellar neuroblastoma: nosology as it relates to medulloblastoma. *Cancer*. 1981;47:772–779.

18. Swenberg JA. Chemical induction of brain tumors. In: Thompson RA, Green JR, eds. *Advances in neurology. Vol. 15. Neoplasia in the central nervous system*. New York: Raven Press; 1976:85.

19. Schiffer D, Giordana MT, Pezzotta S, et al. Cerebral tumors induced by transplacental ENU: study of the different tumoral stages, particularly of early proliferations. *Acta Neuropathol (Berl)*. 1978;41:27.

20. Lantos PL. Chemical induction of tumors in the nervous system. In: Thomas DGT, Graham DI, eds. *Brain tumors. Scientific basis, clinical investigation and current therapy*. London: Butterworths; 1980:85.

21. Stroobandt G, Brucher JM. Etude de tumeurs nerveuses obtenues par l'administration de methylnitrosourée au rat. *Neurochirurgie*. 1968;14:515.

22. Brucher JM, Ermel AE. Central neuroblastoma induced by transplacental administration of methylnitrosourea in Wistar-R rats. An electron microscopic study. *J Neurol*. 1974;208:1.

23. Jones EL, Searle CE, Smith WT. Medulloblastomas and other neural tumors in mice treated neonatally with N-ethyl-N-nitrosourea. *Acta Neuropathol (Berl)*. 1976;36:57.

24. Wechsler W, Rice JM, Vesselinovitch SD. Transplacental and neonatal induction of neurogenic tumors in mice: comparison with related species and with human pediatric neoplasms. *Natl Cancer Inst Monogr*. 1979;51:219–230.

25. Naito M, Aoyama H, Naito J, et al. Morphological and immunohistochemical evidence for the presence of subcortical target cells of N-ethyl-N-nitrosourea-induced cerebellar tumors in rats. *Cancer Res*. 1986;46:5836.

26. Bullard DE, Bigner DD. Animal models and virus induction of tumors. In: Thomas DGT, Graham DI, eds. *Brain tumors. Scientific basis, clinical investigation and current therapy*. London: Butterworths; 1980:51.

27. Mukai N. Human adenovirus-induced embryonic neuronal tumor phenotype in rodents. *Prog Neuropathol*. 1976;3:89–128.

28. Ogawa K. Embryonal neuroepithelial tumors induced by human adenovirus type 12 in rodents. 2. Tumor induction in the central nervous

system. *Acta Neuropathol (Berl)*. 1989;78:232–244.

29. Walker DL, Padgett BL, ZuRhein GM, et al. Human papovavirus (JC). Induction of brain tumors in hamsters. *Science*. 1973;181:674–676.

30. Padgett BL, Walker DL, ZuRhein GM, et al. Differential neurooncogenicity of strains of JC virus, a human polyoma virus, in newborn Syrian hamsters. *Cancer Res*. 1977;37:718–720.

31. London WT, Houff SA, Madden DL, et al. Brain tumors in owl monkeys inoculated with a human polyomavirus (JC). *Science*. 1978;201:1246–1249.

32. Matsuda M, Yasui K, Nagashima K, et al. Origin of the medulloblastoma experimentally induced by human polyomavirus JC. *J Natl Cancer Inst*. 1987;79:585.

33. Takakura K, Inoya H, Nagashima K, et al. Viral neurooncogenesis. *Prog Exp Tumor Res*. 1987;30:10–20.

34. Brinster RL, Chen HY, Messing A, et al. Transgenic mice harboring SV 40 T-antigen genes develop characteristic brain tumors. *Cell*. 1984;37:367–379.

35. Palmiter RD, Chen HY, Messing A, et al. SV 40 enhancer and large T-antigen are instrumental in development of choroid plexus tumours in transgenic mice. *Nature*. 1985;316:457–460.

36. Small JA, Blair DG, Showalter SD, et al. Analysis of a transgenic mouse containing simian virus 40 and v-myc sequences. *Mol Cell Biol*. 1985;5:642–648.

37. Van Dyke TA, Finlay C, Miller D, et al. Relationships between simian virus 40 large tumor antigen expression and tumor formation in transgenic mice. *J Virol*. 1987;61:2029–2032.

38. Theuring F, Götz W, Balling R, et al. Tumorigenesis and eye abnormalities in transgenic mice expressing MSV-SV 40 large T-antigen. *Oncogene*. 1990;5:225–232.

39. Korf H-W, Götz W, Herken R, et al. S-antigen and rhodopsin immunoreactions in midline brain neoplasms of transgenic mice: similarities to pineal cell tumors and certain medulloblastomas in man. *J Neuropathol Exp Neurol*. 1990;49:424–437.

40. Korf H-W, Ekström P. Photoreceptor differentiation and neuronal organization of the pineal organ. In: Trentini GP, De Gaetani C, Pévet P, eds. *Fundamentals and Clinics in Pineal Research*. New York: Raven Press; 1987:35–47.

41. Korf H-W, Klein DC, Zigler JS, et al. S-

antigen-like immunoreactivity in a human pineocytoma. *Acta Neuropathol (Berl)*. 1986; 69:167.

42. Perentes E, Rubinstein LJ, Herman MM, et al. S-antigen immunoreactivity in human pineal glands and pineal parenchymal tumors. A monoclonal antibody study. *Acta Neuropathol (Berl)*. 1986;71:224–227.

43. Korf H-W, Czerwionka M, Reiner J, et al. Immunocytochemical evidence of molecular photoreceptor markers in human cerebellar medulloblastomas. *Cancer*. 1987;60:1763–1766.

44. Bonnin JM, Perentes E. Retinal S-antigen immunoreactivity in medulloblastomas. *Acta Neuropathol (Berl)*. 1988;76:204–207.

45. Mc Allister RM, Isaacs H, Rongey R, et al. Establishment of a human medulloblastoma cell line. *Int J Cancer*. 1977;20:206–212.

46. Jacobsen PF, Jenkyn DJ, Papadimitriou JM. Establishment of a human medulloblastoma cell line and its heterotransplantation in nude mice. *J Neuropathol Exp Neurol*. 1985;44:472–485.

47. Friedman HS, Burger PC, Bigner SH, et al. Establishment and characterization of the human medulloblastoma cell line and transplantable xenograft D283 Med. *J Neuropathol Exp Neurol*. 1985;44:592–605.

48. Friedman HS, Burger PC, Bigner SH, et al. Phenotypic and genotypic analysis of a human medulloblastoma cell line and transplantable xenograft (D341 Med) demonstrating amplification of c-myc. *Am J Pathol*. 1988;130:472–484.

49. Bigner SH, Friedman HS, Oakes WJ, et al. Amplification of the C-MYC gene in medulloblastoma cell lines and xenografts. *Cancer Res*. 1990;50:2347–2350.

50. Trojanowski JO, Friedman HS, Burger PC, et al. A rapidly dividing human medulloblastoma cell line (D283 Med) expresses all three neurofilament subunits. *Am J Pathol*. 1987; 126:358–363.

51. He X, Skapek SX, Wikstrand CJ, et al. Phenotypic analysis of four human medulloblastoma cell lines and transplantable xenografts. *J Neuropathol Exp Neurol*. 1989;48:48–68.

52. Mork SJ, May EE, Papasozomenos SC, et al. Characteristics of human medulloblastoma cell line TE-671 under different growth conditions in vitro: A morphological and immunohistochemical study. *Neuropathol Appl Neurobiol*. 1986;12:277–289.

53. Rouah E, Wilson DR, Armstrong DL, et al. N-myc amplification and neuronal differentiation in human primitive neuroectodermal tumors of the central nervous system. *Cancer Res*. 1989;49:1797–1801.

54. Nisen PD, Zimmerman KA, Cotter SV, et al. Enhanced expression of the N-myc gene in Wilms' tumors. *Cancer Res*. 1986;46:6217–6222.

55. Wasson JC, Saylors RL, Zelter P, et al. Oncogene amplification in pediatric brain tumors. *Cancer Res*. 1990;50:2087–2090.

56. Bigner SH, Vogelstein B. Cytogenetics and molecular genetics of malignant gliomas and medulloblastomas. *Brain Pathol*. 1990;1:12–18.

57. Whelan HT, Nelson DB, Strother D, et al. Medulloblastoma cell line secretes platelet-derived growth factor. *Pediatr Neurol*. 1989; 5:347–352.

58. Fujimoto M, Sheridan PJ, Sharp D, et al. Proto-oncogene analyses in brain tumors. *J Neurosurg*. 1989;70:910–915.

59. Messing A, Pinkert CA, Palmiter RD, et al. Developmental study of SV40 large T antigen expression in transgenic mice with choroid plexus neoplasia. Oncogene Research 1988;3:87–97.

60. Wiestler OD, Brüstle O, Eibl RH, et al. A new approach to the molecular basis of neoplastic transformation in brain. Neuropathol. Appl. Neurobiol. 1992;18:443–453.

61. Wiestler OD, Aguzzi A, Schneemann M, et al. Oncogene complementation in fetal brain transplants. Cancer Res. 1992;52:3760–3767.

CHAPTER 5

Imaging of the Pediatric Posterior Fossa: Normal Anatomy and Brain Tumors

Robert A. Zimmerman

Introduction

Diagnostic imaging of posterior fossa tumors necessitates an understanding of the advantages and disadvantages of the available imaging modalities as well as of the relevant anatomy that they display.[1] The choice today is between computed tomography (CT) and magnetic resonance imaging (MRI).[1] Previously, CT had circumvented the need for both air studies and vertebral or brachial arteriography. In the future, it is likely that MRI, as we currently know it, will broaden its scope to three-dimensional representation, MR angiography, and spectroscopy.

At present, CT is rapid (scans take on the order of seconds and studies take 15 to 25 minutes), special precautions are not necessary relative to the use of monitoring or support equipment, and the technology is widely available, both on an emergent and nonemergent basis. Computed tomography gives a graphic representation of the ventricular size, of the status of the brain tissue, of any mass effect, and following injection of iodinated contrast material, of any abnormality in the blood-brain barrier (BBB). Calcification, hematoma, and fat are well shown and are of sufficient density difference that they are separable from the normal brain, cerebrospinal fluid (CSF), and bone. Studies can be performed not only in the axial plane, but direct coronal sections are possible by positioning the patient, and both coronal and sagittal sections can be reconstructed from axial data. Slice thickness can be varied from 10 mm to 1 mm. However, despite the relative rapidity of the sections, patients who are uncooperative still require sedation. The injection of iodinated contrast material carries the small, but real risk of a contrast reaction. Ultimately, the CT study involves radiation, a process that although not deleterious at the radiation level employed, is still something that is not desirable.[2]

Magnetic resonance produces images in any plane without special positioning of the patient and without degradation of image quality[3] (Figs. 5.1 to 5.3). MR contrast depends on five intrinsic parameters: (a) T1 relaxation of tissue; (b) T2 relaxation of tissue; (c) proton spin density of tissue; (d) flow within vessels, CSF, and within tissue (diffusion); and (e) the intrinsic magnetic field variations of tissue—the so-called magnetic susceptibility. By varying pulse parameters that affect the way in which these five components contribute to the image, various aspects of pathological processes can be emphasized. MR is sensitive to the presence of blood products—acutely, subacutely, and chronically.[4] MR is extremely sensitive to the demonstration of increased water within pathologic tissue. MR is sensitive to differences in the intrinsic magnetic fields of tissues due to the presence of paramagnetic substances such as gadolinium-DTPA (Magnevist), a contrast agent used to demonstrate disturbances of the BBB.[5] MR is sensitive in demonstrating the presence of flow within arteries and veins as well as the lack of flow in such.

Unfortunately, MR examinations are not acquired as a series of single images of short duration, but rather as a multitude of images of

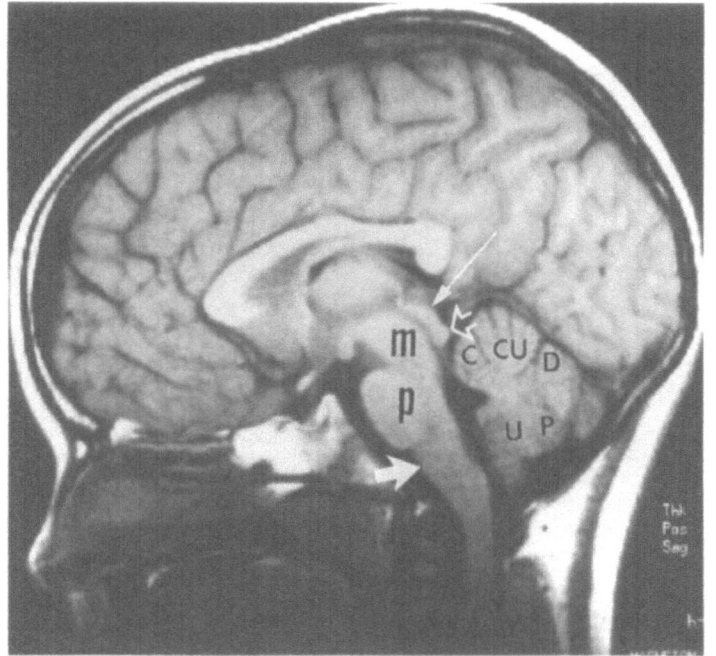

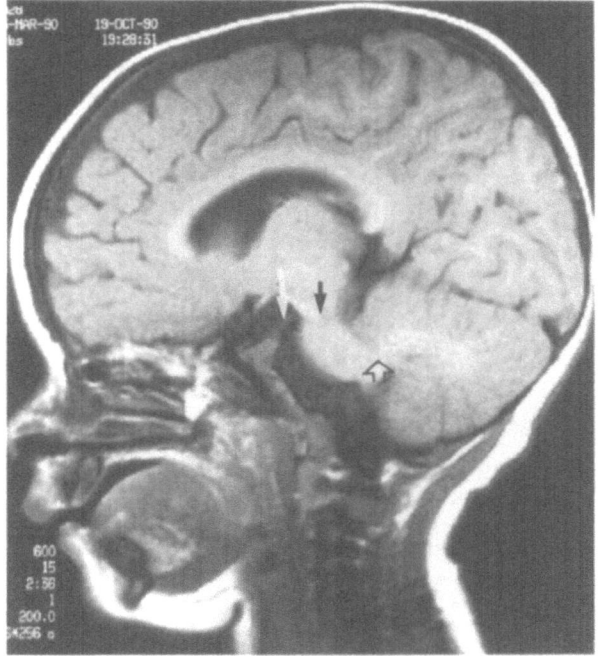

Figure 5.1. Normal sagittal anatomy of the posterior fossa. A: Midline sagittal 5-mm-thick MR section that is T1-weighted shows midbrain (m), pons (p), medulla (short white arrow), superior colliculus (long white arrow), inferior colliculus (open white arrow), central lobule (C), culmen (CU), declive (D), pyramid (P), and uvula (U). Between the superior inferior colliculus and the more inferior structures of the midbrain lies the hypointense course of the aqueduct of Sylvius, leading inferiorly into the fourth ventricle, the triangular-shaped hypointensity between the pons and cerebellar vermis. A portion of the cerebellar tonsil on one side is partially volumed with the section and is identified inferior to the uvula. B: Off-midline sagittal 5-mm-thick T1-weighted MR section shows third cranial nerve (white arrow) extending forward from the interpeduncular cistern toward the cavernous sinus. The cerebral peduncle (black arrow) and middle cerebellar peduncle (open black arrow) are also well shown.

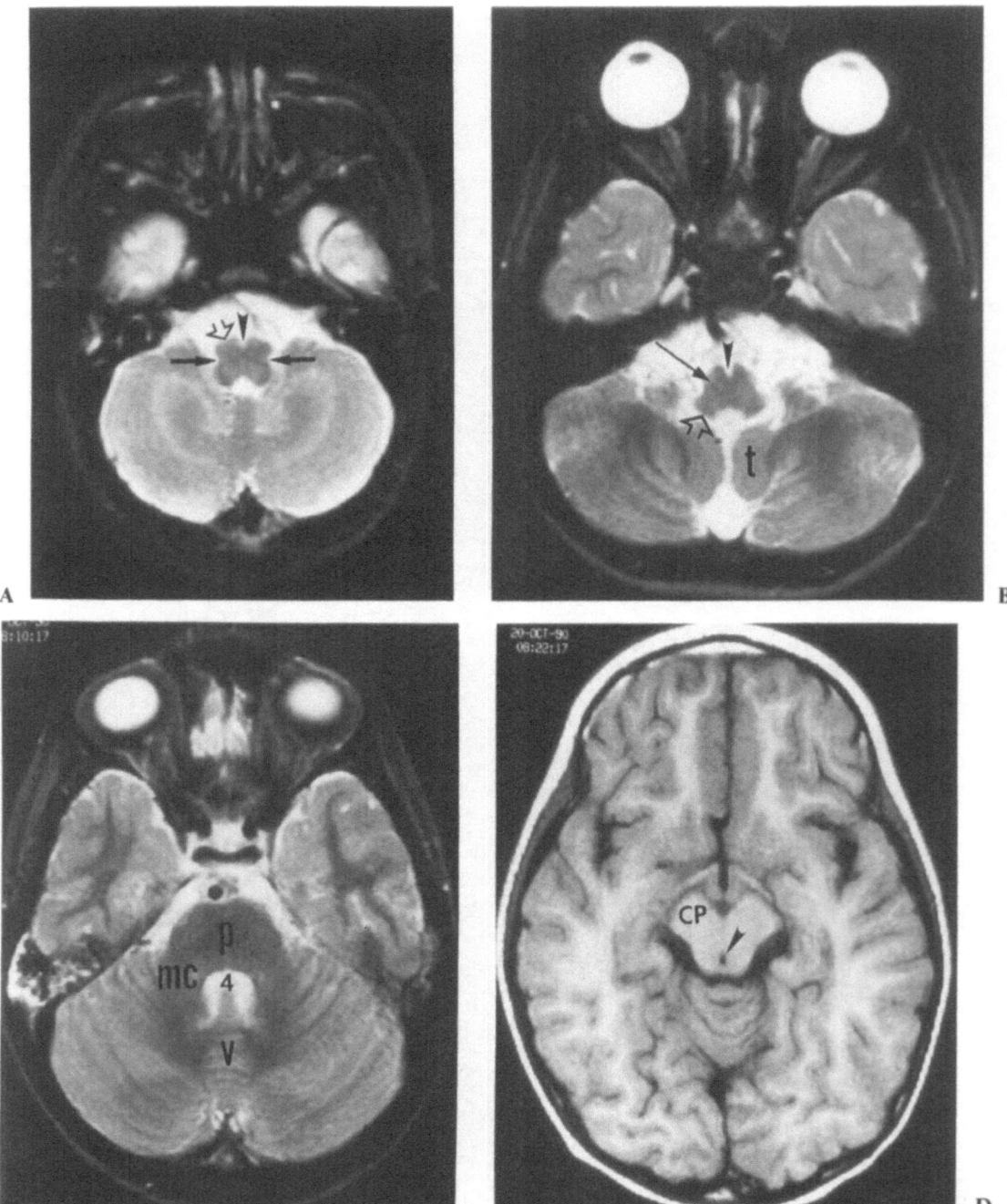

Figure 5.2. Normal axial MR posterior fossa. A: Axial T2-weighted image through the level of the medulla shows the ventral median fissure (arrowhead), the right pyramid (open arrow) and the two ventral lateral sulci (arrows). B: Axial T2-weighted image shows the ventral median fissure (arrowhead), the olivary nucleus (arrow), inferior cerebellar peduncle and restiform body (open arrow), and the left cerebellar tonsil. C: Axial T2-weighted image through the midpons shows the pons (p), middle cerebellar peduncle (mc), fourth ventricle (4), and vermis (V). Cerebellar hemispheres are to either side of the midline vermis. D: Axial T1-weighted section at the level of the midbrain shows right cerebral peduncle (CP) and the aqueduct of Sylvius (arrowhead).

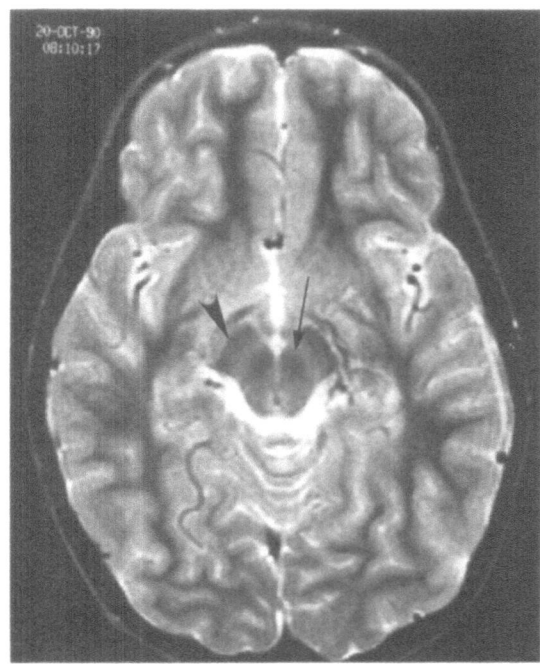

Figure 5.2.E: Axial T2-weighted image at the level of the midbrain shows the substantia nigra on the right (arrowhead) and the red nucleus on the left (arrow).

longer duration, which takes from several to many minutes. If motion occurs during the period of data acquisition, then the image is often degraded or uninterpretable.[3] Thus, adequate sedation or control of motion is a prime necessity in MR imaging.[3] Spatial resolution with MR is comparable to that of CT, and may, in the future, even exceed CT. However, higher spatial resolution is only achieved at the cost of prolonging the time of data acquisition. The environment of the MR scanner is relatively hostile to monitoring and the use of life support systems. Ferromagnetic materials are pulled into the magnet at a speed and with a force such that they can inflict injury on the patient. Thus, care must be exercised within the scanner room. Monitoring devices that use an electron gun, such as an EKG monitor, may have their signal deflected by the magnetic field. Thus, monitoring devices must be utilized that produce intelligible readout. Equipment used to support the patient may produce radiofrequency (RF) signals that in-

terfere with the signals generated and recorded by the MR scanner. Such RF signals will degrade image quality as will any inhomogeneity in the magnetic field introduced within the scanner room by support or monitoring equipment.

Given the advantages and disadvantages of CT and MR, the following conclusions are reached: In the truly emergent situation, CT is easier to do and will show sufficient anatomy and information that an emergency decision can be made as to patient management.[2] Given an emergency patient that has become stable or a nonemergent patient, MR gives a clearer anatomic view and is more sensitive to most pathologic processes that it becomes the diagnostic method of choice.[1] The major exception to this is calcification, which is easily shown on CT, but is often not seen on MR.[6] The paramagnetic contrast agent used with MR, gadolinium-DTPA, is more sensitive than the iodinated contrast material used with CT in demonstrating abnormalities of the BBB, and those of the leptomeninges.[5] In addition, gadolinium-DTPA has a much lower rate of contrast reactions than does the iodinated contrast material.

Normal Anatomy of the Posterior Fossa

Brain Stem

The brain stem is divided into the more cephalad midbrain, larger central pons, and the caudal medulla (Fig. 5.1A).

Midbrain

The midbrain is composed of the smaller dorsal tectum and the larger ventral segment, consisting of the cerebral peduncles, and the central gray substance surrounding the aqueduct (Figs. 5.1A, 5.2D,E, and 5.3C). The cerebral aqueduct, which extends from the posterior third ventricle to the fourth ventricle is seen on axial CT as a focal round hypodensity and on axial MR as a focal round hypointensity (Fig. 5.2D,E). On sagittal MR, the course and size

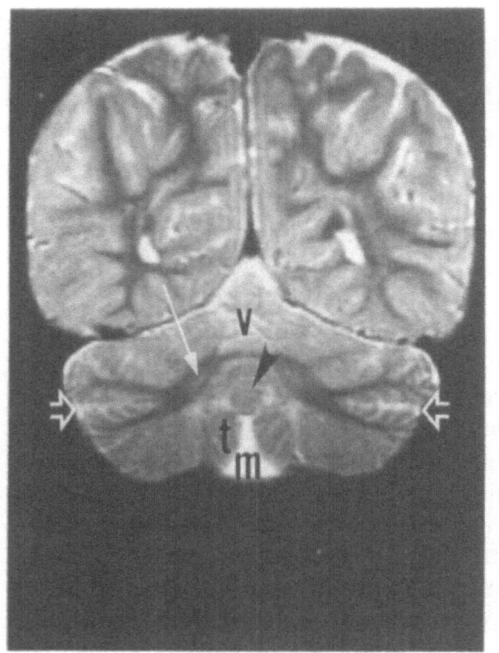

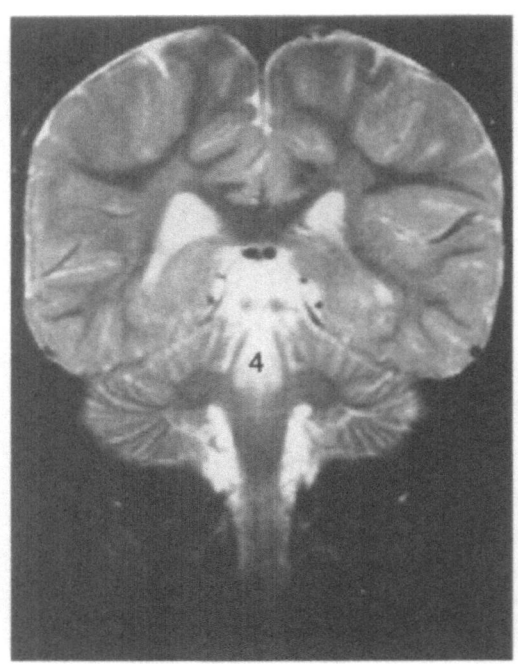

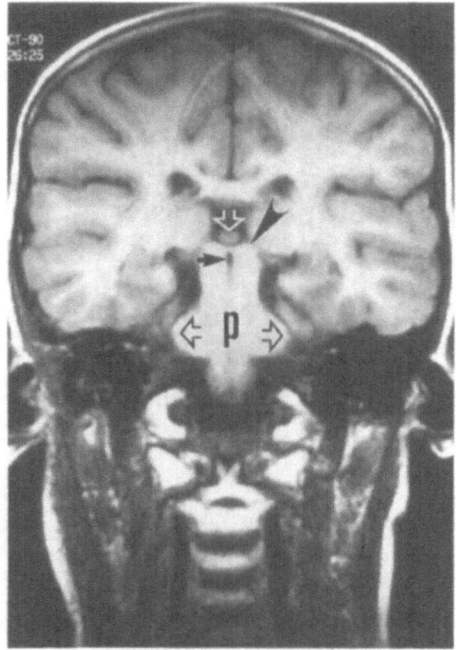

Figure 5.3. Normal coronal MRI anatomy. A: Most posterior coronal T2-weighted image shows the cisterna magna (m), cerebellar tonsil on the right (t), and the vermis in the midline (V), of which the uvula can be distinguished (arrowhead). Within the cerebellum on the right, the dentate nucleus (white arrow) is seen. Two horizontal fissures (open white arrows) divide the inferior from the superior semilunar lobules. B: More anterior coronal T2-weighted section shows the fourth ventricle (4). C: Most anterior coronal T1-weighted section shows pons (p) between the midbrain and the medulla with middle cerebellar peduncles to either side (open arrows). The cerebral aqueduct (short black arrow) lies between and beneath the superior colliculi. The left superior colliculus (arrowhead) is shown. The pineal gland (open white arrow) is above the midbrain.

of the aqueduct is seen (Fig. 5.1A). Anteriorly between the two cerebral peduncles is the interpeduncular fossa containing the posterior perforate substance. The tectum of the midbrain is composed of the superior colliculi, which connect to the ipsilateral lateral geniculate body, and the inferior colliculi, which connect to the auditory cortex (Fig. 5.1A). A layer of pigmented gray matter, the substantia nigra, separates the ventral and dorsal aspect of the cerebral peduncle (Fig. 5.2E). On MR, with aging, the substantia nigra becomes relatively hypointense due to the deposition of iron pigments.[7] The red nucleus also contains iron and is similar in signal intensity[7] (Fig. 5.2E). The red nucleus is dorsal and medial to the substantial nigra.

The third cranial nerve nuclei are located ipsilaterally on each side in front of the cerebral aqueduct. The third cranial nerve emerges in the interpeduncular cistern (Fig. 5.1B), between the cerebral peduncles, to pass to the ipsilateral cavernous sinus and then through the superior orbital fissure to all of the extraocular muscles other than the superior oblique and lateral rectus.[8] It passes between the posterior and superior cerebellar arteries as it proceeds forward. The nucleus of the fourth cranial nerve lies anterior to the aqueduct of Sylvius near the upper part of the inferior colliculus.[8] It projects from the posterior aspect of the brain stem below the inferior colliculus and circles forward through the mesencephalic cistern, passing into the cavernous sinus, through the superior orbital fissure, to innervate the superior oblique muscle within the orbit.[8]

Pons

The pons consists of a large ventral component and a smaller dorsal component, the tegmentum (Figs. 5.1A, 5.2C, and 5.3C). The ventral portion contains transverse strands, which cross the midline forming the middle cerebellar peduncles. The dorsal surface of the tegmentum forms the upper floor of the fourth ventricle. The four nuclei of the fifth cranial nerve (trigeminal) are spread from the level of the in-

ferior colliculus down to the second cervical segment of the spinal cord, but the bulk lies anterior to the floor of the fourth ventricle in the tegmentum of the pons. The motor nucleus lies between the midportion of the floor of the fourth ventricle and the point of exit of the trigeminal nerve from the brain stem. The nerve extends forward from the anterolateral surface of the pons passing through Meckel's cave toward the cavernous sinus.[9] The third division, mandibular (V3) does not enter the cavernous sinus, but passes inferiorly through the foramen ovale. The maxillary division (V2) passes through the cavernous sinus and through the foramen rotundum. The first division, ophthalmic (V1) passes from the cavernous sinus forward through the superior orbital fissure.[9] Cranial nerve V fulfills motor, sensory, and proprioceptor functions.

Sensory fibers take care of the scalp and face, and the mucous membranes of the sinuses, nasal cavity, and mouth. Muscles of mastication, tensors palati and tympani, and the digastric and mylohyoid muscles receive motor innervation. The sixth cranial nerve nucleus is in the ventral aspect of the pons adjacent to the midline at the level of the floor of the fourth ventricle. The abducens (cranial nerve VI) exits the brain stem at the inferior margin of the pons, anteromedially. It runs superiorly and laterally to enter the cavernous sinus.[8] The seventh cranial nerve's three nuclei lie anterolaterally within the pons in front of the floor of the fourth ventricle. The nerve exits at the lateral margin of the pons into the cistern of the cerebellopontine angle as it courses to the internal auditory canal. It is a mixed nerve, consisting of motor, sensory and special function fibers. Cranial nerve VIII, the acoustic nerve, arises from nuclei located in the lateral aspect of the inferior cerebellar peduncle. These are the nuclei that subtend cochlear function. Those that subtend vestibular function lie between the cerebellum and the inferior cerebellar peduncle. The nerve exits the brain stem along the lateral aspect of the pontomedullary juncture to pass forward through the cerebellopontine angle to the internal auditory canal.

Medulla

On the anterior aspect of the medulla is the ventral median fissure (Fig. 5.2A,B), which starts below the pyraminal decussation and ends cephalad at the border with the pons. The pyramid lies between the ventral median fissure and the ventral lateral sulcus (Fig. 5.2A,B). The ventral lateral sulci are two grooves, one on each side (Fig. 5.2A,B). Between the two lateral sulci are the olives with the olivary nuclei. Between the dorsal medial sulcus (present only in the inferior half, ending at the floor of the fourth ventricle) and the dorsal lateral sulcus are the cuneate and the gracile tubercles. The inferior cerebellar peduncles or restiform bodies are diverging prominences on the dorsal aspect of the medulla that form the lateral boundaries of the floor of the fourth ventricle inferiorly (Fig. 5.2A).

The nuclei of the three nerves that compose the glossopharyngeal (cranial nerve IX) lie in the posterolateral portion of the medulla. They pass anterolaterally from the medulla through CSF to the anterior compartment of the jugular foramen. A motor component innervates the stylopharyngeus, whereas a sensory component subtends the posterior oropharynx and soft palate, and a special sensory component functions in taste sensation and discrimination from the posterior third of the tongue.

The nucleus ambiguus and sensory and parasympathetic fibers of the tractus solitarius and dorsal motor nucleus contribute to the 10th cranial nerve, This passes in close proximity to cranial nerves IX and XI within the CSF. The nucleus ambiguus also contributes to the 11th cranial nerve. The anterior horn cells of the first five cervical segments of the spinal cord contribute a spinal component to the 11th cranial nerve. The nucleus of cranial nerve XII extends from the anterior spinal column to the upper portion of the medulla. Within the medulla it is located in a paramedian strip in the floor of the fourth ventricle. Nerve fibers exit between the inferior olivary nucleus and the pyramid. Within the medullary cistern they fuse to form the hypoglossal nerve. The nerve passes through the hypoglossal canal of the occipital bone.

Cerebellum

The cerebellum consists of two hemispheres connected by the more narrow medial portion, the vermis[10] (Figs. 5.1, 5.2, and 5.3A,B). The cerebellum is attached to the brain stem by three cerebellar peduncles, superior (brachium conjunctivum) to the midbrain, middle cerebellar peduncle (brachium pontis) to the pons, and inferior cerebellar peduncle (restiform body) to the medulla (Figs. 5.1B, 5.2C, and 5.3B). The anterior medullary velum is the superior roof of the fourth ventricle. The most superior and anterior lobule of the midline vermis is the lingula (Fig. 5.1A). More posterior in order are the central lobule, culmen, and declive, and more inferior are the folium, tuber, pyramid, and uvale[10] (Fig. 5.1A). the most anterior inferior portion of the vermis is the nodules. Lying to either side of the fourth ventricle, inferior and lateral to the middle cerebellar peduncles and forming the anterior aspect of the lateral recess of the fourth ventricle are the flocculi (Fig. 5.2A). Cerebellar tonsils are portions of the cerebellar hemispheres that lie anteriorly and inferiorly (Figs. 5.1B, and 5.3A).

Posterior Fossa Tumors

The interpretation of the imaging study, whether CT or MR, focuses on the location of the tumor, its extent, and whether or not there is subarachnoid or intraspinal dissemination.[11] With CT, additional information is derived by comparison of the plain study (without contrast) to that following contrast injection. The plain CT study is examined for the density of the tumor tissue, presence or absence of surrounding edema, and whether or not calcification or hemorrhage is present.[12,13] The CT study postcontrast injection is examined for the presence or absence of enhancement at the site of the tumor and whether or not there is intraventricular or subarachnoid tumor dissemination.[12,13]

With MR, the plain examination involves the comparison of the appearance of the tumor on T1-weighted images (T1WI) to those obtained with a longer time to repetition (TR) and a short time to echo (TE) [proton density (PD) image, spin density image, balanced image] and a long TE [T2-weighted image (T2WI)].[12,13] The study is examined for relative hypointensity on T1WI that becomes increased in signal intensity on PDWI and T2WI. This is most often a sign of increased water content within the interstitial space of the tumor.

A relative decrease in signal intensity on the T2WI is seen in tumors that are of high cell density such as primitive neuroectodermal tumors (PNET), lymphomas, and germinomas.[11] Calcification is usually not visible on MR.[6] When it is visible, it is as a focal area of hypointensity. Acute hemorrhage (deoxyhemoglobin) is iso- to hypointense on T1WI and markedly hypointense on T2WI.[14] Subacute hemorrhage (intracellular methemoglobin) is hyperintense (white) on T1WI and markedly hypointense on T2WI.[4] Extracellular methemoglobin is hyperintense on both T1WI and T2WI.[4] Hemosiderin that forms as a result of the breakdown of methemoglobin is iso- to hypointense on T1WI and markedly hypointense on T2WI.[15]

The hypointensity seen on T2WI with deoxyhemoglobin and hemosiderin are due to a magnetic susceptibility effect, in which heterogeneous fields within the affected tissue throw the proton spins out of phase, producing signal loss. The hyperintensity (T1WI) with methemoglobin is due to the paramagnetic effect produced by free electrons, producing a marked shortening of T1 relaxation time (high signal intensity).[4] Flowing blood within arteries and veins appears as a focal round or linear area of hypointensity. This is because the energized protons in flowing blood move out of the slice plane before a signal can be returned. Thus, a grossly hypervascular neoplasm can be identified by an increase in number of flow voids within the tumor bed. The T1-weighted MR

study before the administration of gadolinium-DTPA is then compared to the T1WI after contrast injection.[11] Abnormalities in BBB are demonstrated as areas of high signal intensity due to leakage of gadolinium into the interstitial space of the tumor.[5] Gadolinium produces an increase in signal intensity due to marked T1 shortening related to the presence of free electrons.[5]

Brain Stem Gliomas

Brain stem gliomas most commonly arise within the pons (Fig. 5.4A) from which they then spread in all directions, superiorly into the midbrain, inferiorly into the medulla, and laterally into the cerebellum.[13] Exophytic extension is common, most often anteriorly. The relatively rigid basilar artery can be partially or totally encased by such anterior exophytic tumor growth. A second, but less frequent, group of brain stem tumors arise either in the midbrain or medulla and tend to present a different clinical, histologic, and imaging picture (Fig. 5.4). These tumors are usually well localized, benign histologically, and have more protracted courses.[16]

Most pontine gliomas are either malignant at diagnosis or will be at time of death, which occurs in from 1 to 2 years. On plain CT, most pontine gliomas are either low in density (36%) or isodense (36%).[17] A lesser proportion are of mixed low and isodense components. High-density calcification is unusual, whereas high-density hemorrhage is also unusual at diagnosis but may be found during follow-up.[13] This occurs most often at the site of malignant transformation.

At the time of diagnosis, contrast enhancement is infrequent in malignant pontine gliomas. With progression of the tumor and development of a richer vascular bed, contrast enhancement can be seen, progressively increasing in extent. The corollary of the CT findings on MR are the presence of isointensity to low signal intensity on T1WI and increased signal intensity on PDWI and T2WI (Fig. 5.4A,B). This reflects the water content within the tumor. Contrast enhancement with

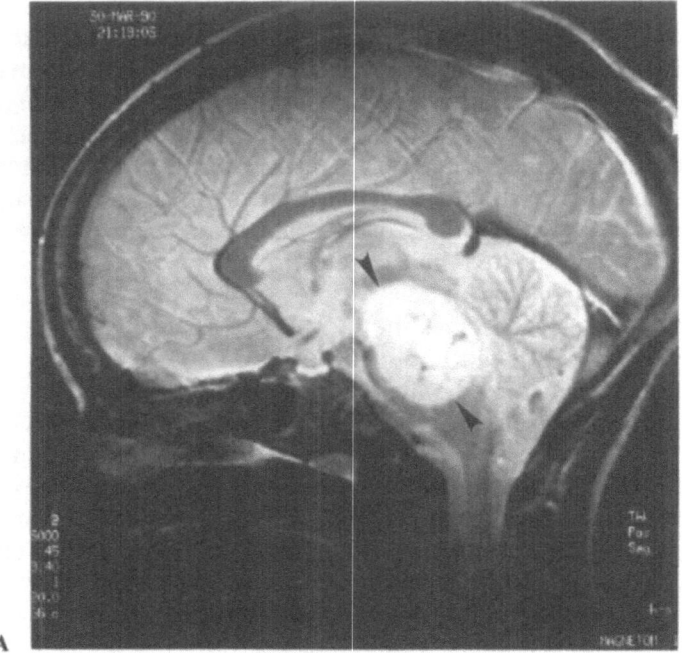

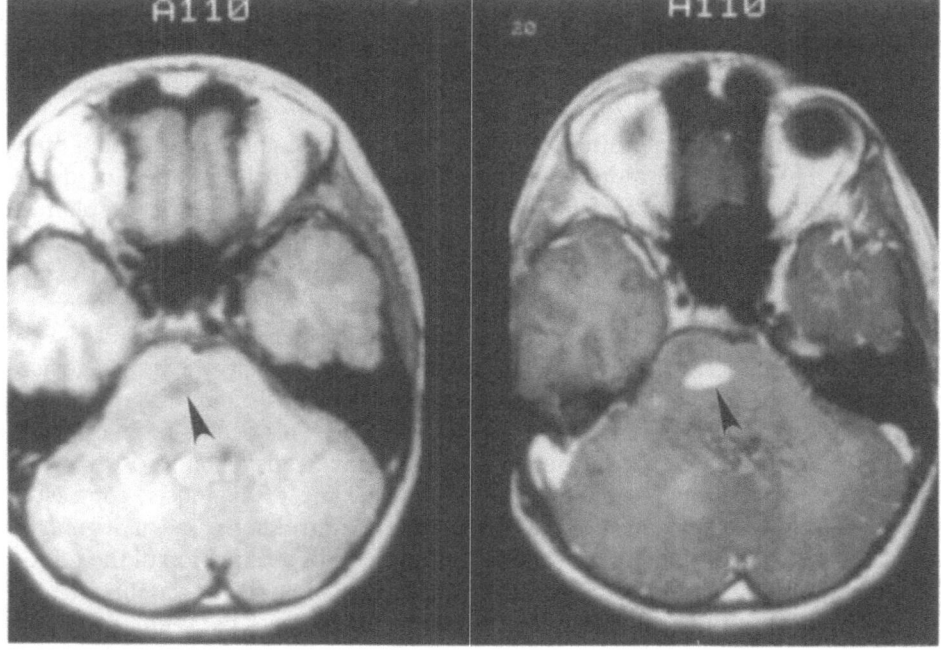

Figure 5.4. Brain stem gliomas. A: Sagittal T2-weighted image shows a high signal intensity mass (arrowheads) expanding the pons, extending into the midbrain. B: Axial T1-weighted image shows an expanded pons, more to the right side, with a focal area of hypointensity (arrowhead). C: Axial T1-weighted image, following gadolinium injection, same patient shown in B. There is focal enhancement (arrowhead). D: Axial T1-weighted image without contrast shows an area of high signal intensity (arrowheads), consistent with methemoglobin, further expanding the right side of the pontine tumor. E: Sagittal T1-weighted image

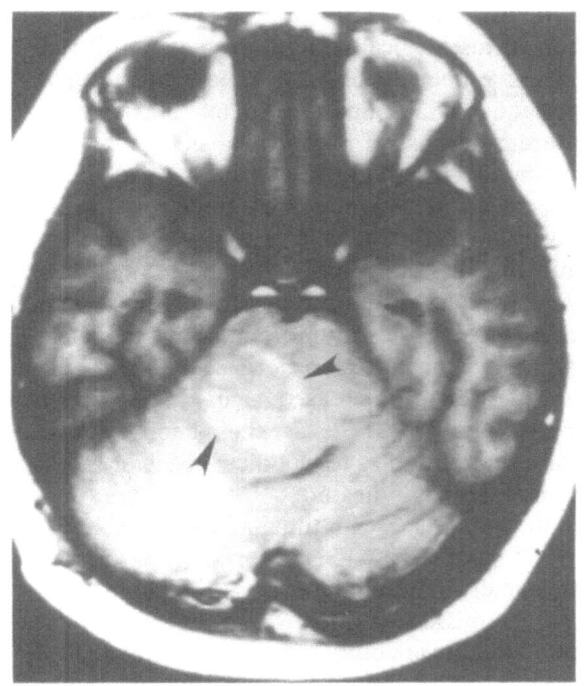
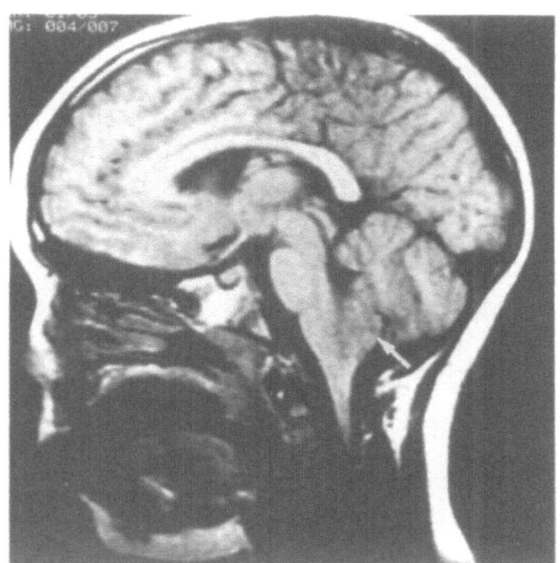

E

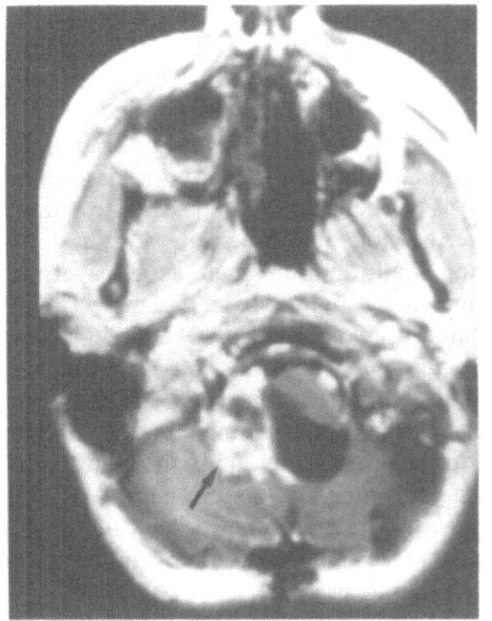

F

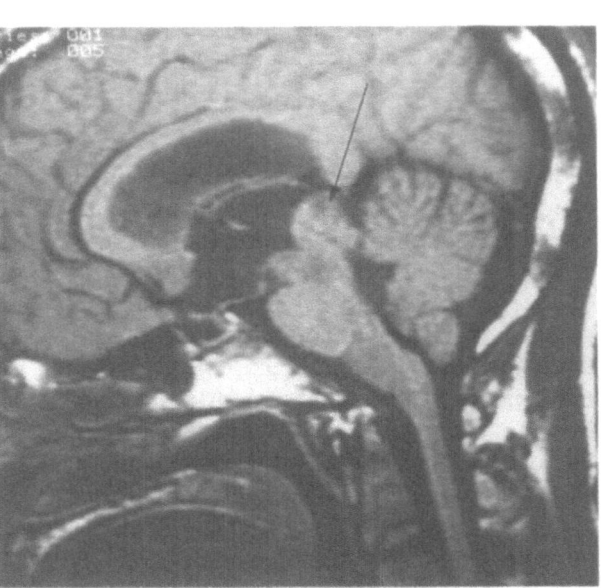

G

shows a dorsally exophytic medullary tumor mass (arrow). F: Axial T1-weighted image postgadolinium in-jection shows a partially solid contrast enhancing exophytic medullary astrocytoma (arrow). There is a cystic component to the left of the midline with compression and rotation of the remaining medulla to the left. G: Sagittal T1-weighted image shows neoplastic enlargement of the tectum of the midbrain (arrow) with obliteration of the aqueduct and hydrocephalic dilatation of the third and lateral ventricles.

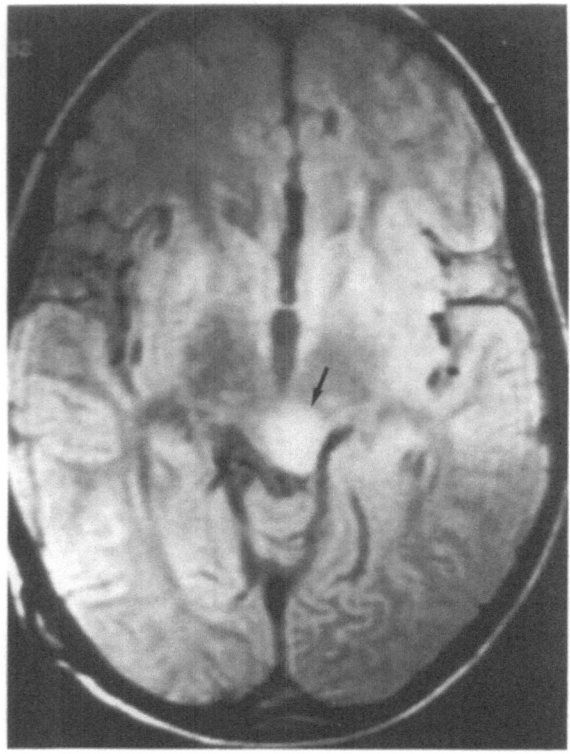

Figure 5.4.H: Axial proton density weighted image shows high signal intensity neoplastic expansion (arrow) of the left side of the midbrain.

gadolinium-DTPA is uncommon early in the course of malignant pontine gliomas. Following hyperfractionation radiation therapy, there is often an initial reduction of up to 50% in size of the tumor.[18] With subsequent recurrence, contrast enhancement and mass effect progressively increase in extent (Fig. 5.4B,C). As the mass enlarges, the enhancement pattern may become ring-like, suggesting central tumor necrosis. Hemorrhage within the tumor is shown both acutely and subacutely by MR. Its appearance on T1WI and T2WI will depend upon the chemical state of the blood products[13] (Fig. 5.4D). Dissemination of tumor into the subarachnoid pathways, although infrequent at diagnosis, may be seen in between one-fifth to one-third of patients at time of death.[19]

Tumors of the midbrain and medulla are often exophytic (Fig. 5.4E,G), may enhance intensely (Fig. 5.4F), and may be cystic (Fig. 5.4F) or solid. These tumors are most often benign histologically. With the advent of MR there has been an increase in the recognition of periaqueductal midbrain tumor masses that present because of hydrocephalus (Fig. 5.4G). In many instances, the patient had been diagnosed in childhood or infancy as having obstructive hydrocephalus on the basis of aqueductal stenosis. MR has shown the previously undiagnosed and untreated tumor mass (Fig. 5.4H). These tumors may not enhance, and may only be seen because of their bulk as an area of increased signal intensity on PDWI and T2WI. So far, their benign course raises a question as to whether biopsy or radiation therapy is indicated.

In comparison with the diagnostic sensitivity of CT and MR, MR is superior in picking up the small symptomatic brain stem glioma that may be missed on CT.[13] This is because of the multiplanar capability of MR and the increased contrast sensitivity to water within the tumor tissue (Fig. 5.4A,H). However, other disease processes may produce similar imaging findings and therefore need to be considered in the differential diagnosis. These include acute disseminated encephalomyelitis, multiple sclerosis, dysmyelinating diseases, and central pontine myelinolysis.[13] When a brain stem mass contains blood products, the differential diagnosis is between a hemorrhagic tumor, an arteriovenous malformation, and an occult vascular malformation such as a cavernous angioma or a hemorrhagic telangiectasia.[13] The differential diagnosis may be aided if other occult vascular malformations are present within the supratentorial space, if there are feeding arteries and draining veins of an arteriovenous malformation, or if there are other high signal intensity abnormalities (PDWI, T2WI) within the supratentorial white matter that are suggestive of the demyelinating and dysmyelinating diseases.

Cerebellar Astrocytomas

Most cerebellar tumors are low-grade pilocytic astrocytomas, whereas fewer are relatively low-grade fibrillary astrocytomas, and even fewer are malignant astrocytomas.[20] The low-grade pilocytic astrocytomas are often partially or totally cystic, with the tumor being either a mural nodule or making up the cyst wall.[12] Histologically more aggressive tumors can infiltrate the cerebellum, extending through the peduncles into the brain stem. Consequently, tumor masses may be localized to the cerebellar hemisphere and vermis or may even be diffuse, involving all of the cerebellum. Cerebellar astrocytomas are most often low density on plain CT[21] (Fig. 5.5A). The tumor is higher in density than is cerebrospinal fluid (CSF).[21] When a tumor cyst is present, the proteinaceous fluid within the cyst is intermediate in density, lower than the solid portion of the tumor, but higher than CSF[21] (Fig. 5.5B). Calcification occurs in 13% to 20% of cerebellar astrocytomas.[12,21] Contrast enhancement of the tumor on CT is often intense (Fig. 5.5B). The part that enhances can be assumed to be tumor.

On MR, both solid and cystic components are hypointense on T1WI (Fig. 5.5C) and hyperintense on PDW and T2WI[12] (Fig. 5.5E). Usually, the proteinaceous cyst fluid is higher in signal intensity than the adjacent tumor on PDWI (Fig. 5.5E). Hemorrhage within the cyst can produce siderosis of the cyst wall lining, appearing as a thin hypointense inner lining on T2WI. Some fibrillary astrocytomas do not enhance on MR, whereas most pilocytic astrocytomas show intense enhancement[5] (Fig. 5.5D). Malignant cerebellar gliomas, although uncommon, appear essentially similar to those seen in the supratentorial space.[11] These tumors are now being seen with an increasing frequency in patients who are long-term survivors posttherapy of posterior fossa primitive neuroectodermal tumors. It is thought that these are radiation-induced neoplasm arising in the residual cerebellar tissue. Dissemination of malignant cerebellar gliomas is not unusual, whereas dissemination of the benign pilocytic cerebellar astrocytoma is. Residual pilocytic astrocytoma left after subtotal resection tends to have a long protracted course during which slow growth occurs. The imaging differential diagnosis of the cerebellar astrocytoma includes pyogenic abscess, tuberculoma, and the occult vascular malformation.[12]

Primitive Neuroectodermal Tumors

The common imaging presentation is that of a midline posterior fossa mass arising in the vermis, extending into the adjacent cerebellar hemisphere, compressing and often obstructing the fourth ventricle[22] (Fig. 5.6A,B,C). The mass is usually slightly increased in density on plain CT[22] (Fig. 5.6A). Following contrast injection, homogeneous enhancement is most often seen[22] (Fig. 5.6B). However, cystic or necrotic areas can be present. Calcification on CT occurs in 10% to 15% of cases.[12,23] Occasionally, the mass does not enhance and may be more cystic than usual.

With MR, the mass is hypointense on T1WI (Fig. 5.6C), slightly hyperintense on PDWI (Fig. 5.6D), but relatively hypo- to isointense on T2WI[12] (Fig. 5.6E). This is sufficiently different from the cerebellar astrocytoma (which is high in signal intensity on T2WI) that the primitive neuroectodermal tumor should not often be mistaken for a cerebellar astrocytoma. It is thought that the etiology of the signal intensity on T2WI is related to the highly cellular nature of the tumor, its relatively low interstitial water content, and its relatively high degree of vascularity. Contrast enhancement of the tumor is the rule with MR (Fig. 5.6F), but again there are a few exceptions. Dissemination of the tumor intracranially and intraspinally may be found at time of diagnosis. At time of recurrence and death, dissemination is frequent[24] (Fig. 5.6G,H). Myelography with follow-up CT had been the gold standard for the evaluation of spinal dissemination.[25] At present, gadolinium-enhanced T1WI surpasses myelography for intraspinal disease and for intracranial dissemination.[25]

Ependymoma

Posterior fossa ependymomas arise from the ependymal lining of the fourth ventricle or along the course of the tela choroidea that extends from the lateral recesses of the fourth ventricle into the cerebellopontine angle cistern (CPL). Ependymomas tend to extend in a plastic-like fashion from the fourth ventricle, through the recesses and around the brain stem, enveloping the adjacent cranial nerves

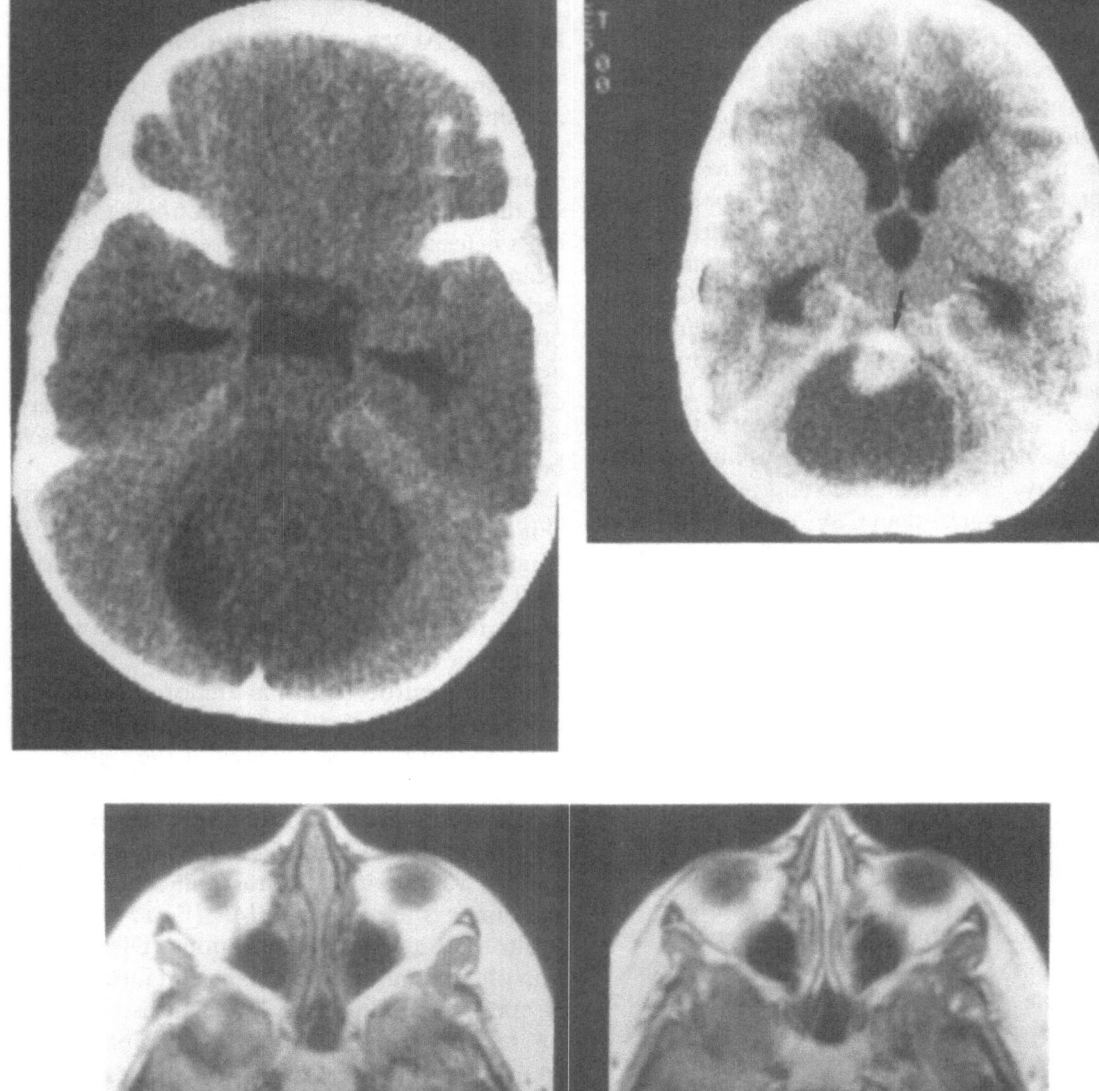

Figure 5.5. Cerebellar astrocytomas. A: Axial CT without contrast shows a hypodense posterior fossa mass. The temporal horns are dilated because of obstructive hydrocephalus. B: Axial postcontrast CT shows an enhancing mural tumor nodule (arrow) of a cystic cerebellar astrocytoma. The cyst fluid is higher in density than CSF in the obstructed third and lateral ventricles. C: Axial T1-weighted image without contrast shows a hypointense mass in the left cerebellar hemisphere compressing and displacing the fourth ventricle (open arrow). D: Same patient as in C. Axial T1-weighted image postgadolinium shows enhancement of the tumor in the wall of a centrally cystic cerebellar astrocytoma.

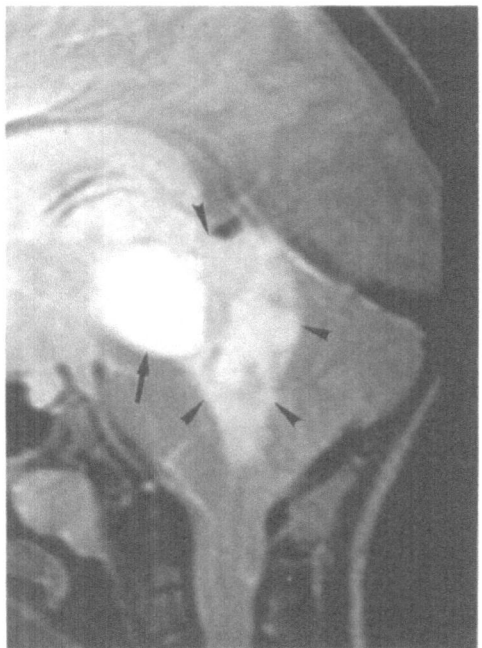

Figure 5.5.E: Sagittal proton density–weighted image shows an anterior superior vermian tumor mass that markedly compresses the upper brain stem. A tumor cyst is present (arrow), and is higher in signal intensity than the adjacent solid tumor (arrowheads).

and blood vessels. On CT, the density is frequently mixed, due to the presence of calcification, old areas of bleeding, and tumor matrix[26] (Fig. 5.7A). Contrast enhancement, although frequent, is absent in a significant but small percentage. On MR the tumor is lowest in signal intensity on T1WI, except at sites of intrinsic subacute hemorrhage (methemoglobin), which are higher in signal intensity[12] (Fig. 5.7B). Interspersed calcification and tumor blood vessels contribute to a mixed signal intensity seen on PDWI and T2WI[12] (Fig. 5.7C). These calcifications and blood vessels can produce hypointensities. Subacute hemorrhage in the form of extracellular methemoglobin produces hyperintensity on PDWI and T2WI as does most of the tumor tissue. A small percentage of ependymomas do not enhance with gadolinium. A consequence of this is that their sites of dissemination do not enhance. Thus, recognition of residual, recurrent, or disseminated ependymoma, may be difficult.

Choroid Plexus Tumors

Tumors of the fourth ventricle that arise from the choroid plexus are either benign choroid plexus papillomas or malignant choroid plexus carcinomas. The papillomas are seen most often in the adolescent, whereas the carcinomas are seen in the infant. Invasion of the adjacent cerebellum and dissemination of tumor within the subarachnoid space is a characteristic of the carcinoma. Hydrocephalus is frequent with both at presentation. On CT, the papilloma is dense, often calcified, and attached along the posterior aspect of the fourth ventricle (Fig. 5.8A). Tumor may extend through the lateral recess of the fourth ventricle into the cerebellopontine angle, or may arise from the choroid that normally lies in that location.[27] The fourth ventricular expansion due to obstruction is frequent and resulting hydrocephalus may or may not have a component due to overproduction of CSF. Marked contrast enhancement occurs on CT.

Vertebral arteriography is less frequently done than before. When it is performed, the posterior inferior cerebellar arteries and their choroidal branches are found to be dilated, producing a diffuse tumor stain seen in the arterial phase and lasting into the venous phase. Choroid plexus carcinomas may or may not have calcification, arise within the fourth ventricle, and invade the adjacent walls.

On CT, a necrotic center produces inhomogeneous contrast enhancement of a thick, irregular wall. The spread of the tumor into the adjacent subarachnoid spaces or up through the aqueduct into the supratentorial ventricular system should be looked for.

On MR, the choroid plexus papilloma is seen on T1WI as an iso- to hypointense papillary mass. This tumor is relatively hypointense to CSF and to the adjacent brain on PDWI and T2WI. This signal intensity is attributed to the presence of calcification and a rich vascularity. Intense enhancement occurs following gadolinium injection (Fig. 5.8B). The choroid plexus carcinoma may not be as hypointense as the papilloma on PDWI and T2WI. Its enhancement is also intense. The T1WI postgadolinium should be examined for the possibility of dis-

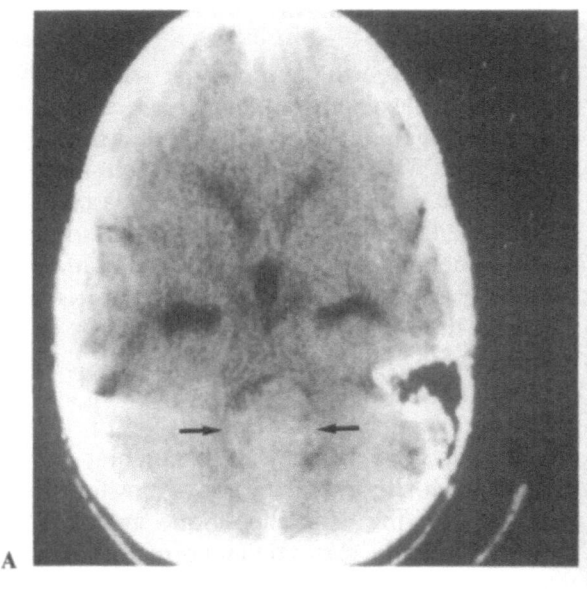

A

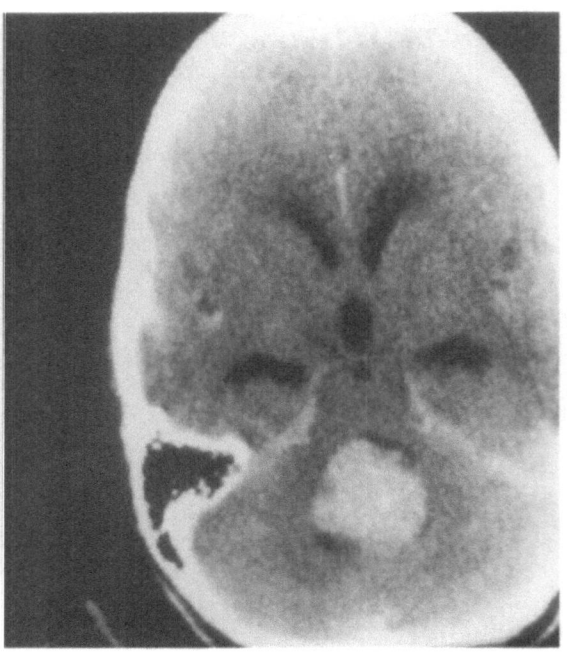

B

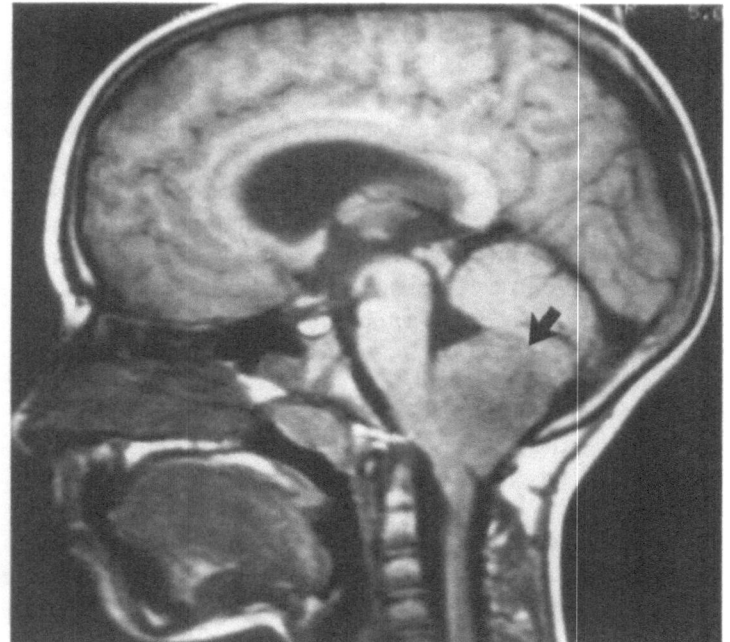

C

Figure 5.6. Primitive neuroecto-dermal tumors. A: Axial CT without contrast shows a mass (arrows) of increased density in the vermis that projects into the fourth ventricle. Hydrocephalus is present with dilatation of the temporal horns. B: Same patient as in A. Axial CT postcontrast shows marked enhancement of the tumor mass. C: Sagittal T1-weighted image shows a hypointense mass (arrow) projecting forward from the inferior vermis producing obstruction of the fourth ventricle with resultant hydrocephalus.

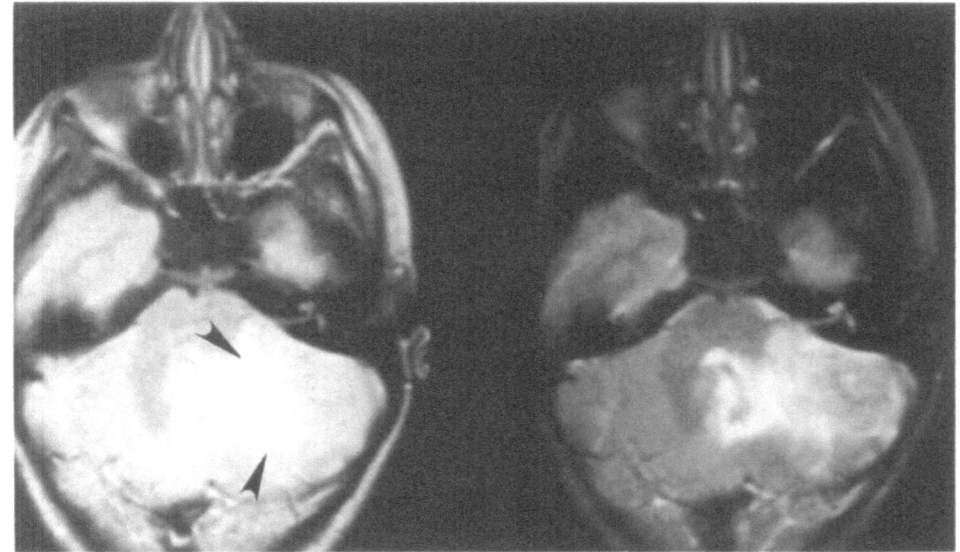

D   E

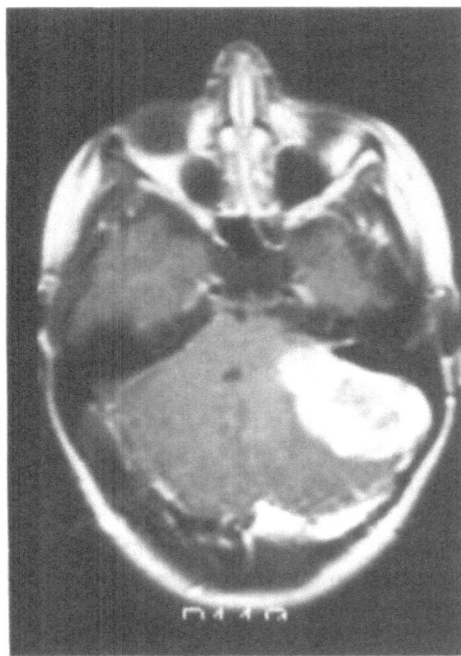

Figure 5.6.D: Axial proton density–weighted image shows a high signal intensity mass (arrowheads) in the left cerebellum. E: Axial T2-weighted image in the same patient as in D shows that the mass has become iso- to hypointense. F: Axial T1-weighted image after gadolinium injection shows marked tumor enhancement. This is the same case as in D and E.

F

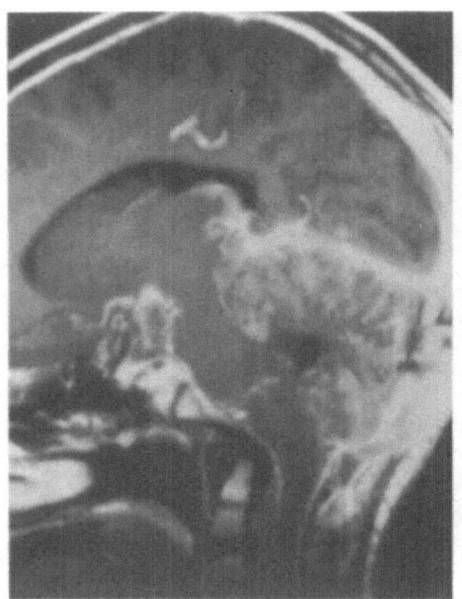
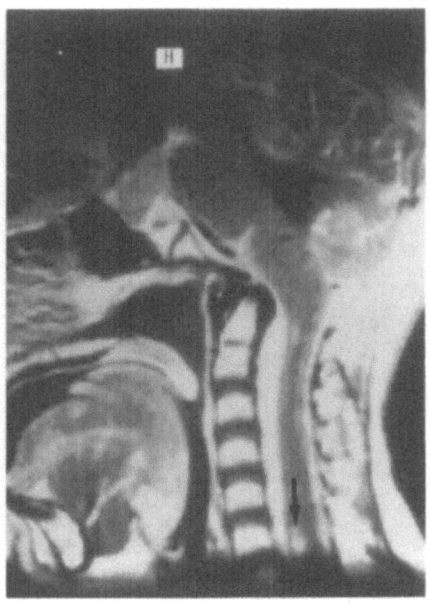

G   H

Figure 5.6.G: Sagittal T1-weighted image postgadolinium shows marked subarachnoid space enhancement outlining the cerebellar sulci and the interpeduncular cistern as well as coating the brain stem and upper cervical cord. This is secondary to dissemination of primitive neuroectodermal tumor, 3 years after diagnosis and treatment. H: Sagittal T1-weighted image of the upper cervical cord and posterior fossa after gadolinium in the same patient shown in G, shows marked enhancement of tumor coating the cervical spinal cord with intramedullary invasion (arrow).

semination. Invasion of the adjacent cerebellum and brain stem can be shown on multiplanar MR using gadolinium injection, or even on T2WI by the presence of edema within the brain at the site of invasion.

Congenital Inclusion Tumors

At the time of closure of the neural tube, portions of the developing germinal layers of the embryo may become trapped. Inclusion of these tissues leads to the formation of such masses as lipomas, dermoids, and teratomas. In the posterior fossa, lipomas are most frequent in the tectum of the midbrain and, to a lesser extent, within the cerebellopontine angle.[28] Dermoids may be associated with an overlying occipital dermal sinus track that provides continuity for the spread of infection inward from the skin. Teratomas occur in the midline, from the pineal down through the choroidal region. They are found in infancy, and can grow to a huge size at presentation.

On CT the lipoma (fat) is hypodense, lower in density than CSF, but higher than air. The lipoma measures in the range of −100 to −50 Hounsfield units.[28] The dermoid also frequently contains fatty tissue. In addition, it contains other components of variable densities, which may include teeth of high density. Teratomas have multiple components from all three germinal layers, and consequently have a very variable spectrum of densities ranging from fat to bone.[28] Malignant teratomas tend to be large, invasive, and very heterogeneous.

On MR, the lipoma is high in signal intensity on T1WI, and progressively less intense from PDWI to T2WI. Comparison of the lipoma to the scalp fat shows precisely the same change in signal intensity. The dermoid is bright on T1WI where there is fat, and of different signal intensity where there is other soft tissue. For instance, at the site of teeth there is hypointensity on T1WI, PDWI, and T2WI. Teratomas are of variable signal intensity, depending on the components within the tumor (Fig.

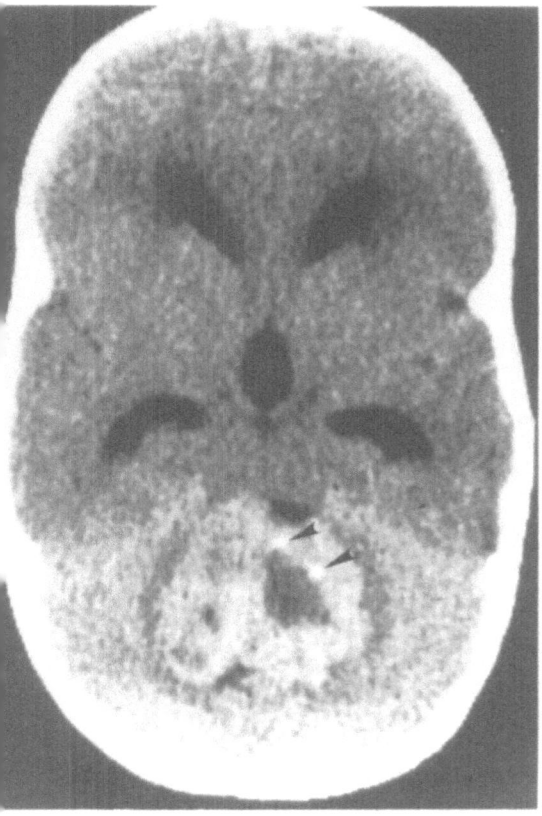

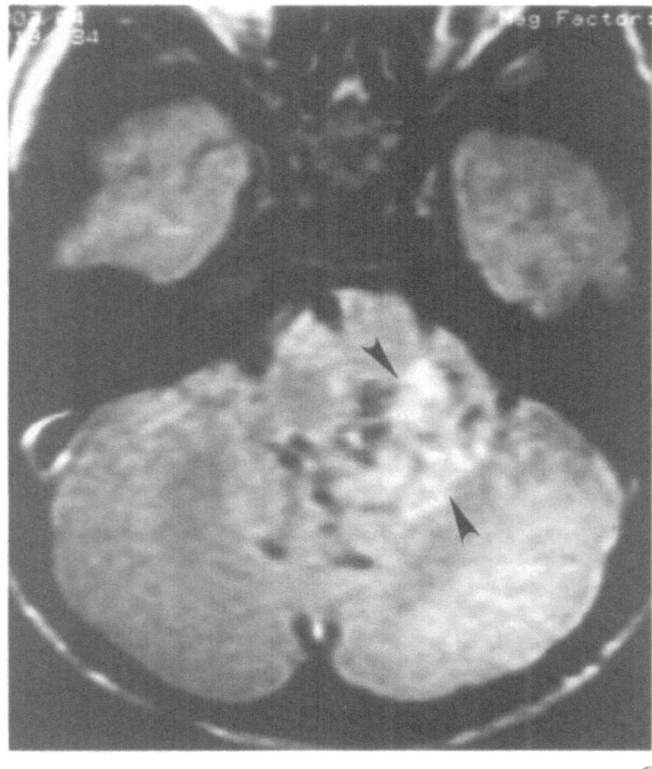

C

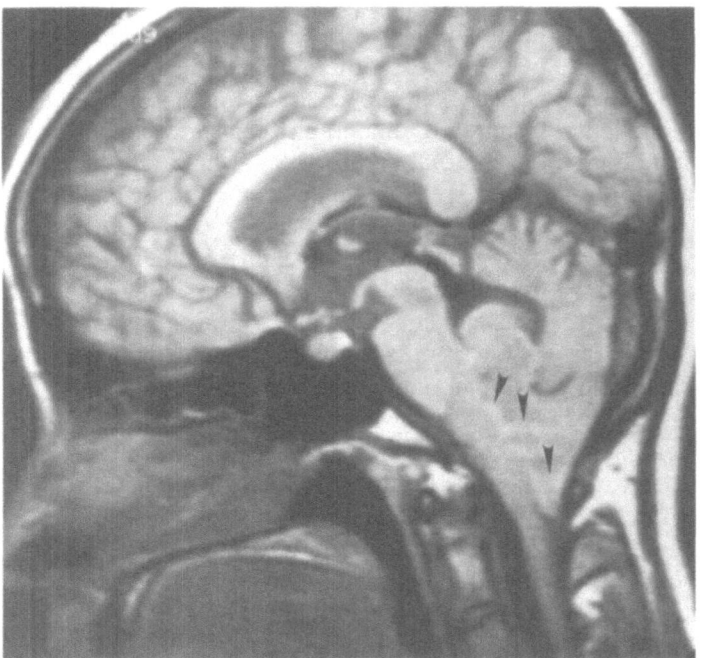

B

Figure 5.7. Ependymomas. Axial CT without contrast shows a mixed density tumor mass in the region of the fourth ventricle producing obstructive hydrocephalus. Two denser areas (arrowheads) are flecks of calcification. B: Sagittal T1-weighted image shows an intra–fourth ventricular mass extending through the foramen Magendie that is filling the cisterna magna. Note that there are areas of increased signal intensity (arrowheads) consistent with methemoglobin within the tumor. C: Axial proton density–weighted image shows a mass (arrowheads) of increased signal intensity within the left lateral recess of the fourth ventricle. There are a multitude of hypointensities in and around the mass that are consistent with either blood vessels or calcifications.

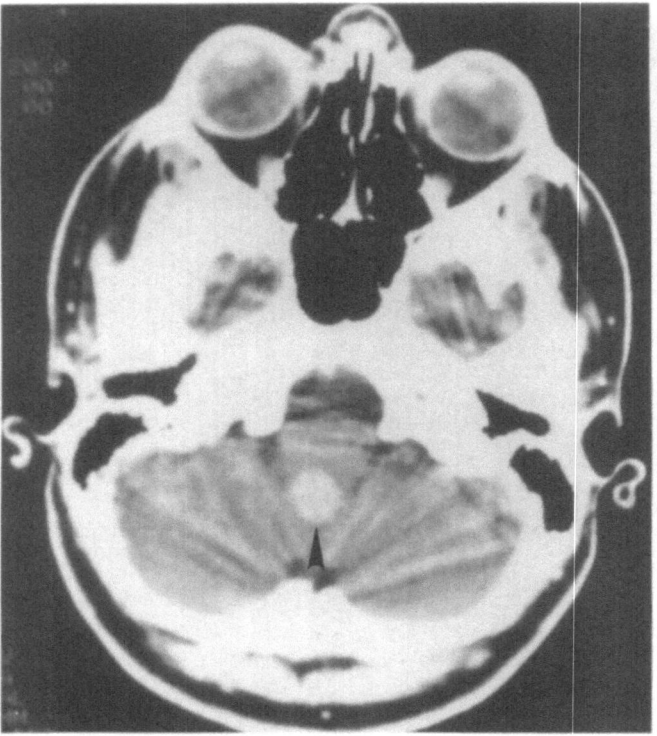

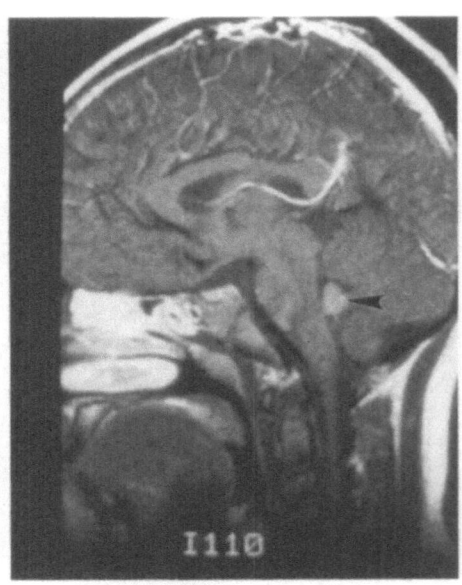

B

A

Figure 5.8. Choroid plexus papillomas. A: Axial CT postcontrast enhancement shows a hyperdense midline mass (arrowhead) in the inferior aspect of the fourth ventricle. B: Sagittal T1-weighted image post gadolinium shows enhancement of a mass (arrowhead) in the fourth ventricle.

5.9A,B). On T1WI, most of the tissue is iso- to hypointense. Exceptions are areas of fat or areas of methemoglobin from prior bleeding (Fig. 5.9A). On PDW and T2WI, the tumor again is quite variable (Fig. 5.9B). Malignant teratomas show contrast enhancement on both CT and MR (Fig. 5.9C). Dermoids may show enhancement when they are infected. Lipomas do not enhance.

Acoustic Neuromas

Acoustic neuromas presenting in childhood occur almost exclusively in the clinical setting of type 2 neurofibromatosis.[29] Their synchrony, the rate at which they present, is variable. Thus, one tumor may present before the other. In type 2 neurofibromatosis, cutaneous stigmata are often not present. Consequently, one should be suspicious of an acoustic neuro-

ma in any child or adolescent. Other tumors, meningiomas, cord ependymomas, and even neuromas of other cranial nerves or spinal nerve roots are common in these patients.[29] Computed tomography can show expansion of the internal auditory canal, and an intracanalicular or extracanalicular contrast-enhancing soft tissue mass. Because these tumors may be quite small at their inception, the best method of study is with MR. MR allows imaging, in the axial and coronal plane, with thin sections. On T1WI, a mass is sought along the course of the eighth cranial nerve. On PDWI and T2WI the acoustic neuroma may be increased in signal intensity or even isointense. If isointense and small, it is difficult to recognize. On T1WI following gadolinium injection, acoustic neuromas enhance intensely (Fig. 5.10). Thus, the best method of identifying an acoustic neuroma is the postgadolinium T1WI.

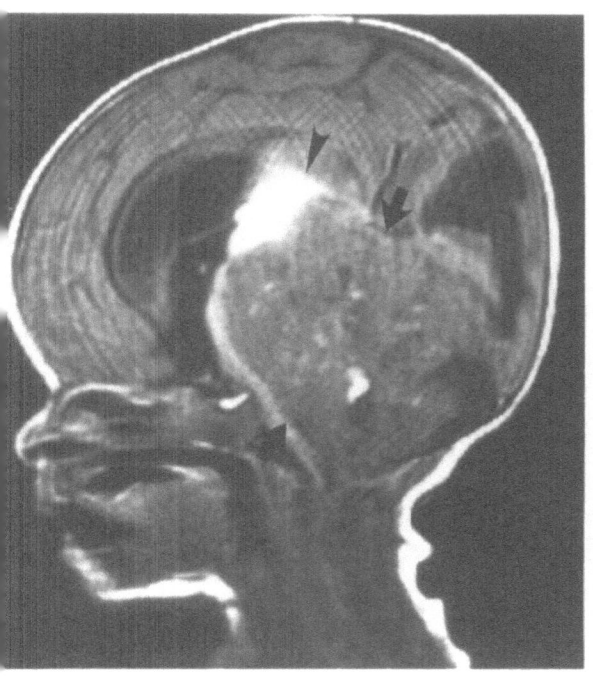
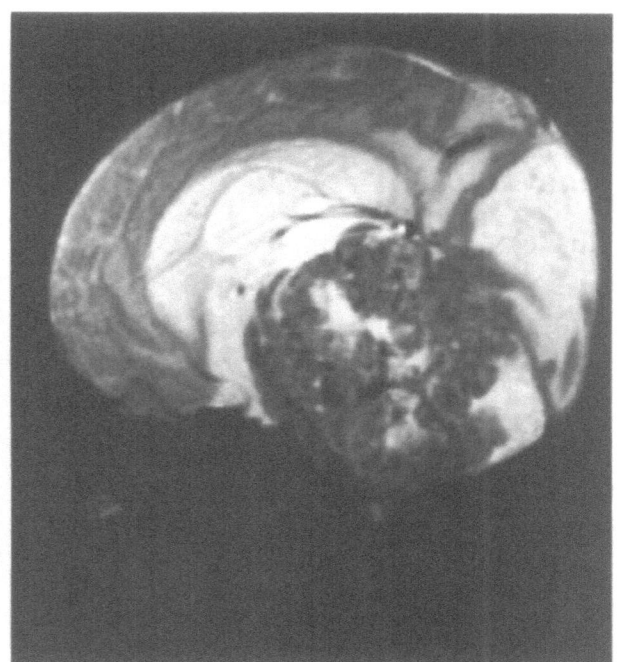

B

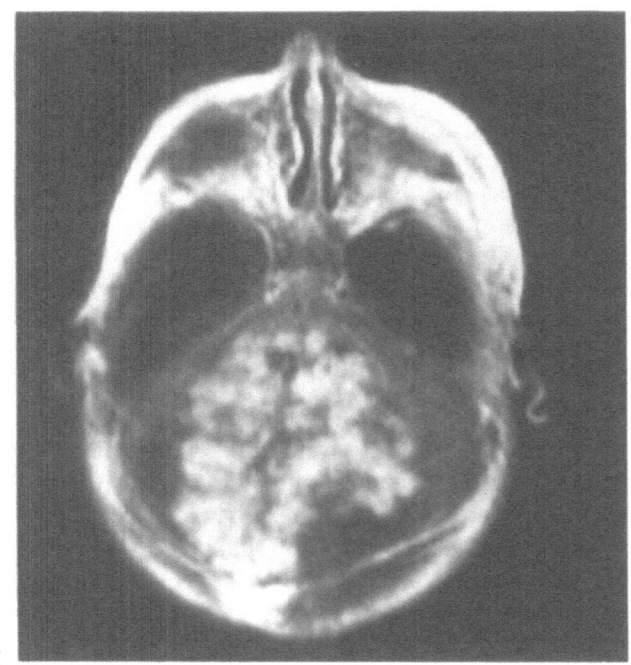

Figure 5.9. Malignant teratoma. A: Sagittal T1-weighted image shows a very large mixed signal intensity mass (arrows) occupying almost all of the posterior fossa, extending into the supratentorial space through the tentorial incisura. On the anterior superior margin there is high signal intensity methemoglobin (arrowhead). Hydrocephalus is present. B: Sagittal T2-weighted image shows the mass to be of mixed low and high signal intensity. C: Axial T1-weighted image post-gadolinium injection shows marked contrast enhancement with the tumor having a multilobulated pattern.

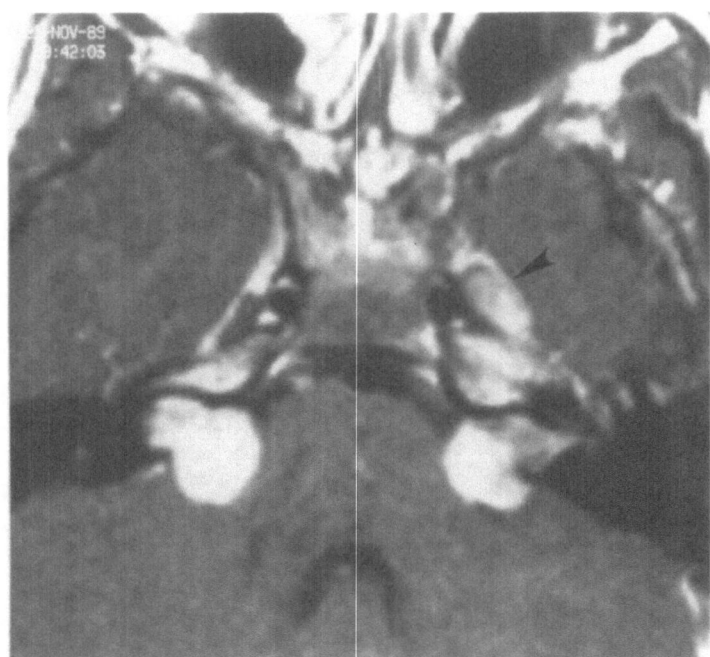

Figure 5.10. Acoustic neuromas. Axial T1-weighted image post gadolinium shows bilateral contrast enhancing acoustic neuromas projecting out of the internal auditory canals into the cerebellopontine angle cisterns. There is enlargement of the left cavernous sinus by a mass (arrowhead) that is consistent with a fifth nerve neuroma. The patient also had a C1-C2 cervical meningioma.

Metastatic Disease

The two most frequent tumors to hematogenously metastasize to the cranial vault and dura of a child are neuroblastoma and Ewing's sarcoma.[30] The bony destruction is best evaluated by CT, with and without contrast. Soft tissue and bone windows should be used. MR becomes valuable in demonstrating compression of flow within the dural venous sinuses (Fig. 5.11), a situation that has been known to produce venous hypertension, increased intracranial pressure, and papilledema. Postgadolinium T1WI are effective in showing penetration of the dura by tumor. Such penetration is unusual with neuroblastoma. Rhabdomyosarcoma of the temporal bone can extend through the osseous structures and dura to invade the posterior cranial fossa. The combination of CT for bone destruction and gadolinium-enhanced T1WI for dural invasion gives the maximum information.

Benign Tumors of the Cranial Vault

The most frequent benign tumor of the cranial vault in the child is histiocytosis. Epidermoid tumors and hemangiomas occur. Sharp edges and a lytic lesion involving the inner and outer tables of the skull with a contrast-enhancing soft tissue mass on CT bespeaks the probability of histiocytosis. Epidermoids rarely extend from the intradiploic space into the posterior fossa during childhood and epidermoids within the subarachnoid space are rarely encountered in childhood, being more frequent in adults. Hemangiomas of the bone are relatively uncommon, expand the cranial vault, and primarily affect the external table, with a picture of vascular channels, often in a spokewheel arrangement. These masses can be highly vascular, supplied most often by external carotid and meningeal branches. Again, these tumors of the osseous vault infrequently affect the intracranial structures. Computed tomog-

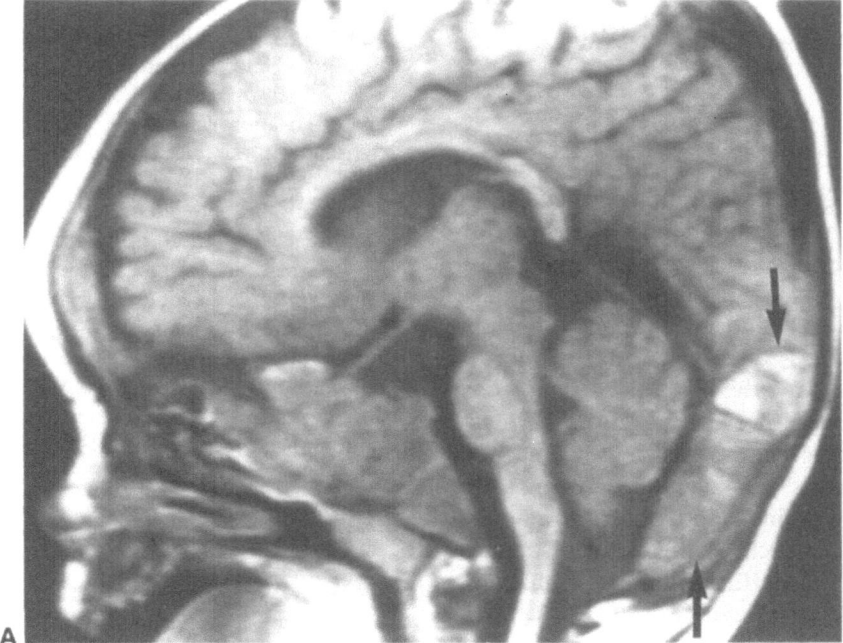

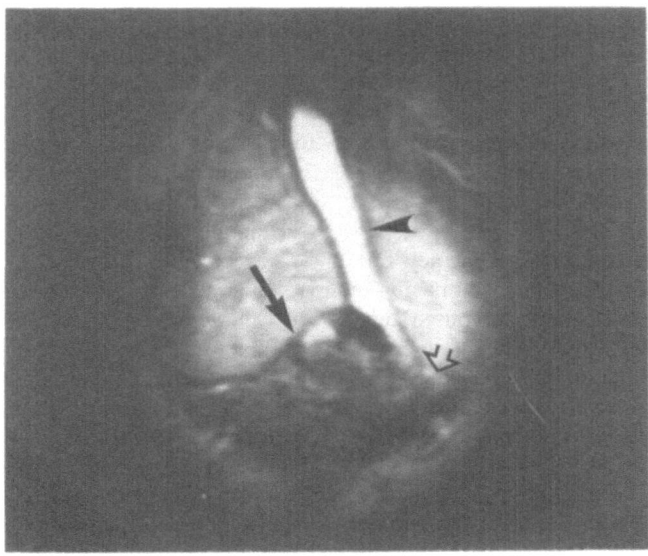

Figure 5.11. Neuroblastoma. A: Sagittal T1-weighted image shows a partially hemorrhagic mass (arrows) behind the torcula along the posterior wall of the posterior fossa. B: Coronal gradient echo image demonstrates high signal intensity flow in the superior sagittal sinus (arrowhead) that comes down to and abuts a hypointense tumor mass (arrow). flow goes off to the left transverse sinus (open arrow) which is compressed. flow into the right transverse sinus is obstructed.

raphy is the best mode of evaluation for the intraosseous lesions of the cranial vault.

Summary

Except for the identification of calcification and the speed of examination, MR is superior to CT in the evaluation of pediatric posterior fossa tumors. Bony destructive processes necessitate both CT and MR when extension beyond the dura is questioned. No method is perfect in predicting the histological characteristics of tumors. However, based on the location and imaging characteristics, an educated imaging diagnosis can be made. As imaging becomes more refined and other parameters are added to it, such as magnetic resonance spectroscopy and perfusion-diffusion imaging, greater specificity will evolve.

References

1. Zimmerman RA, Bilaniuk LT. CT and MR: diagnosis and evolution of head injury, stroke, and brain tumors. *Neuropsychology*. 1989;3: 191–230.
2. Gibby WA, Zimmerman RA. X-ray computed tomography, In: Mazziotta, Gilman, eds. *Contemporary Neurology*. Philadelphia, PA: F.A. Davis; 1991: in press.
3. Zimmerman RA, Bilaniuk LT, Hackney DB. Applications of magnetic resonance imaging in diseases of the pediatric central nervous system. *Magn Reson Imaging*. 1986;4:11–24.
4. Zimmerman RA, Bilaniuk LT, Hackney DB, Goldberg HI, Grossman RI. Head injury: early results of comparing CT and high-field MRI. *AJNR*. 1986;7:757–764.
5. Zimmerman RA, Gusnard DA, Bilaniuk LT. Gadolinium DTPA-enhanced MR evaluation of pediatric brain tumors. In: Bleyer, Packer, Pochedly, eds. *New Trends in Pediatric Neuro-Oncology*. New York: Raven Press; 1990.
6. Atlas SW, Grossman RI, Hackney DB, Gomori JM, Campagna N, Goldberg HI, Bilaniuk LT, Zimmerman RA. Calcified intracranial lesions: detection with gradient echo acquisition rapid MR imaging. *AJNR* 1988;9:253–259.
7. Braffman BH, Grossman RI, Goldberg HI, Stern MB, Hurtig HI, Hackney DB, Bilaniuk LT, Zimmerman RA. MR imaging of Parkinson disease with spin-echo and gradient-echo sequences. *AJNR*. 1988;9:1093–1099.
8. Braffman BH, Zimmerman RA, Rabischong P. Cranial nerves III, IV, VI: a clinical/radiologic/anatomic approach to the evaluation of their dysfunction. *Semin Ultrasound*. 1987;8(3):185–213.
9. Hufnagel TJ, Savino PJ, Zimmerman RA, Sergott RC. Painful ophthalmoplegia caused by neurotropic malignant melanoma. *Can J Ophthalmol*. 1990;25(1):38–41.
10. Courchesne E, Press GA, Murakami J, et al. Cerebellum in sagittal plane—anatomic-MR correlation: 1. The vermis. *AJNR*. 1989;10:659.
11. Zimmerman RA. Pediatric supratentorial tumors. *Semin Roentgenol*. 1990;25(3):225–248.
12. Gusnard DA. Cerebellar neoplasms in children. *Semin Roentgenol*. 1990;25(3):263–278.
13. Smith RR. Brain stem tumors. *Semin Roentgenol*. 1990;25(3):249–262.
14. Gomori JM, Grossman RI, Goldberg HI, Zimmeman RA, Bilaniuk LT. Intracranial hematomas: imaging by high-field MR. *Radiology*. 1985;157:87–93.
15. Gomori JM, Grossman RI, Bilaniuk LT, Zimmerman RA, Goldberg HI. High-field MR imaging of superficial siderosis of the central nervous system. *J Comput Assist Tomogr*. 1985;9(5):972–975.
16. Krischer J, Kun L, Packer R, Zimmerman R, Freeman C, Wara W, Albright L, Allen J, Hoffman H. MR characteristics of brain stem gliomas: correlation with survival statistics in a three-center study. *J Neurosurg*. Submitted.
17. Bilaniuk LT, Zimmerman RA, Littman P, et al. Computed tomography of brain stem gliomas in children. *Neuroradiology*. 1980;134:89–95.
18. Smith RR, Zimmerman RA, Packer RJ, et al. Pediatric brainstem glioma: post-radiation MR follow-up. *Neuroradiology*. 1990;32:265–271.
19. Packer RJ, Allen J, Nielson S, et al. Brainstem glioma: clinical manifestations of meningeal gliomatosis. *Ann Neurol*. 1983;14:177–182.
20. Russell DS, Rubinstein LJ. *Pathology of Tumours of the Nervous System*. Baltimore: Williams & Wilkins; 1989:149–152.
21. Zimmerman RA, Bilaniuk LT, Bruno L, et al. Computed tomography of cerebellar astrocytoma. *AJR*. 1978;130:170–174.
22. Zimmerman RA, Bilaniuk LT, Pahlajani H. Spectrum of medulloblastomas demonstrated by computed tomography. *Radiology*. 1978;126: 137–141.
23. Ramondi A, Tomita T. Medulloblastoma in

childhood: comparative results of partial and total resection. *Childs Brain*. 1979;5:310–328.

24. Heideman RL, Packer RJ, Albright LA, Freemen CR, Rorke LB. Tumors of the central nervous system. In: Pizzo PA, Poplack DG, eds. *Principles and Practice of Pediatric Oncology* (Ch. 24). Philadelphia, PA: J.B. Lippincott; 1989.

25. Kramer ED, Rafto S, Packer RJ, Zimmerman RA. Comparison of myelography with computed tomography follow-up vs. gadolinium magnetic resonance imaging for subarachnoid metastatic disease in children. *Neurology*. 1990; submitted.

26. Swartz JD, Zimmerman RA, Bilaniuk LT. Computed tomography of intracranial ependymomas. *Radiology*. 1982;143:97–102.

27. Zimmerman RA, Bilaniuk LT. Computed tomography of choroid plexus lesions. *CT: J Comput Tomogr*. 1979;3(2):93–103.

28. Zimmerman RA, Bilaniuk LT. Cranial CT of epidermoid and congenital fatty tumors of maldevelopmental origin. *CT: J Comput Tomogr*. 1979;3:40–50.

29. Zimmerman RA. The phakomatoses. In: Ishibashi Y, Hori Y, eds. *Tuberous Sclerosis and Neurofibromatosis: Epidemiology, Pathophysiology, Biology and Management*. Germany: Elsevier Science; 1990.

30. Zimmerman RA, Bilaniuk LT. Computed tomography of primary and secondary craniocerebral neuroblastoma. *Am J Neuroradiol*. 1980;1:431–434.

CHAPTER 6

Ventricular Shunts and Drainage in the Management of Posterior Fossa Tumors

Jens Haase

The symptomatology of posterior fossa tumors in children is based on local tumor growth and subsequent compression or distortion of the brain stem, which often leads to a secondary hydrocephalic state with increased intracranial pressure.[1-6] Among younger patients the hydrocephalus leads to increased head circumference, whereas among older children late development of papilledema will be the result.[2]

In the beginning of the neurosurgical era, children came for posterior fossa tumor operations in an absolutely devastated state.[1,3,7-10] Severe papilledema, blindness, and low body weight and electrolyte disturbances due to long-term vomiting, resulting from increased intracranial pressure, represented the usual clinical situation.[1,9] Thus, morbidity and mortality following operations were extremely high and Cushing[1] stated: "It is the hydrocephalus that is responsible for the most serious symptoms of all from a standpoint of useful life after a successful operation: namely blindness"—the result of long-lasting papilledema.

With the development of ventriculography and pneumoencephalography, the diagnosis of posterior fossa tumors changed from a purely clinical one with a late diagnosis to a much earlier one.[7] The grade of hydrocephalus was clearly shown, and when performing ventriculography intracranial pressure was monitored and thereafter often relieved by removal of cerebrospinal fluid (CSF).[4,7] Surgeons in earlier days used an occipital burr hole for the ventriculography.[7] This was later used for peroperative puncture of the lateral posterior horn before opening of the dura, whereby the hydrocephalic state was treated with sub-sequent decrease of the intracranial pressure.[7,8,11] Exploration of the posterior fossa could thus be carried out in a much easier way.[7]

In earlier days the severely edematous posterior fossa contents under high pressure, with the added pressure from brain spatulas and the "blinded" explorations of the fossa, had resulted in the majority of the disastrous results.[7,8] Incomplete removal of tumors was common and led to obstructive postoperative swelling and subsequent deterioration of the clinical state.[8] These observations led to Torkildsen's[12] use of a shunting procedure in cases of centrally located tumors. He placed a tube from the posterior horn to the cisterna magna to treat the hydrocephalus; however, the success rate of the Torkildsen shunt was not high. With the development of the ventriculoatrial shunt system preoperative shunting first became a reliable operative procedure.[8,13-15] In the years prior to that, extraventricular drainage through a frontal burr hole had been used before permanent operations, with excellent results.[11,12,16,17]

In the 1990s, when we discuss whether to shunt or not it must be based on the actual diagnostic situation. The diagnosis of posterior fossa tumors is no longer based on ventriculography[2,15] but on computed tomography (CT) and/or magnetic resonance imaging (MRI) scanning.[5,6] Today we have a precise anatomical location of the tumor and an exact evaluation of the degree of hydrocephalus, and thus we can more precisely design the needed operative procedure.[5,6] The tumors can be approached through small craniectomies or craniotomies and with the adjuvant modern equipment such as ultrasound aspiration, laser manipulation, and microsurgical techniques the majority of tumors can be completely removed without any major exploration in the posterior fossa.[4,7] The CT and MRI scans have also led to a much earlier diagnosis and the severe cases with papilledema and blindness are virtually not seen today.

The following sections discuss issues relevant to the treatment of hydrocephalus.

Clinical Status of the Patient

Among children with clinical signs of prolonged, increased intracranial pressure and severe papilledema, a gradual release of intracranial pressure is still to be advocated. We know that we can achieve a normalization of cerebral blood flow, a decrease of cerebral venous outflow, and a normalization of an anatomically distorted brain stem. This results in the relief of vomiting and with further IV feeding restoration of electrolyte disturbances can be achieved. The added risks of a major operation and general anesthesia are thus lowered. However, once again it must be emphasized that this clinical situation is very uncommon today.

Tumor Location

Tumors of the midline, in the vermis and in the fourth ventricle, and major cystic cerebellar tumors are easily removed through small craniotomies. Major solid tumors with severe distortion of the brain stem may lead to problems if the dura is opened and the intracranial pressure at the same time is still severely increased. In these cases pre- or perioperative control of the intracranial pressure seems necessary.

Type of Operative Procedure Used for Direct Tumor Approach

The induction of general anesthesia will always lead to an increase of the intracranial pressure.[18] This will be of specific importance

among patients with an imbalanced pressure/volume curve.[9] It has been reported that bleeding within tumors and cases of downward or upward herniations of the contents of the posterior fossa may result from this imbalance.[3,19] With the opening of the dura a sudden release of intracranial pressure may lead to both bleeding and herniation, with the patients in the prone or sitting positions.[7,18] Protrusion of the cerebellar tissue, however, will be more pronounced with the patient in the sitting position, whereas the decrease of intracranial venous pressure in the sitting position reduces the risk of sudden intracranial pressure decrease.[18] The importance of a specific pediatric neuroanesthesia must be emphasized.

Tumor Type

Some tumors always seed as part of their natural history, such as medulloblastomas and ependymomas.[20,21] Gjerris et al.[21] found, with ultracentrifugation of ventricular CSF, tumor cells in 9 out of 12 children with medulloblastomas. Generalized spread of medulloblastomas has been reported outside the central nervous system (CNS), in cases both with and without preoperative shunting.[22]

Spread is never seen with astrocytomas. Although it has never been proven what the real risk of extracerebral spread is with and without shunting, the postoperative treatment, radiation and/or chemotherapy, and the tumor type must be carefully determined before deciding whether or not to shunt.

Type of Shunting Procedure for the Treatment of Secondary Hydrocephalus

We use either extraventricular temporary drainage or a permanent shunt system.

Extraventricular Drainage

Through a frontal burr hole a ventricular catheter is inserted in the lateral ventricle and immediate drainage of CSF with resulting lowering of the intracranial pressure can be achieved. The ventricular catheter is connected through tubing to a glass bottle and the height of the fluid in the bottle indicates the intracranial pressure. The bottle is placed at bedside and elevated to a pressure difference of around 25 cm of water, and following that slowly reduced to about 10 cm of water within the first day or two. The method is extremely reliable; it makes rapid changes and adjustment of the intracranial pressure possible, but it also harbors some hazards such as infection, disconnection, and problems of nursing.

Perioperative use of shunting procedure with the patient in a sitting position may lead to subdural and epidural bleeding and may thus be dangerous in cases with severe hydrocephalus.

Permanent Shunt System

An ordinary ventriculoatrial shunt was the first type to be used in these cases. However today the majority of authors prefer ventriculoperitoneal shunting for the treatment of hydrocephalus, whether it is based on tumors or not. The morbidity of shunting is not negligible as it includes infections, disconnections, obstructions, subdural effusions, and epidural hematomas.[4,23] Besides that, there is no safe way of testing the shunt system when in place to assure having control of changes of intracranial pressure unless an epidural pressure monitor is added.[24]

Discussion

True "Incidence" of Hydrocephalus Related to Posterior Fossa Tumors

The true incidence of hydrocephalus in connection with posterior fossa tumors is not well defined,[2,5,6] as the majority of figures in the literature are not incidence figures but prevalence figures. (Incidence is the number of events occurring in a stable, well-defined population within a certain time period, e.g., 1 year. Prevalence is the number of events occurring in a certain time period.) The prevalence seems to be from 40% to 90% except for tumors of the brain stem.[4,10,14] A time incidence study can be found in Denmark through the work by Gjerris.[25] In an earlier series Raimondi and Tomita[4] found among 117 children, 110 with cerebellar and fourth ventricle tumors and hydrocephalus. In the Danish tumor series, shunting preoperatively was done in 4%.[26]

True "Incidence" of Hydrocephalus Postoperatively

This is a very important issue, as there is no need to use a shunt postoperatively if the child does not develop hydrocephalus. In Papo et al.'s[16] series, postoperative shunting was necessary in 25% of the survivors. In this series it was also shown that 40.7% of the children under 10 years of age needed a permanent shunt compared with only 10.7% of children who were 10 years or older. Cabanes et al.[27] stated that despite the knowledge of the development of postoperative hydrocephalus, little concerning this complication had been reported in the literature. They found that local arachnoidal adhesions or surgical bleeding may be part of the mechanism involved in the pathogenesis. A kind of aseptic meningitis was found by Carmel et al.[28] in 70% of their cases following operations without preoperative shunting. Other authors have found figures as low as 14%.[17,29–31] Thus, the exact figures are not known today.

If we therefore follow the procedure of preoperative shunting of all children with posterior fossa tumors, as suggested by the Toronto group,[32] we must accept that in many of these cases the procedure is not necessary and that the complication rate related to the shunting procedure will add morbidity to the results. It is worthwhile looking into Shalit et al.'s[33] study in which only 13.5% of the patients needed a definite shunt. Shunting is by no way an innocuous procedure.[23,33]

Complications of Shunting

Ventriculoatrial and ventriculoperitoneal shunting carries a long list of complications including infection, disconnection, obstruction, subdural effusion, epidural hematomas, and bowel perforations.[23] The use of preoperative shunting, as mentioned earlier, has also been criticized due to the possibility of seeding tumor cells.[20] Hoffman and coworkers[20] demonstrated metastatic spread beyond the CNS through ventricular peritoneal shunts in patients with medulloblastomas and advocated the use of a Millipore filter incorporated in the shunt to prevent this. However, their reported results have never been confirmed by other authors.[4,6]

Albright and Reigel[10] found in a retrospective study that children with CSF shunts before tumor removal had significantly better postoperative conditions than children without shunts. The operative mortality of children without treatment of their hydrocephalus before tumor surgery was 12.8% compared with 3.7% among children with preexistent shunts. Their conclusion that all children should be shunted is not based on a control study; however, their conclusion led to the general advocation of preoperative shunting.

Epstein and Murali[19] warned of the hazards of shunting by calling attention to upward herniation of the posterior fossa contents and hemorrhage occurring within tumors after shunting. They concluded that a 10% incidence (prevalance) of upward herniation with pre-shunting was found, a result that has never been confirmed by later authors.[4,34] O'Brien[34] found in his series of 53 consecutive pre-shunted posterior fossa tumors among children no cases of upward herniation, and Raimondi and Tomita[4] found only 3%.

Vaquero et al.[35] discussed the intratumoral hemorrhage and suggested that it was based on a too rapid change between the pressures of the supra- and infratentorial compartments. O'Brien[34] again emphasized that spontaneous intratumoral hemorrhage without any kind of treatment can also be found. Further, O'Brien discussed the problems of intracranial pressure changing during induction of anesthesia, an imbalance problem that was pointed out by Gulliksen and Haase[36] when encountering epidural hematomas following ventriculoperitoneal shunt revisions. To reduce the chance of a sudden imbalance, a changeable shunt system was introduced whereby slow re-duction of intracranial pressure could possibly be achieved by changing the pressure/flow characteristics of the shunt (Sophy). No scientific proof of the benefit of the system has been given in the literature. In major textbooks, McLone[5] and Schut et al.[6] both criticize the use of perioperative permanent shunt systems.

Complications of Extraventricular Drainage

In Shalit et al.'s[33] series, the frequency of infection was 8.1% with extraventricular drainage of a mean of 9 days. When keeping the extraventricular drainage for periods no longer than 4 or 5 days, the true frequency of infection is very low. If a proper operative technique is used as in Sundbärg et al.'s[37] series, the infection rate even with prolonged drainage can be kept under 4%.[16,37,38] Problems such as disconnection, height of bottle, and other nursing problems are all anecdotal and there is no scientific series demonstrating exact frequency of these complications.

Conclusion

Today, preoperative control of increased intracranial pressure is not documented as being necessary to any large degree. Eventual shunting must be related to specific conditions where lowering of the increased intracranial pressure is necessary for rehydration, and for technical reasons when carrying out the posterior fossa explorations. This seems to be the only case among children under the age of 5 years or among those harboring major solid tumors. In cases where a control of increased intracranial pressure must be achieved for a short period, extraventricular drainage can be used without major risk. Modern CT and MRI scanning facilitate both early operations and controlling the development of eventual postoperative intracranial hydrocephalus. In many intensive care units routine epidural pressure monitoring is also used in the postoperative phase of all tumor cases, where it can be documented whether a postoperative shunt is needed or not.

References

1. Cushing H. Experiences with the cerebellar medulloblastomas. *Acta Pathol Microbiol Scand.* 1930;7:1–86.
2. Matson DD. *Neurosurgery of Infancy and Childhood.* 2nd ed. Springfield, IL: Charles C. Thomas; 1969.
3. Raimondi AJ, Yashon D, Matsumoto S, et al. Increased intracranial pressure without lateralizing sings: the midline syndrome. *Neurochirurgia.* 1967;10:197–209.
4. Raimondi AJ, Tomita T. Hydrocephalus and infratentorial tumors. Incidence, clinical picture, and treatment. *J Neurosurg.* 1981;55:174–182.
5. McLone DG. Cerebellar astrocytomas. In: Wilkins RH, Rengachary SS, eds. *Neurosurgery.* New York: McGraw-Hill; 1985;1:754–757.
6. Schut L, Bruce DA, Sutton LN. Medulloblastomas. In: Wilkins RH, Rengachary SS, eds. *Neurosurgery.* New York: McGraw-Hill; 1985;1:758–762.
7. Bucy PC. Exposure of the posterior cerebellar fossa. *J Neurosurg.* 1966;24:820–832.
8. Hekmatpanah J, Mullan S. Ventriculo-caval shunt in the management of posterior fossa tumors. *J Neurosurg.* 1967;26:609–613.
9. Plum F, Posner JB. *The Diagnosis of Stupor and Coma.* 2nd ed. Contemporary Neurology Series, Vol. 10. Philadelphia: FA Davis; 1972.
10. Albright L, Reigel DH. Management of hydrocephalus secondary to posterior fossa tumors. *J Neurosurg.* 1977;46:52–55.
11. Poppen JL. Ventricular drainage as a valuable procedure in neurosurgery. Report of a satisfactory method. *Arch Neurol Psychiatry.* 1943;50:587–589.
12. Torkildsen A. Should extirpation be attempted in cases of neoplasm in or near the third ventricle of the brain? Experiences with a palliative method. *J Neurosurg.* 1948;5:249–275.
13. Elkins CW, Fonseca JE. Ventriculovenous anastomosis in obstructive and acquired communicating hydrocephalus. *J Neurosurg.* 1962;18:139–144.
14. Abraham J, Chandy J. Ventriculo-atrial shunt in the management of posterior fossa tumors. Preliminary report. *J Neurosurg.* 1963;20:252–253.
15. Jane JA, Kaufman B, Nulsen F, et al. The role of angiography and ventriculovenous shunting in the treatment of posterior fossa tumors. *Acta Neurochir (Wien).* 1973;28:13–27.
16. Papo I, Caruselli G, Luongo A. External ventricular drainage in the management of posterior fossa tumors in children and adolescents. *Neurosurgery.* 1982;10:13–15.
17. Rappaport ZH, Shalit MN. Perioperative external ventricular drainage in obstructive hydrocephalus, secondary to infratentorial brain tumours. *Acta Neurochir (Wien).* 1989;86:118–121.
18. Newfield P, Cottrell JE. *Handbook of Neuroanesthesia: Clinical and Physiologic Essential.* 3rd ed. Boston/Toronto: Little, Brown; 1989.
19. Epstein F. Murali R. Pediatric posterior fossa tumors: Hazards of the "preoperative" shunt. *Neurosurgery.* 1978;3:348–350.
20. Hoffman HJ, Hendrick EB, Humphreys RP. Metastasis via ventriculo-peritoneal shunt in patients with medulloblastoma. *J Neurosurg.* 1976;44:562–566.
21. Gjerris F, Klinken L, Haase J, Bang F. Tumour cells in the ventricular cerebrospinal fluid in children with medulloblastoma. International Society for Paediatric Neurosurgery, Scientific Meeting, Philadelphia, 1982.
22. Simesen K, Haase J, et al. Knoglemetastaser fra cerebellart medulloblastom (with English summary). *Ugeskr Laeger.* 1984;146:1129–1140.
23. Haase J, Bang F, Tange M. Danish experience with the one-piece-shunt. *Childs Nerv Syst.* 1987;3:93–96.
24. Chapman PH, Cosman E, Arnold M. Telemetric ICP monitoring after surgery for posterior fossa and third ventricular tumors. *J Neurosurg.* 1984;60:649–651.
25. Gjerris F. *Intracranial Tumors in Childhood—Incidence and Long-Term Prognosis.* Thesis Lægeforeningens Forlag, Copenhagen 1979.
26. Gjerris F. Clinical aspects and long-term prognosis of infratentorial intracranial tumours in infancy and childhood. *Acta Neurol Scand.* 1978;57:31–52.
27. Cabanes J, Vazquez R, Rivas A. Hydrocephalus after posterior fossa operations. *Surg Neurol.* 1978;9:42–46.
28. Carmel PW, Frazer RAR, Stein BM. A septic meningitis following posterior fossa surgery in children. *J Neurosurg.* 1974;41:44–48.
29. Scatliff JH, Kummer AJ, Frankel SA, et al. Cystic enlargement and obstruction of the fourth ventricle following posterior fossa surgery. The postoperative Dandy-Walker syndrome. *Am J Roentgenol.* 1962;88:536–542.
30. Stein BM, Tenner MS, Fraser RAR. Hydrocephalus following removal of cerebellar

astrocytomas in children. *J Neurosurg.* 1972; 36:763–768.

31. Gross P, Goat M, Knoblic OE. Disorders of CSF circulation after interventions in the area of the posterior cranial fossa with prior shunt operation. *Adv Neurosurg.* 1978;5:199–202.

32. Park TS, Hoffman HJ, Hendrick EB, et al. Medulloblastoma: clinical presentation and management. Experience at the Hospital for Sick Children, Toronto 1950–1980. *J Neurosurg.* 1983;58:543–552.

33. Shalit MN, Ben Ari Y, Eynan N. The management of obstructive hydrocephalus by the use of external continuous ventricular drainage. *Acta Neurochir (Wien).* 1979;47:161–172.

34. O'Brien MS. Comment. *Neurosurgery.* 1978;3:350.

35. Vaquero J, Cabezudo JM, De Sola RG, Nombela L. Intratumoral hemorrhage in posterior fossa tumors after ventricular drainage. *J Neurosurg.* 1981;54:406–408.

36. Gulliksen G, Haase J. Epidural haematoma following a shunt revision. *Acta Neurochir (Wien).* 1977;36:107–109.

37. Sundbärg G, Kjällquist Å, Lundberg N, et al. Complications due to prolonged ventricular fluid pressure recalling in clinical practise. In: Dietzh BM, ed. *Intracranial Pressure.* New York/Heidelberg/Berlin: Springer-Verlag; 1972: 348–352.

38. Smith RW, Alksne JF. Infections complicated in use of external ventriculostomi. *J Neurosurg.* 1976;44:567–570.

CHAPTER 7

What a Neurosurgeon Should Know About Anesthesia for Posterior Fossa Tumors

H. von Gösseln and D. Suhr

In neurosurgery, microsurgical techniques have led to a distinct improvement of the prognosis for intracranial, infratentorial operations. It can therefore be expected that the anesthetist will use all existing possibilities to provide the neurosurgeon with optimal conditions for operating on the patient.

Special problems can arise for the anesthetist due to the neurological disease itself, the effects of anesthesia on brain functions, and special demands on the neurosurgeon relative to the patient's position. Whereas the most favorable operative approaches for the extirpation of tumors in the posterior fossa have been clearly defined in the past, there are different opinions regarding the most desirable position for the patient during these neurosurgical procedures. Namely, the discussions involve some variation of the prone and modified lounging positions. Since the decision for or against a given position is predominantly dependent on the risks involved, the two most frequently encountered complications of the lounging position, venous air embolism and arterial hypotension, will be discussed with reference to new publications. This seems to be especially interesting since studies by Black et al.[1] have suggested a relationship between the postoperative neurological outcome and the different positions of patients during surgery.

In regard to the introduction of new hypnotic drugs and methods (total intravenous anesthesia) one also must evaluate whether these substances in neuroanesthesia are additive or alternative.[2,3] Apart from this discussion about different substances and anesthesiological methods, the following points are set as goals for good neuroanesthesia[4]: The cerebral blood flow and energy supply must always meet the energy and oxygen needs of the brain. Anesthesiological procedures should not influence autoregulation, which might be impaired locally by a tumor or the operation itself. Stable hemodynamics without hypertonic or hypotonic phases should prevent brain edema or ischemia. The physiological reactivity of the brain vessels to changes of arterial carbon dioxide concentrations should be maintained. The applied anesthetics must not lower the threshold for cerebral convulsions. Slowed awakening and a deterioration in the patient's consciousness postoperatively are clinical signs of complications, e.g., postoperative hemorrhage. In order to evaluate the neurological status of a patient early after the operation, anesthetics should be used that are easy to control in their actions.

One must always be aware that anesthetics affect reversibly, and in different ways, the functions of the central nervous system. The influence on cerebral blood flow, brain metabolism, and intracranial pressure play an important role in neuroanesthesia in improving the intra- and postoperative neurological outcome. Herein, we discuss briefly some basic principles that may assist judgment regarding the differences of anesthesiological procedures.

Basic Principles

Because of the anatomy of the skull, the intracranial pressure (ICP) is an expression of the volume of the brain, the cerebrospinal fluid

(CSF), and the blood in the cerebral vasculature. Causes for an elevation of the ICP include tumors, infections, edema, trauma, and hemorrhage. Apart from these primary factors, the ICP is influenced by anesthesiological procedures, e.g., intubation. All anesthesiological methods must be designed to keep the ICP normal and to bring about a decrease in the event of elevation.

If one of the intracranial components (brain, blood, CSF) increases in volume, the ICP is bound to be elevated unless one of the other components decreases in volume simultaneously. These methods of compensation are known to be insufficient in the presence of acute space-occupying lesions, which means that an increase in volume rapidly leads to an elevation of the ICP. After the critical threshold has been reached, the compliance of the system (brain and fluid-filled compartments) is reduced. An additional disturbance of the venous return, or the application of drugs that may increase the cerebral blood flow (CBF) by vasodilatation, leads to grave consequences. As a result, local and general cerebral ischemia, which are especially dangerous with regard to vital brain stem functions, may develop.

If the ICP is elevated, anesthetics with vasoconstrictive effects are to be favored over those causing cerebrovascular dilatation.[5] Of course, apart from this the application of other measures (osmotherapy, drainage of CSF, vasoconstriction by hyperventilation, corticoids, diuretics, barbiturates) to reduce the ICP must be considered on an individual case basis.

A protection for the brain against ischemia during anesthesia can be achieved over two pathways, sufficient CBF and/or reduction of cell metabolism that leads to a reduced oxygen need. Since increases in blood glucose concentration following brain cell ischemia leads to a less successful neurological outcome, the use of glucose-containing infusions should be strictly limited, only given after special indications.[6]

The supply of the brain cells with oxygen requires adequate CBF and cerebral perfusion pressure (CPP), corresponding to the difference between mean arterial pressure (MAP) and the ICP. The CBF is not changed if the MAP is not less than 50 mm Hg and not more than 150 mm Hg, since the arterioles in the brain can alter their diameters—the phenomenon of autoregulation. Within this range of blood pressure values the CBF of adults is 45 to 55 ml/min/100 g brain tissue, corresponding to 15% of the cardiac minute volume. In contrast to the white matter (20 ml/min/100 g), the gray matter of the brain receives much more blood—75 to 80 ml/min/100 g.[7] Typical signs of ischemia can be found in the electroencephalogram (EEG) as soon as the general CBF is reduced to less than 22 ml/min/100 g.[7]

When outside the range of 50 to 150 mm Hg, the brain perfusion in normotensive patients follows the cerebral perfusion pressure passively. It needs to be mentioned that for patients with arterial hypertension, autoregulation occurs within other ranges so that these patients require a higher MAP in order to have an adequate CBF than normotensive patients.[8] Whether a low MAP may cause ischemia depends on its cause (hypovolemia with consecutive vasoconstriction, drug-induced hypotension).

As Ernst et al.[9] has shown in animal experiments, there is a potential risk in the sitting position for a decrease in CBF during elevated ICP. Opinions differ about the CBF at normal ICP. There was no reduction of CBF in animals, whereas patients reacted with a decreased blood flow in the sitting position.[9,10] These findings do not correspond to those of another study in which the CBF and the MAP of 15 anesthetized patients in the sitting position increased.[11]

The ability of brain vessels to autoregulate may be inhibited by either perifocal or general brain edema, decreased arterial oxygen concentration, hypercapnia, brain trauma, or inhalational anesthetics [halothane, enflurane >1 MAC (minimal alveolar concentration)]. In this situation the CBF is solely determined by the CPP, and hyperemia and ischemia are possible.[5]

The carbon dioxide concentration of the arterial blood (pCO_2) is generally considered to be the most important factor influencing the CBF. The CBF value changes per mm Hg by about 1 to 2 ml/min/100 g.[8] A decrease in CBF (about 50%) can be achieved by hyperventilation with hypocapnia (pCO_2 20 mm Hg), an increase (about two fold) by hypoventilation with hypercapnia (pCO_2 70 to 80 mm Hg).[8]

These reactions are of great clinical importance. They occur within a few minutes as a result of localized changes of the pH value, which controls the tone of the vascular smooth muscle.[5] Vasodilatation during hypoxia (CBF elevated at pO_2 <60 mm Hg) and vasoconstriction with a decrease in blood flow (10%) after application of 100% oxygen are also assumed to be initiated by changes in the local hydrogen ion concentration.[5] The blood flow in the brain is influenced by the rate of metabolism of its cells, i.e., their oxygen need. Cerebral convulsions increase the CBF, whereas the global CBF is reduced to less than 40 ml/min/100 g during coma.[5]

Nerve cells need a continuous supply of oxygen and glucose and the general metabolic activity is measured as the cerebral metabolic rate for oxygen ($CMRO_2$). This oxygen need equals 3 to 3.5 ml/min/100 g in conditions of rest, i.e., 20% of the total requirement.[7] Glucose is the main substrate for the production of energy in brain cells. They are therefore dependent on a continuous supply of 5 mg/min/100 g.[8] More than 90% of the glucose is aerobic metabolized and only a low percentage anaerobic to lactate. Under anaerobic conditions, these cells cannot meet their energy demand. They react to a shortage of oxygen or glucose very rapidly with an impairment of their function, i.e., deterioration in the patient's consciousness, even as far as coma.

Drugs in Use for Anesthesia

Now that we have reviewed the basic principles that are generally to be kept in mind during anesthesia for intracranial operations, we can describe the drugs used for induction and/or maintenance of narcosis. Of main interest are the effects on CBF, $CMRO_2$, and the ICP.

Intravenous Hypnotics

Barbiturates

Methohexital and thiopental have been successfully used for years in neuroanesthesia for the induction, and less frequently for the maintenance, of narcosis. Among the desired effects are predominantly dose-dependent decreases of ICP, CBF, and $CMRO_2$. High doses that lead to an isoelectric EEG reduce the CBF by about 50%.[8] Autoregulation and the physiological reactability to changes of the arterial carbon dioxide concentration (pCO_2) are, however, maintained. The main disadvantage, especially after repeated applications, is the slow awakening of the patient.[12] In comparison to thiopental, methohexital has advantages because of a shorter duration of action and fewer effects on cardiovascular parameters. The commonly used dosage for the initiation of a narcosis only causes a shallow anesthesia, so that an intubation without combination with other drugs often leads to an elevation in blood pressure and tachycardia.

Etomidate

The effect of this short-acting hypnotic on ICP, CBF, and $CMRO_2$ is qualitatively that of barbiturates but quantitatively less pronounced.[2] The reaction of arterioles to pCO_2 changes is not influenced.[13] The effect on the autoregulation has not yet been studied.[2] Alterations of the heart rate, myocardial contractility, stroke volume index, blood pressure, and peripheral resistance are less significant than after the injection of barbiturates. In contrast to barbiturates, etomidate does not influence the oxygen consumption of the myocardium (barbiturates +50%) and increases the coronary blood flow by reduction of the vessel's resistance only about 20% (barbiturates +50%). There have been no reports of postoperative convulsions caused by etomidate.[2] However, because of the unfavorable effect on cortisone synthesis, this substance is only appropriate to induce an anesthesia, not to maintain it.[12,14]

Ketamine

This substance, the only intravenous hypnotic drug, causes anesthesia and analgesia (dissociative anesthesia). Ketamine stimulates the $CMRO_2$ and CBF, also causing vasodilatation of the brain vessels.[7] The result of this effect is an elevation of the ICP independently from the initial value.[15,16] The cerebral autoregulation and the vascular reaction to changes in pCO_2 are not influenced.[16]

Ketamine presumably stimulates the cardiovascular system via central activation of the sympathetic nervous system, thereby causing tachycardia, hypertonia, and elevation of both the cardiac output and myocardial oxygen consumption.[8] Ketamine is thought to be an unsuitable agent for neurosurgical procedures.[5]

Propofol

This new hypnotic drug reduces, dose-dependently, the ICP, so that it may be considered as an alternative to barbiturates and etomidate.[17,18] With higher dosages, typical EEG waves (burst suppression) similar to those with barbiturates indicate a deep state of anesthesia.[5] The neurological outcome after incomplete ischemia has proven better in animal experiments with propofol in comparison to N_2O-fentanyl.[19] According to studies by Stephan et al.[20] and Vandesteene et al.,[21] propofol reduces the CBF, $CMRO_2$ and glucose metabolism under normocapnia or hypocapnia. The reactivity of the arterioles to pCO_2 is not influenced. After a bolus application plus an infusion, a reduction of the CBF of 51% and $CMRO_2$ of 36% has been measured.[20] Ravussin et al.[22] found a reduction of the CPP of 10%, and lumbar cerebrospinal fluid pressure (CSFP) of 32%, after bolus injection. Dosages that produce an isoelectric EEG in animals reduce the CBF without restricting autoregulation. This reduction of the CBF involves the cortex and supratentorial region, but not the mesencephalon or spinal cord.[23]

Patients often react with arterial hypotension and changes in heart rate to bolus injections of propofol.[24] These reactions are thought to be caused by a reduction of the peripheral resistance and the cardiac index. Although propofol has no influence on the sensitivity of the baroreceptors, it still causes the reflex counterregulation (tachycardia) to be only moderate in spite of low blood pressure.[25] The reactions of the circulatory system to intubation stimulus are less severe when using propofol than barbiturates or etomidate.[26] In order to reduce the described decrease of the MAP, lower dosages than originally recommended should be used for the induction of anesthesia. For the maintenance of the narcosis, continuous application is recommended.[27,28] Because of its rapid metabolism, the patient awakes within a short period of time even after long operations.[26]

Benzodiazepines

These substances affect the ICP, $CMRO_2$, and CBF in a way similar to barbiturates.[2] A dose of 0.15 mg/kg body weight reduces the ICP 30% to 34%.[29,30] The reactions of the vessels to different carbon dioxide concentrations is not suppressed.[31] If a respiratory depression with hypercapnia is avoided, midazolam is useful as an intravenous hypnotic for patients with an elevated ICP. When comparing the cerebral effects with those of barbiturates and narcotics, midazolam takes an intermediate position.[2] Benzodiazepines have only a slight effect on the cardiovascular system, e.g., blood pressure, heart rate, myocardial contractility, myocardial oxygen consumption, and coronary blood flow.[8] Because of its short duration of action (1.5 to 2.5 hr), the use of midazolam is, in comparison to other benzodiazepines, favorable in anesthesia.

Opioids

Despite contradictory statements, we may assume that opioids (fentanyl, alfentanil, sufentanil) cause a reduction of the $CMRO_2$, CBF, and ICP.[32-35] The extent of these changes are dependent on the interaction with other anesthetics used in narcosis. Fentanyl showed no effect on autoregulation and pCO_2 reactivity of brain vessels in animal experiments.[36] Since data on alfentanil, in the past, resulted only from animal studies, and corresponded to those of fentanyl, this opioid seems unlikely to affect CBF, $CMRO_2$, pCO_2 reactivity of the vessels, and autoregulation.[2,7,37] Recent studies support the hypothesis that sufentanil does not influence the CBF, pCO_2 reaction, and autoregulation.[38,39] Clinical observations have led to the decision to use opioids for neuroanesthesia if hypocapnia is secured by controlled ventilation.[7,40,41]

Inhalational Anesthetics

Halothane, enflurane, and isoflurane cause cerebral vasodilatation, possibly an elevation of the intracranial pressure, and decreased cerebral metabolism. All the effects of volatile anesthetics are dose-dependent. Since these three substances influence cardiovascular function and cerebral autoregulation, appropriate conditions have to be considered for comparisons, i.e., a constant MAP and equipotential concentrations in the gas mixture (MAC values). Under these conditions the CBF was increased 18% by isoflurane, 37% by enflurane, and 191% by halothane.[42,43]

The reduction of the $CMRO_2$ in equivalent gas concentrations is more pronounced under enflurane and isoflurane in comparison to halothane.[43,44] Whether or not an elevation of the ICP after the application of isoflurane can be reliably suppressed cannot be predicted. Because of his observations, Grosslight et al.[45] suggest refraining from the use of isoflurane when the ICP is elevated. This contradicts the studies of Murphy et al.,[42] which show no effect on the MAC values by isoflurane in the range of 0.6 to 1.1, but only when the MAC value exceeds 1.6. These results correspond to studies showing an elevation of the ICP in hypocapnic patients if the inspiratory concentration of isoflurane was 2.0%.[46]

Today, opinions vary greatly regarding the use of isoflurane during intracranial hypertension.[7,8,47] Changes of CBF, $CMRO_2$, and ICP while using halothane are reduced in combination with barbiturates or benzodiazepines and hypocapnia. Still, one should evaluate individually the indications for halothane or enflurane in neuroanesthesia. The reaction of the brain vessels to changes in pCO_2 is not influenced by halothane, enflurane, and isoflurane.[48,49] In contrast to this, all three substances show a dose-dependent effect on the autoregulation.[42,44] Depending on its inspiratory concentration, nitrous oxide (N_2O) elevates the $CMRO_2$ and CBF.[50–52] The increase

of the CBF presumably is not only due to vasodilatation, but also to the variations in metabolism in different regions of the brain. This results in an increase in blood flow in the frontal cortical brain areas, with a simultaneous decrease in blood flow in the occipital cortical regions. The N_2O-dependent elevation of the intracranial pressure can be suppressed by barbiturates, benzodiazepines, or hyperventilation.[53–55] Nitrous oxide reduces the brain protecting effect of barbiturates or benzodiazepines on the cerebral metabolism, which can be measured by oxygen and glucose consumption.[54,56] Baughman et al.[57] showed, in their experimental studies, that the secondary neurological defects under ischemic conditions were more severe when N_2O was used during anesthesia.

Muscle Relaxants

The nondepolarizing muscle relaxants vecuronium, atracurium, and pancuronium have no disadvantageous effects on the ICP, independent of the initial value.[58] The use of pancuronium needs to be limited if the MAP increases because of a vagolytic effect.[7] Because of its rapid onset and excellent muscle relaxation, succinylcholine is commonly used as a depolarizing substance for intubation. Even though it may sometimes cause an elevation of the ICP, for unknown reasons, the observations of Minton et al.[59] have shown that this undesired reaction can be prevented by a preceding injection of vecuronium. With appropriate precautions like precurarization, hyperventilation, sufficient depth of anesthesia, and blood pressure monitoring, it may safely be used for intubation.[7]

Preoperative Evaluation

During the preoperative visit the anesthetist should familiarize himself with the symptoms of the neurological disease as well as those of any other existing important illness. Of special interest are signs of elevated ICP, lesions of cranial nerves with dysphagia, dehydration with altered electrolytes, and cardiopulmonary impairment. If the operation is elective, these symptoms should be treated accordingly. Any possible interaction of drugs taken regularly by the patient (e.g., antihypertensive agents, beta-blockers) with anesthetics should be considered carefully. The selection of drugs for premedication is best done for each patient individually in order to initiate a "stress-free" anesthesia. For the treatment of fearful patients, benzodiazepines have been especially successful. Because of the possible respiratory depression, opiates are not indicated when the ICP is elevated.

Induction of Anesthesia

The induction of anesthesia for intracranial operations should not allow changes of blood pressure and/or elevation of the intracranial pressure (e.g., coughing during the intubation). For adults, a combination of intravenous hypnotics and opioids has proven especially appropriate, whereas the use of an inhalation mask (volatile anesthetics with a N_2O/O_2 mixture) is preferred for small children. Aside from the actual intracranial pressure, correct ventilation should be closely monitored, for any mistakes here will lead to serious consequences. Therefore, it is essential to compensate the unavoidable respiratory depression after the use of hypnotics with manual ventilation in order to guarantee normocapnia. Intubation should be followed, in general, by controlled hyperventilation, to induce hypocapnia. Some side effects need to be noted: a high mean airway pressure can hinder the venous return from the brain, elevate the ICP, and reduce the cardiac minute volume. The same effect is produced by ventilation with positive end-expiratory pressure (PEEP) without elevating the head and the upper part of the body. On the other hand, extreme hyperventilation should be prevented because hemoglobin gives off less oxygen to tissues during the state of respiratory alkalosis. Laryngoscopy and intubation should be performed with equally great caution, for they can lead to an elevation of blood pressure and, with insufficient relaxation, to coughing and defense ac-

tions. The ICP can also be elevated if autoregulation of the cranial vessels is disturbed.

Several possibilities exist to reduce these undesired effects during intubation: application of an opioid, prior to the use of hypnotic drugs; use of a higher dose of thiopental, to deepen the anesthesia; or, use of a volatile anesthetic. The intravenous injection of a local anesthetic (lidocaine) or a short-acting beta-blocker (esmelol) may be considered an alternative in reducing the reactions to the stimulus of intubation.[60,61]

The secure fixation of the endotracheal tube after verification of its position is very important, because any dislocation before or during the operation can have serious consequences (brain swelling, hypoxia, cardiac arrest). The correct position of the endotracheal tube must be verified after each change of the patient's position, because complications may result from a deviation into either of the main bronchi. Other unexpected problems during the controlled ventilation period (e.g., obstruction of the tube by secretions, cuff hernia) can only be handled effectively if the anesthetist has free access to the tube at any given time (Fig. 7.1).

Monitoring During Anesthesia

The following measures have been proven valuable for intraoperative monitoring: electrocardiogram (ECG), continuous measurement of the arterial blood pressure, and superior vena cava pressure. During operations where the patient is in a lounging position, the tip of the catheter must be located within the right atrium in order to be able to aspirate any invaded air during air embolism. Additionally, there should be continuous measurement of the end-expiratory CO_2 concentration, body temperature, diuresis, and the arterial oxygen saturation (oximetry). It is advisable to check the muscle relaxation with a neurostimulator to ensure sufficient relaxation on one hand and the ability to evaluate intraoperatively function of the cranial nerves (e.g., N. VII) on the other. Regular arterial blood gas analyses are an additional measure of control for ventilation and oxygenation of the patient.

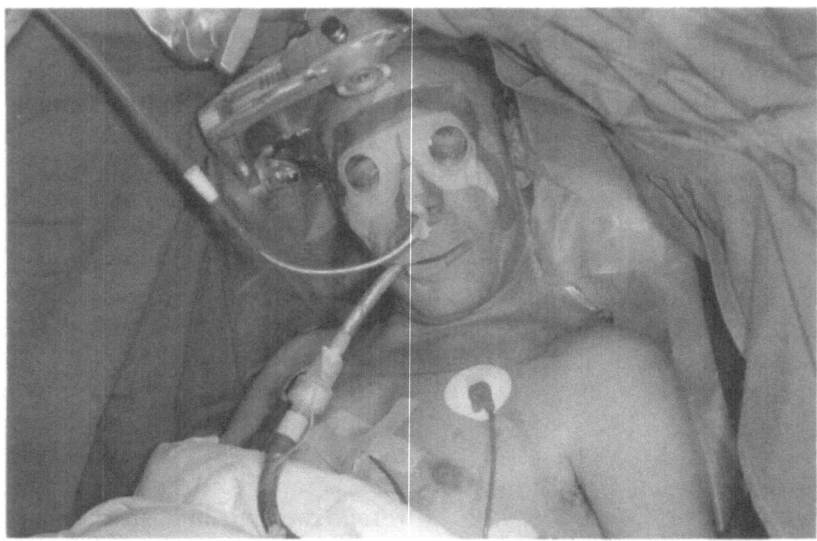

Figure 7.1. Free access to the endotracheal tube.

Performance of Anesthesia

The induction and maintenance of anesthesia are closely related. As there are different suggestions for the use of drugs and methods for its initiation, there are different opinions about the maintenance of anesthesia as well. According to the authors there are a number of different anesthesiological methods to allow operations in the posterior fossa. Important is the continuous attention to the relationship between cerebral circulation, metabolism, autoregulation, pCO_2 reaction, and the anesthesia in every single individual. Because of the often rapid reaction of the brain to anesthesiological measures, we assume the performance of the anesthesia to be equal in importance to the choice of the individual drugs themselves. For intracranial operations, we give preference to total intravenous anesthesia (TIVA) where the dosage of drugs is closely adjusted to the needs of the patient and the different stages of the operation. Muscle relaxation and controlled ventilation are used for every patient, so that coughing, elevation of ventilation pressure, or brain swelling may safely be prevented.

For operations of tumors in the posterior fossa, preference is given to the lounging position, and ventilation is by PEEP (10 cm H_2O).

Control of the relaxation with an appropriate monitor prevents an overdose of muscle relaxants. Supplementation of infusions and plasma expanders are determined by fluid losses, length of operation, hemodynamic parameters, diuresis, and laboratory data.

Since this procedure (TIVA) is surely not common in neuroanesthesia, we shall discuss it from an anesthesiological standpoint in the following paragraphs.

In the past in different centers patients have been operated in the sitting position and with spontaneous respiration, so that respiratory changes functioned as signs of alarm during surgical procedures on the brain stem.[2,62] In general, patients received nitrous oxide and an inhalational anesthetic. The uncontrolled spontaneous respiration and the thereby elevated arterial pCO_2 concentration could also elevate the CBF, thus impairing the conditions of the operation by leading to brain swelling. In accordance with several studies, we can assume that the hemodynamic parameters (blood pressure, heart rate) and the ECG are more suitable for monitoring than the respiratory parameters (tidal volume, respiratory rate and rhythm) while operating close to vital areas of the brain stem.[62,63]

In contrast to halothane or enflurane,

neuroleptanesthesia (NLA) has been chosen (favorable cerebral effects, only slight impairment of the cardiovascular system) as the most often used method in neuroanesthesia for many years now. This consists of ventilation with an oxygen/nitrous oxide mixture and an injection of opioids and droperidol. The induction of this form of anesthesia is usually by an intravenous hypnotic. A disadvantage of this procedure is the possibility of hypertonic reactions of the circulatory system, caused by insufficient reflex suppression, which may not be compensated intraoperatively simply by elevating the opioid dosage. One solution to this problem is the application of a low-dose inhalational anesthetic and the injection of a benzodiazepine instead of droperidol, a procedure known as balanced anesthesia.

There is no doubt that this procedure, or the adequate modifications of it, have led to good results in neuroanesthesia. A discussion about alternative methods was started because the previously mentioned procedures still contained substances that increased the CBF and possibly elevated the ICP. Even though this rarely caused problems, it should be given on an individual basis.

According to recent publications, it seems sensible to the authors generally not to use N_2O when the ICP is elevated.[4,51,52,64,65] Since N_2O during brain ischemia impairs the neurological outcome, one should consider eliminating the use of N_2O in those procedures that present some risk of cerebral ischemia.[66]

In the case of a pneumocephalus, N_2O can increase the volume of the air-filled spaces for physical reasons, two- to fourfold and, thus, elevate the pressure accordingly if volume equalization is not achieved in time. Even though these problems have been seen by different authors, only in a few cases can they be eliminated simply by banning N_2O from anesthesia.[67,68] Because of these still unanswered questions, a new method—total intravenous anesthesia—deserves special consideration. This technique is based on the exclusive use of intravenously applied substances (analgesics, hypnotics, relaxants) and refraining from the use of N_2O and volatile anesthetics.[4,22,26,69,70] Now anesthetics are

fully eliminated as the cause for elevation of the CBF since no drug can cause vasodilatation or a stimulation of the brain metabolism. If opioids or hypnotics with a short half-life (e.g., alfentanil, propofol) are applied continuously, the ability to control this procedure during long operations can be compared to that of inhalational anesthetics.[26,71]

Hypertensive reactions of the circulatory system as a sign of insufficient reflex suppression are rarely seen. The risk of hypotension due to the patient's position is diminished by low-dosage propofol. The advantage of propofol is its very short half-active life, as compared to the longer half-active lives of benzodiazepines and barbiturates.[72] These are especially profound if barbiturates or benzodiazepines have to be given in high dosages when refraining from N_2O and volatile anesthetics, in order to assure that the patient remains anesthetized during the operation. Of course, there is the possibility to inject a specific antagonist (flumazenil) in order to reduce the sedation caused by benzodiazepines postoperatively, but not without the risk of a short-lasting elevation of CBF and ICP in comparison with the intraoperative values (as measured in dogs to be 44% to 56% or 180% to 217%).[73,74] The antagonist has no effect on these parameters when the patient is awake, so one may observe a "neurogenic transmitted awakening reaction."[30] The appropriate end of the infusion (propofol, alfentanil) allows early neurological evaluation, even after long-lasting operations.

Special Anesthesiological Aspects of Operations in the Posterior Fossa

Lounging Position

For many years now there have been different and opposing viewpoints regarding positioning for posterior fossa neurosurgical procedures.[1,2,63,67,75-77] The generally accepted advantages of the lounging position are favorable surgical approach, remarkable diminution in pooling of blood, better venous return, diaphragm mobility, and ability to perform intraoperative monitoring of the facial musculature after facial nerve stimulation in the cerebellopontine angle.[1,67,77]

Complete exposure and visualization of all structures in the posterior fossa and operating continuously in a clean field are the most significant advantages to the surgeon and the patient. With the steady use of irrigation, it is possible to guarantee a clear surgical field and to reduce the amount of suction, which might traumatize the delicate and important structures of the area.[78,79]

Special attention must be given to the detailed analysis by Black et al.,[1] in which the intrinsic relationships between the perioperative complications and long-term results on one hand, and the positions for posterior fossa surgery on the other, were examined. For example, the caudal cranial nerves could be better preserved functionally in those patients operated in the lounging position, whereas palsies of the facial nerve occurred more often in patients positioned horizontally.

Air embolism and reduction of blood pressure have been reported as intraoperative complications of the lounging procedure. Tension pneumocephalus, postoperative bleeding, and edema of the soft tissues of the neck, are recog-

nized untoward events that may occur with the patient in the lounging position.[80]

Additionally, other rarely seen complications have been described: lesions of the brachial plexus, peroneal nerve, and sciatic nerve; and traumatization of the cervical part of the medulla, followed by tetraplegia and damage to joints and skin. Authors with great experience do not accept these as "lounging or sitting position" complications. Rather, they have shown convincingly that such untoward events occurred independently of the position.[1,67]

Bringing patients into a lounging position can cause reduction in blood pressure because of blood pooling in the lower extremities and the abdomen, for the adequate regulation through baroreceptors is suppressed by anesthetics. Studies by Black et al.[1] have shown hypotensive reactions to be equally as frequent in patients with horizontal positioning during the operation. Comparative measurements of the CBF have, as already mentioned, led to contradictory data. Therefore it now seems impossible to come to a valid conclusion concerning the reactions of the CBF in the lounging position.[10,11] The frequency of reactions of the circulatory system during positioning of the patient can be reduced if the following measures

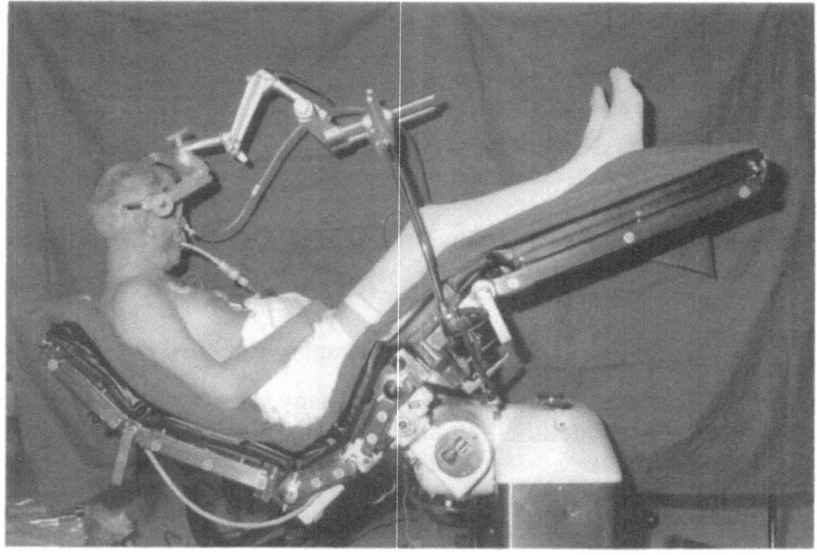

Figure 7.2. Lounging position.

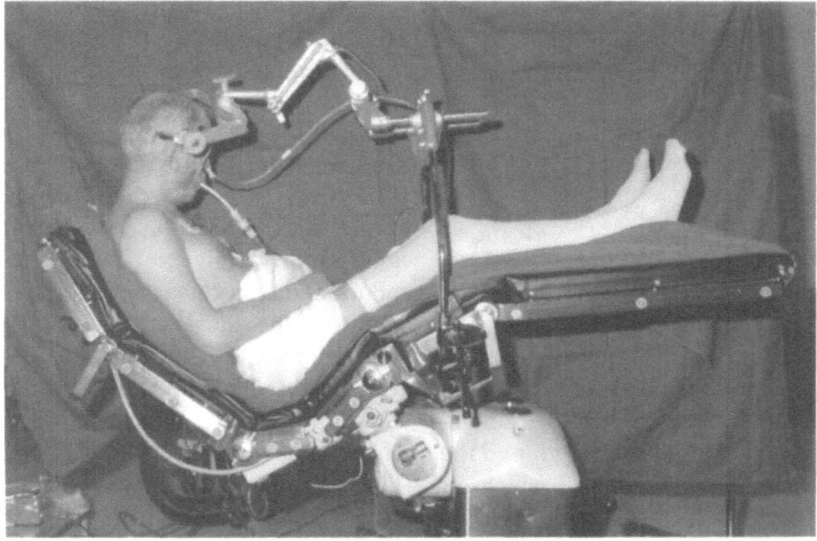

Figure 7.3. Sitting position.

are taken: slow elevation, lounging instead of sitting position (Figs. 7.2 and 7.3), sufficient infusion of electrolytic solutions and plasma expanders, and compression stockings.

In comparison to other positions, we have rarely found disturbances in the relation between ventilation and perfusion of the lungs.

Prone and Semiprone Position

Because of the risk of air embolism, some neurosurgeons prefer patients for posterior fossa operations to be placed in a prone, or park-bench position. Many studies have proven that the horizontal position cannot reliably eliminate the risk of venous air embolism (VAE) in children or adults.[1,81,82] Traumatization of the eyes, brachial plexus, and peripheral nerves, and edema of the face and soft tissues of the neck, as well as dislocation of the endotracheal tube, can be caused by incorrect placement of the patient or movement during surgery in any of the above positions. Concerning the anesthetist, the park-bench position has no advantage over the lounging position because of irregular ventilation and perfusion of the lungs. When comparing different forms of positioning, one must not forget to evaluate

the intraoperative blood loss and subsequent need for transfusions. According to the studies of Black et al.,[1] 13% of the patients undergoing surgery in an horizontal position needed transfusions in comparison to 3% of the patients in the lounging position.

Regardless of the surgeon's decision regarding special positioning of the patient, controlled ventilation should be preferred to spontaneous respiration in order to prevent hypoxia and brain swelling as a result of hypoventilation.

Venous Air Embolism

Numerous publications in the past years have reported the risk and frequency of venous air embolism (VAE) during posterior fossa surgical procedures with patients in the lounging position (Table 7.1). Independent of the difference between the reported observations based on a variety of diagnostic procedures, the morbidity and mortality are quite low.[1,67] Embolism can occur during surgical procedures by invading air entering into opened veins of the neck muscles and the bone, or into the emissary and bridging veins.

Table 7.1. Frequency of venous air embolism.

Study	No. of patients	Frequency
Hey, 1983	207	11%
Standefer, 1984	488	7%
Matjasko, 1985	554	23.5%
Young, 1986	255	30%
Black, 1988	579	45%
Lodrini, 1989	417	33%

Whether or not the entrance of air into an opened vein or sinus results in complications depends on three factors: persistence of a patent foramen ovale (20% to 25% of the population), the rate at which air has entered, and the total amount of air.[83,84] The rate at which air penetrates the vascular tree in a patient in the lounging position relates to the vascular surface, the pressure gradient between surgical field and the right atrium, and the flow velocity of the blood, with this latter ranging between −3 and 30 cm/sec, depending on the pulse phase.[85] The amount of air in the right heart chambers and in the pulmonary arteries, which may cause a fatal outcome, cannot be determined from existing, diverse reports.[86] Changes in pumonary gaseous interchange and pathological x-rays of the lungs following a VAE were rare and disappeared within a short time.[87]

In animal experiments, Adornato et al.[88] has shown that the slow infusion of air causes a pressure rise in the pulmonary arteries, a reduction of the peripheral resistance, a compensatory increase in cardiac output, and a moderate arterial hypotension. A bolus injection of air reduced the pressure in the pulmonary arteries, and led to changes in the electrocardiogram and shock.

Serious consequences of venous air embolism can be avoided by early recognition, diagnosis, and corresponding therapy.[1,77] Among the methods of diagnosing air embolism in a sitting position, the Doppler ultrasound examination has become of great importance because of its high sensitivity. The minimal amount of air that can be registered with the Doppler device ranges between 0.02 and 0.24 ml/kg of body weight.[89,90] A deviation of sensitivity values is due to differing measur-

ing conditions. Critics of this method have argued that technical problems may arise due to positioning of the transducer and sometimes during bipolar coagulation.

Today, two different types of ultrasonic Doppler devices are known, one where the transducer is placed on the patient's thorax above the right atrium and the other where it is located within the esophagus. The first-mentioned transducer needs to be securely fastened to the thorax, for any dislocation can lead to the loss of the signal.[62] A higher sensitivity is possible with transesophageal echocardiography (TEE), which may detect amounts of air as low as 0.01 ml/kg of body weight.[91] TEE can also specifically localize small air bubbles in the right and/or the left atrium.[92,93] It is possible to prove paradox air embolism in patients with persisting foramen ovale, using this method. For now, the high costs are limiting the expanded use of these devices in neurosurgery. Due to their lower sensitivity (0.4 to 0.6 ml/kg of body weight), the value of end-expiratory CO_2 concentration, transcutaneous pCO_2, and the Swan-Ganz catheter are not ideal for the early diagnosis of air embolism.[90,94,95]

An addition to the registration of the pressure in the pulmonary artery can be seen in the continuous measurement of the mixed-venous saturation with a fiberoptic system, which allows the evaluation of hemodynamic reactions as a result of air embolism. Time will tell if this method can supply relevant data for the early diagnosis of air embolism.[96] According to our opinion, there are real advantages in using capnometry. Air in the atrium is identified by Doppler sound changes. When air passes into the pulmonary capillaries there are capnographic alterations, as described by Müller et al.[97] These alterations were caused by the increase of the physiological dead space and changes in perfusion by embolized air bubbles. So, they allow an evaluation of the severity according to the CO_2 reduction. This sudden CO_2 decrease is characteristic for VAE and is thereby easy to distinguish from other changes in the capnogram, e.g., caused by hypothermia, diminishing muscle relaxation, hypovolemia, or technical defects. The combination of Doppler and capnography are theoretically superior to monitor stages of air penetration, practical, convenient, and reliable.

As animal experiments and clinical studies have shown, the transcutaneous measurement of the oxygen tension is also appropriate for monitoring.[95] The measured values react promptly to the invasion of air into opened veins, and thereby cause changes in the ventilation/perfusion index in the lung. Since the correlation between these data is very good, it can be instantly evaluated if ventilation with oxygen and refraining from the use of N_2O are appropriate to prevent hypoxia. The anesthetist must bear in mind that the transcutaneous measurement of oxygen is subject to tissue perfusion. Thus, a reduction of the heart minute volume, obstruction of the blood flow, or a vasoconstriction might produce values that are characteristic for VAE.

A quantitative evaluation of the penetrated air volume is only possible with mass spectrometry. Nevertheless, the sensitivity of this method, in animal experiments, has been lower than that of the Doppler monitoring device.[98]

Arterial hypotension, heart murmur (mill wheel murmur), and ECG changes as signs of right ventricular strain are only seen after larger volumes have penetrated and are of no relevance to the early diagnosis.[94]

The therapeutic recommendations for VAE are compression of the jugular veins, interruption of the supply of nitrous oxide, aspiration of air by means of the atrial catheter, inclination of the surgical table cranialward, and increase of the end-expiratory pressure.[80] An increase in pressure in the veins of the surgical field is achieved as with no other procedure through compression of the neck veins.[99,100] Because of the known physical characteristics, N_2O expands the volume of air bubbles within the veins two to four times and, therefore, the supply must be stopped at once.[101,102]

As the median pressure in the confluens sinuum in the supine position is 6 cm H_2O, dropping to 0 cm H_2O after lifting the upper trunk 25°, and is −13 cm H_2O in the upright position,[103] the upper trunk should be raised just enough to allow head fixation in the Mayfield head ring, being sure that the patient's chin does not contact his sternum (Figs. 7.4 and 7.5). Similar findings, with a fall in the superior sagittal sinus pressure proportional to the changes in the position, were described by Grady et al.[99] in children. It is well known that patients operated in the supine position may suffer air embolism. This has been reported in

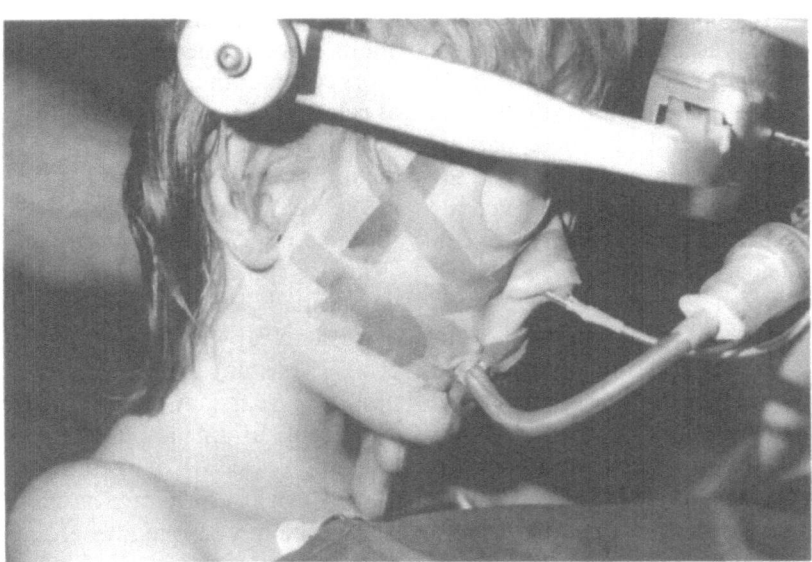

Figure 7.4. Position for proper venous return.

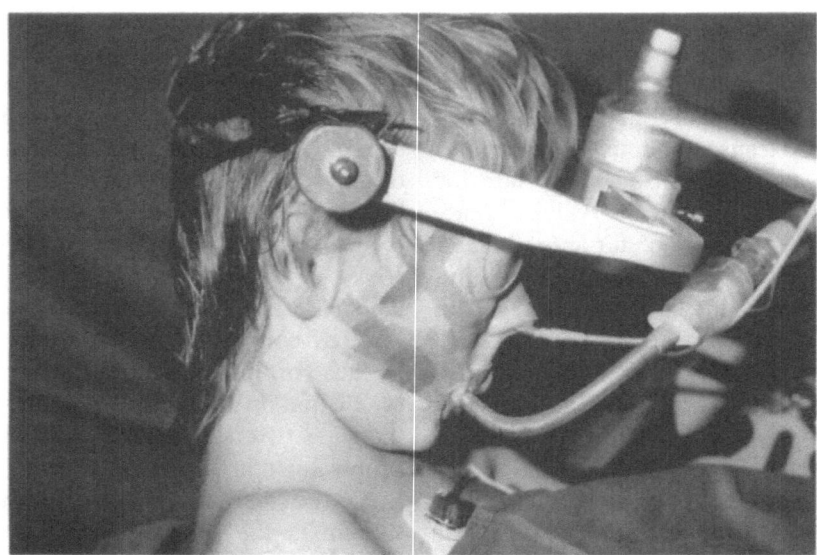

Figure 7.5. Incorrect positioning (chin contacts the sternum).

children operated for craniostenosis (66%), and in adults operated for different lesions in 11% to 12% of the cases.[1,81,82]

Apparently, raising the head above the plane of the cardiac chambers is enough to create a negative pressure in the operative field.

In the sitting position with 10 cm PEEP, there are reductions in the mean arterial pressure (14%), stroke volume (15%), and cardiac output (15%). No changes occurred in heart rate or in systemic vascular resistance.[104–106] Colohan et al.[107] and Voorhies et al.[108] have shown that pre- and intraoperative fluid therapy plays an important role in these parameters. Therefore, infusion with plasma expanders is indicated so that the venous pressure increases and the gradient between surgical field and heart decreases.

The observations of Voorhies et al.,[108] who used PEEP values of 10 to 20 cm H_2O, of increased venous pressure in the surgical field with corresponding PEEP values, are not in agreement with newer studies.[99,103,109] In these studies, a rise of pressure in the sagittal sinus did not occur regularly in all patients. Clinical experience observing the operative field reveals greater sinus pressure using PEEP ventilation.

Contrary to other authors[62,110,111] who used PEEP for prevention of VAE, Bedford et al.[112] and Perkins-Pearson et al.[113] have considered another aspect of this problem.. They were able to measure, in a percentage of their patient population operated in the sitting position, a right atrium pressure (RAP) that was higher than the wedge pressure (PCWP) of the pulmonary capillaries.[104,112,113] Presuming that this PCWP represents the pressure in the left atrium (LAP), and that 20% to 30% of the adults have a patent foramen ovale, the authors consider the risk of systemic air embolism as relevant. In other studies, the same authors observed that during the operation the gradient between PCWP and RAP decreased during ventilation with PEEP, and that even RAP surpassed PCWP.[106] With volume substitution (Ringer's solution), the reduction of PCWP did not occur.[107,114]

It is unclear why this observation by Perkins et al.[114] has not been further discussed in the past few years. A patent foramen ovale is significant, as air may enter the coronary and cerebral vessels. Volumes between 0.05 and 0.5 ml can cause a myocardial ischemia.[84,93] The problem with the interpretation of the results of Bedford et al.[112] and Perkins-Pearson et al.[113] could lie either in the methodology or the assumption that PCWP always represents LAP. Also, the fact that systemic air embolism seldom occurs, and that conventional monitoring often fails to register it, makes the evaluation difficult.[115,116]

In animal experiments it was observed that RAP and LAP increase with ventilation with PEEP, without changes in the difference between the pressure values. Air penetration causes pressure increases in the pulmonary artery and an increase of the pulmonary vascular resistance without a gradient change.[117] The significance of a patent foramen ovale for the relationship between RAP/LAP gradient and the appearance of systemic air embolism were studied by Oliver et al.[118] on animals with an iatrogenically produced atrial septal defect. Neither the influence of the ventilation protocol [zero end-expiratory pressure (ZEEP)/ PEEP] nor the pressure difference between RAP and LAP played a role in causing systemic emblism. In the study of Black et al.[119] the appearance of systemic air embolism in the presence of an atrial septal defect does not correlate with the gradient in the mean pressure values in the atrium. The ventilation patterns do not have an effect on the origin of systemic air embolism. The discrepancy between the rare cases of systemic air embolism and the relatively frequent persistence of a patent foramen ovale must still be clarified. Zasslow et al.[120] have pointed out that a positive end-expiratory pressure of up to 10 cm H_2O in patients in the lounging position does not change the difference between RAP and PCWP.

Changes in Cardiovascular System During Surgery

In different phases during posterior fossa surgery, changes of heart rate, cardiac rhythm, and/or blood pressure can be registered. They can occur during the insertion of the cerebellar spatula and/or during the preparation and extirpation of the tumor. Hypertension, hypotension, tachycardia, bradycardia, arrhythmia, and asystole have been described.[121–123]

Possible causes for the elevation of the blood pressure during the retraction of the cerebellum may be pain reactions, ischemia of the cerebellum or the brain stem, and perhaps the stimulation of the vasomotor center.[124] We can assume that anesthetics in addition to their well-known peripheral effect can also influence the cardiovascular centers of the brain stem. These centers are in immediate association with cells that control the respiratory system, and with nuclei of caudal cranial nerves on the floor of the fourth ventricle.[62]

With these anatomical relationships in mind, it is not surprising that the extirpation of tumors in the posterior fossa can lead to sudden cardiovascular reactions. Bradycardia and hypotension are signs of irritation of cranial nerve nuclei IX and X (nucleus ambiguus) and/ or of the depressor area.[123] Manipulation close to the pressor area or the sensory nucleus of N. V causes tachycardia, hypertension, and sometimes extrasystoles. This nucleus also contains nociceptive neuronal projections of nerves V, VII, IX, and X (tractus solitarius).

In studies by Rupp et al.[124] involving 26 patients who were treated for trigeminal neuralgia by vascular decompression, every patient reacted to the insertion of the cerebellar spatula with an elevation of the blood pressure. Since there is an obvious relationship between the changes in blood pressure and the anesthetics (isoflurane, halothane, sufentanil), the author seems entitled to reflect on how the anesthetist can influence the cardiovascular reactions by choice of anesthesia. Assuming that the preparation close to the brain stem or on the floor of the fourth ventricle is done with utmost precaution, we have after several years of observation come to the decision to consider it legitimate to reduce the range of circulatory reactions by choice of an adequate form of anesthesia. In our own study involving 120 patients who underwent posterior fossa tumor surgery in the lounging position, the total intravenous anesthesia (propofol, alfentanil with no N_2O) has been most efficient in comparison to neuroleptanesthesia. Because of the stability of hemodynamic parameters the use of other drugs like vagolytics, sympathomimetic, and beta-blockers may be reserved for individual cases only. We found no disadvantages for the patient in respect to the cardiovascular and/or respiratory functions while using this concept.

Postoperative Complications

After the completion of the operation, patients must be equally closely monitored as in the initial phase of the anesthesia, and as during the entire surgical procedure. The patient should be awakened without stress, anxiety, coughing, or shivering, since these reactions can increase the ICP or the oxygen need of the organism. If the body temperature should have dropped during the operation, it is advisable to ventilate the patient until normal values have been reached so that the increased oxygen need can be met. Anesthesia with opioids can lead, in the early postoperative phase, to a depression of the respiratory system, which, untreated, may in turn lead to an increase in CBF. Until these drug-induced side effects have passed, a short-lasting ventilation is advantageous, for it will reliably prevent hypercapnia. The risk of postoperative respiratory depression can be diminished by using short-acting opioids and hypnotics, which are easy to control. Since the autoregulation of the vessels in the surgical field may be impaired, the elevation of the blood pressure may cause brain edema. The patient should only be extubated if hemodynamically stable, sufficient spontaneous respiration is achieved, fluid and blood volume are well balanced, and there are no problems to be expected from the operation site. With today's existing possibilities of careful postoperative ventilation, there are no advantages in the use of antagonists (naloxone, flumazenil), which may lead to undesired side effects, elevation of blood pressure, cerebral blood flow, and $CMRO_2$.[125,126] If the extubation should be followed by respiratory problems, reintubation and assisted ventilation should not be delayed, considering of the close relationship between brain stem and respiration.

The necessity for early postoperative evaluation of the patient (which is stressed by the neurosurgeons) needs to be acknowledged especially if postoperative ventilation is advisable, due to intraoperative problems (severe arrhythmia and blood pressure changes, brain edema). Selecting a short-acting sedative is advantageous here.

Independent of anesthetics, respiratory problems may result from edema or ischemia in the surgical field. Problems may also be caused by increases of the ICP due to hydrocephalus or swelling of the tongue, or the soft tissues of the neck after extubation. Here, we have found inadequate positioning of the patient or disturbances of the venous return to be responsible. This agrees with the findings of Frost,[127] who described swelling of the tongue caused by incorrect positioning of the oropharyngeal tube.

The problems of pneumocephalus, which can also develop in supine operating positions, have already been mentioned. Often, its signs are postoperative lethargy, which therefore can be more easily diagnosed clinically when short-acting anesthetics are used.

Lesions of the caudal cranial nerves cause long-term complications if combined with dysphagia or loss of laryngeal reflexes. Because of the close relationship of the cardiovascular centers to nuclei of the caudal cranial nerves, functional lesions of these nerves are to be expected following severe intraoperative hemodynamic reactions.

Conclusion

Anesthesia for posterior fossa surgery shows some specific differences from regular neuroanestheia and, thus, should be of special interest to neurosurgeons. The exact knowledge of available substances, their rational selection in regard to the existing pathological changes and the close cooperation between surgeon and anesthetist are the requirements for a good neurological outcome for the patient. Our own experiences with more than 1,000 patients who underwent posterior fossa tumor surgery in the lounging position have proven that these considerations lead to good results.

References

1. Black S, Ockert DB, Oliver WC, et al. Outcome following posterior fossa craniectomy in patients in the sitting or horizontal positions. *Anesthesiology*. 1988;69:49–56.
2. Drummond JC. Changing practices in neuroanaesthesia. *Can J Anaesth*. 1990;37:4/Slxxxix–Sxcix.
3. Van Hemelrijck J, Tempelhoff R, Jellish WS, et al. Comparison of thiopental-isoflurane-N_2O, propofol-N_2O, and propofol alone for neuroanesthesia. *Anesthesiology*. 1990;73:A167.
4. Van Aken H, Van Hemelrijck J, Merckx L, et al. Totale intravenöse Anästhesie mit Propofol und Alfentanil im Vergleich zur balancierten Anästhesie in der Neurochirurgie. *Anästh Intensivther Notfallmed*. 1990;25:54–58.
5. Zattoni J, Siani C. Neurosurgical anaesthesia. *J. Drug Dev*. 1989;2(suppl 2):87–94.
6. Sieber FE, Smith DS, Traystman RJ, et al. Glucose: A reevaluation of its intraoperative use. *Anesthesiology*. 1987;67:72–81.
7. Drummond JC, Shapiro HM. Cerebral physiology. In: Miller RD, ed. *Anesthesia*. New York, Edinburgh, London, Melbourne: Churchill Livingstone; 1990:621–658.
8. Larsen R, ed. *Anästhesie*. München, Wien, Baltimore: Urban & Schwarzenberg; 1987:619–671.
9. Ernst PS, Albin MS, Bunegin L. Intracranial and spinal cord hemodynamics in the sitting position in dogs in the presence and absence of increased intracranial pressure. *Anesth Analg*. 1990;70:147–153.
10. Werner C, Kochs E, Reimer R, et al. Einfluß von Lagerungsveränderungen auf die zerebrale Hämodynamik unter Allgemeinanästhesie. *Anaesthesist*. 1990;39:429–433.
11. Nelson RJ, Lovick AH, Pickard JD, et al. Changes in cerebral blood flow during anaesthesia and surgery in the sitting position. *J Neurol, Neurosurg Psychiatry*. 1987;50:971–975.
12. Bendriss P, Pick K, Stoiber HP, Dabadie P. Neurosurgical sedation. *J Drug Dev*. 1989;2(suppl 2):95–96.
13. Cold GE, Eskesen V, Eriksen H, et al. CBF and $CMRO_2$ during continuous etomidate infusion supplemented with N_2O and fentanyl in patients with supratentorial cerebral tumour. A dose-response study. *Acta Anaesthesiol Scand*. 1985;29:490–494.
14. Crozier TA, Beck D, Wuttke W, et al. Abhängigkeit der Kortisolsynthesehemmung in vivo von der Etomidatplasmakonzentration. *Anaesthesist*. 1988;37:337–339.
15. Belapavlovic M, Buchthal A. Modification of ketamine-induced intracranial hypertension in neurosurgical patients by pretreatment with midazolam. *Acta Anaesthesiol Scand*. 1982;26:458–462.
16. Shapiro HM, Wyte SR, Harris AB. Ketamine anesthesia in patients with intracranial pathology. *Br J Anaesth*. 1972;44:1200–1204.
17. Weinstabl C, Mayer N, Plattner H, et al. Impact of propofol on intracranial dynamics in head trauma ICU patients. *Anesthesiology*. 1990;73:A1217.
18. Hartung HJ. Intrakranielles Druckverhalten bei Patienten mit Schädel-Hirn-Trauma nach Propofol- bzw. Thiopental-Applikation. *Anaesthesist*. 1987;36:285–287.
19. Kochs E, Hoffman WE, Werner C, et al. The effects of propofol on neurologic outcome from incomplete cerebral ischemia in the rat. *Anesthesiology*. 1990;73:A719.
20. Stephan H, Sonntag H, Schenk HD, et al. Einfluß von Disoprivan auf die Durchblutung und den Sauerstoffverbrauch des Gehirns und die CO_2-Reaktivität der Hirngefäße beim Menschen. *Anaesthesist*. 1987;36:60–65.
21. Vandesteene A, Trempont V, Engelman E, et al. Effect of propofol on cerebral blood flow and metabolism in man. *Anaesthesia*. 1988;43(suppl):42–43.
22. Ravussin P, Guinard JP, Ralley F, et al. Effect of propofol on cerebrospinal fluid pressure and cerebral perfusion pressure in patients undergoing craniotomy. *Anaesthesia*. 1988;43(suppl):37–41.
23. Werner C, Hoffmann WE, Segil LJ, et al. Effects of propofol on cerebral and spinal cord blood flow autoregulation in rats. *Anesthesiology*. 1990;73:A694.
24. Podlesch I. Disoprivan—ein neues intravenöses Hypnotikum. *Fortschr Anaesth*. 1988;2:1–31.
25. Sebel PS, Lowdon JD. Propofol: A new intravenous anesthetic. *Anesthesiology*. 1989;71:260–277.
26. Ravussin P, Berger-Bayer M, Nydegger M, et al. Thiopentone-isoflurane vs propofol in neuroanesthesia for intracranial surgery. *Anesthesiology*. 1988;69:A577.
27. Mangez JF, Menguy E, Roux P. Constant rate propofol sedation in the head injured patient.

Preliminary data. *Ann Fr Anesth*. 1987;6:336–337.

28. Bendriss P, Stoiber HP, Bendriss-Brusset AC, et al. Propofol effects on EEG and relationship with plasma concentration during neurosurgery. *Anesthesiology*. 1990;73:A203.

29. Forster A, Juge O, Morel D. Effects of midazolam on cerebral blood flow. *Anesthesiology*. 1982;56:453–455.

30. Forster A, Juge O, Louis M, et al. Effects of a specific benzodiazepine antagonist (RO 15-1788) on cerebral blood flow. *Anesth Analg*. 1987;66:309–313.

31. Forster A, Juge O, Morel D. Effects of midazolam on cerebral hemodynamics and cerebral vasomotor responsiveness to carbon dioxide. *J Cereb Blood Flow Metab*. 1983;3:246–249.

32. Bailey PL, Stanley TH. Narcotic intravenous anesthetics. In: Miller RD, ed. *Anesthesia*. New York, Edinburgh, London, Melbourne: Churchill Livingstone; 1990:281–366.

33. Vernhiet J, Renou AM, Orgogozo JM, et al. Effects of diazepam-fentanyl mixture on cerebral blood flow and oxygen consumption in man. *Br J Anaesth*. 1978;50:165–169.

34. Keykhah MM, Smith DS, Carlsson C, et al. Influence of sufentanil on cerebral metabolism and circulation in the rat. *Anesthesiology*. 1985;63:274–277.

35. Milde LN, Milde JR. The cerebral hemodynamic and metabolic effects of sufentanil in dogs. *Anesthesiology*. 1987;67:A570.

36. Hoffman WE, Werner C, Segil LJ, et al. Fentanyl with nitrous oxide does not alter cerebral autoregulation or blood flow compared to unanesthetized rats. *Anesthesiology*. 1990;73:A603.

37. McPherson RW, Krempasanka E, Eimerl D, et al. Effects of alfentanil on cerebral vascular reactivity in dogs. *Br J Anaesth*. 1985;57:1232–1238.

38. Murkin JM, Farrar JK, Tweed WA. Sufentanil anaesthesia reduces cerebral blood flow and cerebral oxygen consumption. *Can J Anaesth*. 1988;35:S131.

39. Mayer N, Weinstabl C, Podreka I, et al. Sufentanil does not increase cerebral blood flow in healthy human volunteers. *Anesthesiology*. 1990;73:240–243.

40. Shupak RC, Harp JR. Comparison between high-dose sufentanil-oxygen and high-dose fentanyl-oxygen for neuroanesthesia. *Br J Anaesth*. 1985;57:375–381.

41. From RP, Warner DS, Todd MM, et al. Anesthesia for craniotomy: A double-blind comparison of alfentanil, fentanyl, and sufentanil. *Anesthesiology*. 1990;73:896–904.

42. Murphy FL, Kennell EM, Johnstone RE, et al. The effects of enflurane, isoflurane and halothane on cerebral blood flow and metabolism in men. Abstracts of scientific papers, ASA Meeting. 1974:61–62.

43. Todd MM, Drummond JC, Shapiro HM. Comparative cerebrovascular and metabolic effects of halothane, enflurane and isoflurane. *Anesthesiology*. 1982;57:A332.

44. Todd MM, Drummond JC. A comparison of the cerebrovascular and metabolic effects of halothane and isoflurane in the cat. *Anesthesiology*. 1984;60:276–282.

45. Grosslight K, Foster R, Colohan AR, et al. Isoflurane for neuroanesthesia: risk factors for increases in intracranial pressure. *Anesthesiology*. 1985;63:533–536.

46. Sainz JJG, Camiruaga JAE, Cano FF, et al. Effects of isoflurane on intraventricular pressure in neurosurgical patients. *Br J Anaesth*. 1988;61:347–349.

47. Michenfelder JD. Cerebral blood flow and metabolism. In: Cucchiara RF, Michenfelder JD, eds. *Clinical Neuroanesthesia*. New York, Edinburgh, London, Melbourne: Churchill Livingstone; 1990:1–40.

48. Madsen JB, Cold GE, Hansen ES, et al. Cerebral blood flow, cerebral metabolic rate of oxygen and relative CO_2-reactivity during craniotomy for supratentorial cerebral tumors in halothane anaesthesia. A dose-response study. *Acta Anaesthesiol Scand*. 1987;31:454–457.

49. Young WL, Prohovnik I, Correll JW, et al. Cerebral blood flow reactivity to CO_2 during halothane or isoflurane anesthesia for carotid endarterectomy. *Anesthesiology*. 1990;73:A204.

50. Albin MS, Bunegin L, Gelineau J. ICP and CBF reactivity to isoflurane and nitrous oxide during normocarbia, hypocarbia and intracranial hypertension. In: Miller JD, Teasdale GM, Rowan JO, et al., eds. *Intracranial Pressure, VI*. Berlin, Heidelberg, New York, Tokyo: Springer-Verlag; 1986:719–724.

51. Hansen TD, Warner DS, Todd MM. Nitrous oxide is a more potent cerebral vasodilator than either halothane or isoflurane. *Anesthesiology*. 1988;69:A537.

52. Kaieda R, Todd MM, Warner DS. The effects of anesthetics and $PaCO_2$ on the cerebrovascular, metabolic, and electroencephalographic responses to nitrous oxide in the rabbit. *Anesth Analg*. 1989;68:135–143.

53. Phirman JR, Shapiro HM. Modification of nitrous oxide-induced intracranial hypertension by prior induction of anaesthesia. *Anesthesiology*. 1977;46:150–151.

54. Hoffman WE, Miletij DJ, Albrecht RF. The effects of midazolam on cerebral blood flow and oxygen consumption and its interaction with nitrous oxide. *Anesth Analg*. 1986;65:729–733.

55. Misfeldt BB, Jorgensen PB, Rishoj M. The effect of nitrous oxide and halothane upon the intracranial pressure in hypocapnic patients with intracranial disorders. *Br J Anaesth*. 1974;46:853–858.

56. Sakabe T, Kuramoto T, Kumagae S, et al. Cerebral responses to the addition of nitrous oxide to halothane in man. *Br J Anaesth*. 1976;48:957–962.

57. Baughman VL, Hoffman WE, Thomas C, et al. The interaction of nitrous oxide and isoflurane with incomplete cerebral ischemia in the rat. *Anesthesiology*. 1989;70:767–774.

58. Stirt JA, Maggio W, Haworth C, et al. Vecuronium: effect on intracranial pressure and hemodynamics in neurosurgical patients. *Anesthesiology*. 1987;67:570–572.

59. Minton MD, Grosslight KR, Stirt JA, et al. Increases in intracranial pressure from succinylcholine: Prevention by prior nondepolarizing blockade. *Anesthesiology*. 1986;65:165–169.

60. Yukioka H, Yoshimoto N, Nishimura K, et al. Intravenous lidocaine as a suppressant of coughing during tracheal intubation. *Anesth Analg*. 1985;64:1189–1192.

61. Cucchiara RF, Benefiel DJ, Matteo RS, et al. Evaluation of esmelol in controlling increases in heart rate and blood pressure during endotracheal intubation in patients undergoing carotid endarterectomy. *Anesthesiology*. 1986;65:528–531.

62. Walters FJM. Anaesthesia for posterior fossa surgery. *Curr Anaesth Crit Care*. 1990;1:83–89.

63. Cucchiara RF. Monitoring and anesthetic management of the anesthetized sitting patient. In: Popp AJ, Nelson LR, Bourke RS, et al., eds. *Seminars in Neurological Surgery*. New York: Raven Press; 1985:1–6, 112.

64. Jung R, Reinsel R, Galicich J, et al. Impact on CSF pressure in brain tumor patients: isoflurane vs N_2O. *Anesthesiology*. 1990;73:A193.

65. Turner JM. Anaesthesia for intracranial surgery. *Curr Anaesth Crit Care*. 1990;1:77–82.

66. Van Aken H, Gerling W. Lachgas: Nebenwirkungen und Gefahren. In: Lawin P, Anger C, eds. *Anästhesiologische Praxis, Alte Fragen—Neue Antworten*. Stuttgart, New York: G. Thieme Verlag; 1990:45–53.

67. Standefer MW, Bay JW, Trusso R. The sitting position in neurosurgery: A retrospective analysis of 488 cases. *Neurosurgery*. 1984;14:649–658.

68. Hemstad JR, Domino KB, Lam AM, et al. Effect of nitrous oxide on ICP following cranial-dural closure. *Anesthesiology*. 1990;73:A177.

69. Steegers PA, Foster PA. Propofol in total intravenous anaesthesia without nitrous oxide. *Anaesthesia*. 1988;43(suppl):94–97.

70. Van Hemelrijck J, Tempelhoff R, Jellish WS, et al. Use of EEG for determining propofol requirement during neuroanesthesia. *Anesthesiology*. 1990;73:A202.

71. Merckx L, Van Hemelrijck J, Van Aken H, et al. Total intravenous anaesthesia using propofol and alfentanil infusion in neurosurgical patients. *Anesthesiology*. 1988;69:A576.

72. Vuyk J, Hennis PJ, Burm AGL, et al. Comparison of midazolam and propofol in combination with alfentanil for total intravenous anesthesia. *Anesthesiology*. 1990;73:A325.

73. Fleischer JE, Milde JH, Moyer TP et al. Cerebral effects of high-dose midazolam and subsequent reversal with RO 15-1788 in dogs. *Anesthesiology*. 1988;68:234–242.

74. Artru AA. Flumazenil reversal of midazolam in dogs: dose-related changes in cerebral blood flow, metabolism, EEG, and CSF pressure. *J Neurosurg Anesth*. 1989;1:46–55.

75. Young ML, Smith DS, Murtagh F, et al. Comparison of surgical and anesthetic complications in neurosurgical patients experiencing venous air embolism in the sitting position. *Neurosurgery*. 1986;18:157–161.

76. Albin MS. The paradox of paradoxic air embolism-PEEP, Valsalva, and patent foramen ovale. Should the sitting position be abandoned? *Anesthesiology*. 1984;61:222–223.

77. Matjasko J, Petrozza P, Cohen M, et al. Anesthesia and surgery in the seated position: Analysis of 554 cases. *Neurosurgery*. 1985;17:695–702.

78. Samii M, Wild K von. Operative treatment of lesions in the region of the tentorial notch. *Neurosurg Rev*. 1981;4:3–10.

79. Samii M, Penkert G, Bini W. Komplikationen bei Eingriffen im Kleinhirnbrückenwinkel. In: Bock WJ, Schirmer M, eds. *Komplikationen*

bei neurochirurgischen Eingriffen. München, Bern, Wien, San Francisco: W. Zuckschwerdt Verlag; 1988:49–57.

80. Wiedemann K, Krier C. Einleitung und Durchführung der Anästhesie bei Eingriffen in sitzender Position. In: Ahnefeld FW, Dick W, Schuster HP, eds. *Anästhesie in der Neurochirurgie.* Berlin Heidelberg New York: Springer; 1983:98–113.

81. Albin MS, Carroll RG, Maroon JC. Clinical considerations concerning detection of venous air embolism. *Neurosurgery.* 1978;3:380–384.

82. Harris MM, Yemen TA, Davidson A, et al. Venous air embolism during craniectomy in supine infants. *Anesthesiology.* 1987;67:816–819.

83. Guggiari M, Lechat P, Garen-Colonne C, et al. Early detection of patent foramen ovale by two-dimensional contrast echocardiography for prevention of paradoxical air embolism during sitting position. *Anesth Analg.* 1988;67:192–194.

84. Hills BA, Butler BD. Air embolism: Further basic facts relevant to the placement of central venous catheters and Doppler monitors. *Anesthesiology.* 1983;59:163.

85. Schalk H von. Luftembolie. In: List WF, Osswald PM, eds. *Komplikationen in der Anästhesie.* Berlin, Heidelberg, New York: Springer; 1987:447–454.

86. Panning B. Die sogenannte venöse Luftembolie. *Anaesthesist.* 1987;36:111–115.

87. Toth C, Mendelsohn DS, Tausk HC, et al. Respiratory complications of venous air embolism during neurosurgery. *Anesthesiology.* 1990; 73:A198.

88. Adornato DC, Gildenberg PL, Ferrario CM, et al. Pathophysiology of intravenous air embolism in dogs. *Anesthesiology.* 1978;49:120–127.

89. Brechner Th, Brechner VL. An audible alarm for monitoring air embolism during neurosurgery. *J Neurosurg.* 1977;47:201–204.

90. Glenski JA, Cucchiara RF, Michenfelder JD. Transesophageal echocardiography and transcutaneous O_2 and CO_2 for detection of venous air embolism. *Anesthesiology.* 1986;64:541–545.

91. Furuya H, Suzuki T, Okumura F, et al. Detection of air embolism by transesophageal echocardiography. *Anesthesiology.* 1983;58:124–129.

92. Cucchiara RF, Nugent M, Seward JB, et al. Air embolism in upright neurosurgical patients. Detection and localisation of two-

dimensional transesophageal echocardiography. *Anesthesiology.* 1984;60:353–355.

93. Furuya H, Okumura F. Detection of paradoxical air embolism by transesophageal echocardiography. *Anesthesiology.* 1984;60:374–377.

94. Gildenberg PL. O'Brien RP, Britt WJ, et al. The efficacy of Doppler monitoring for the detection of venous air embolism. *J Neurosurg.* 1981;54:75–78.

95. Glenski JA, Cucchiara RF. Transcutaneous O_2 and CO_2 monitoring of neurosurgical patients: Detection of air embolism. *Anesthesiology.* 1986;64:546–550.

96. Khoury A, Cagny-Bellet A, Tondriaux A, et al. Continuous monitoring of mixed venous oxygen saturation during sitting neurosurgical procedures. *Anesthesiology.* 1990;73:A184.

97. Müller H, Brähler A, Gerlach I, et al. Diagnostische und prognostische Bedeutung hämodynamischer und respiratorischer Parameter bei venöser Luftembolie. *Anaesthesist.* 1984;33:493–498.

98. Matjasko J, Petrozza P, Mackenzie CF. Sensitivity of end tidal nitrogen in venous air embolism detection in dogs. *Anesthesiology.* 1985;63:418–423.

99. Grady D, Bedford RF, Parks TS. Changes in superior sagittal sinus pressure in children with head elevation, jugular venous compression and PEEP. *J Neurosurg.* 1986;65:199–202.

100. Toung TJK, Miyabe M, McShane AJ, et al. Effect of PEEP and jugular venous compression on canine cerebral blood flow and oxygen consumption in the head elevated position. *Anesthesiology.* 1988;68:53–58.

101. Mehta M, Sokoll MD, Gergis SD. Effects of venous air embolism on the cardiovascular system and acid balance in the presence and absence of nitrous oxide. *Acta Anaesthesiol Scand.* 1984;28:226–231.

102. Munson ES, Merrick HC. Effect of nitrous oxide on venous air embolism. *Anesthesiology.* 1966;27:783–787.

103. Iwabuchi T, Sobata E, Suzuki M, et al. Dural sinus pressure as related to neurosurgical positions. *Neurosurgery.* 1983;12:203–207.

104. Bedford RF, Perkins-Pearson NAK. PEEP for treatment of venous air embolism. *Anesthesiology.* 1982;57:A379.

105. Marshall WK, Bedford RF, Miller ED. Cardiovascular responses in the seated position—impact of four anesthetic techniques. *Anesth Analg.* 1983;62:648–653.

106. Perkins NAK, Bedford RF. Hemodynamic

consequences of PEEP in seated neurological patients—implications for paradoxical air embolism. *Anesth Analg*. 1984;63:429–432.

107. Colohan ART, Perkins NAK, Bedford RF, et al. Intravenous fluid loading as a prophylaxis for paradoxical air embolism. *J Neurosurg*. 1985;62:839–842.

108. Voorhies RM, Fraser RAR, Poznak A van. Prevention of air embolism with positive end-expiratory pressure. *Neurosurgery*. 1983;12: 503–506.

109. Lodrini S, Montolivo M, Pluchino F, et al. Positive end-expiratory pressure in supine and sitting positions: Its effect on intrathoracic and intracranial pressures. *Neurosurgery*. 1989;24: 873–877.

110. Hey O, Fischer F, Reinery G, et al. Erkennung und Verhütung von Luftembolien während neurochirurgischer Eingriffe in sitzender Position. In: Ahnefeld FW, Dick W, Kilian J, et al., eds., *Anästhesie in der Neurochirurgie*. Berlin, Heidelberg, New York; Springer; 1983:197–209.

111. Lee DS, Lichtmann MW, Weintraub HD. Effect of PEEP on air embolism during sitting neurosurgical procedures. *Anesth Analg*. 1981;60:262.

112. Bedford RF, Marshall WK, Butler A, et al. Cardiac catheters for diagnosis and treatment of venous air embolism. *J Neurosurg*. 1981;55:610–614.

113. Perkins-Pearson NAK, Marshall WK, Bedford RF. Atrial pressures in the seated position. *Anesthesiology*. 1982;57:493–497.

114. Perkins NAK, Bedford RF. Intravenous fluid loading: Prophylaxis for paradoxical air embolism. *Anesthesiology*. 1983;59:A389.

115. Cuchiara RF, Seward JB, Nishimura RA, et al. Identification of a patent foramen ovale during sitting position craniotomy by transesophageal echocardiography with positive airway pressure. *Anesthesiology*. 1985;63:107–109.

116. Cucchiara RF, Nishimura RA, Black S. Failure of preoperative echo testing to prevent paradoxical air embolism: Report of two cases. *Anesthesiology*. 1989;71:604–607.

117. Pearl RG, Larson P. Hemodynamic effects of positive end-expiratory pressure during continuous venous air embolism in the dog. *Anesthesiology*. 1986;64:724–729.

118. Oliver S, Cucchiara RF, Nishimura R, et al. Parameters affecting the occurrence of paradoxical air embolism. *Anesthesiology*. 1987; 67:A435.

119. Black S, Cucchiara RF, Nishimua RA, et al. Parameters affecting occurrence of paradoxical air embolism. *Anesthesiology*. 1989;71:235–241.

120. Zasslow MA, Pearl RG, Larson P, et al. PEEP does not affect left atrial–right atrial pressure difference in neurosurgical patients. *Anesthesiology*. 1988;68:760–763.

121. Meridy HW, Creighton RE, Humphreys RP. Complications during neurosurgery in the prone position in children. *Can Anaesth Soc J*. 1974;21:445–452.

122. Artru AA, Cucchiara RF, Messich JM. Cardiorespiratory and cranial-nerve sequelae of surgical procedures involving the posterior fossa. *Anesthesiology*. 1980;52:83–86.

123. Drummond JC, Todd MM. Acute sinus arrhythmia during surgery in the fourth ventricle: An indicator of brain-stem irritation. *Anesthesiology*. 1984;60:232–235.

124. Rupp SM, Wickersham JK, Rampil IJ, et al. The effect of halothane, isoflurane, or sufentanil on the hypertensive response to cerebellar retraction during posterior fossa surgery. *Anesthesiology*. 1989;71:660–663.

125. Shupak RC, Harp JR, Stevenson-Smith W, et al. High-dose fentanyl for neuroanesthesia. *Anesthesiology*. 1983;58:579–582.

126. Keykhah MM, Smith DS, Englebach I, et al. Effects of naloxone on cerebral blood flow and metabolism. *Anesthesiology*. 1983;59: A309.

127. Frost EAM. Some inquiries in neuroanesthesia and neurological supportive care. *J Neurosurg*. 1984;60:673–686.

CHAPTER 8

Basic Techniques in Approaching Posterior Fossa Tumors

Anthony J. Raimondi

It is impossible to state categorically what the single, most important aspect of an operative procedure is—diagnosis, anatomic localization, blood control, flap selection, exposure, or head and body position. It is realistic, however, to assert that if the surgeon positions the patient's head and body properly—taking into consideration the location of the lesion, the planned skin incision, and bone flap—he will, throughout the operation, be oriented anatomically and will always have the lesion at the center of his operative field.

Positioning for pediatric neurosurgery varies considerably with the age of the child (newborn, infant, toddler, juvenile), the number of surgeons (one surgeon alone, surgeon and assistant, etc.), the location of the anesthesiologist and amount of monitoring equipment he brings into the working area, and the target area.

These variables are generally not applicable to neurosurgical operative procedures on adolescents and adults owing to their uniform size, the constant relationship between brain and skull, and the lack of anatomical considerations such as open fontanels and sutures, relatively larger basal cisterns, continuity of the periosteum with the outer layer of the dura at the sutures, and the presence of ossification centers, all of which assume primary importance. Therefore, this chapter is organized to present to the reader general and specific considerations concerning age, individual body positions, relative position of surgeon vis-à-vis patient, and position of the head.

General Discussion

Age

The relative sizes of the surgeon's hands and the head of the newborn, infant, toddler, and adolescent put into relief the remarkable differences in dimension of skull and brain in the different pediatric age groups. This range in overall head size is expressive of a proportionate range in individual anatomical structures (lobes of the brain) or compartments (basal cisterns), since they vary individually, and disproportionately, from the newborn to the toddler.

The head of a premature newborn may be so small as to fit within the palm of the surgeon's hand (Fig. 8.1A), whereas that of a term newborn rests comfortably within the fully cupped adult hands (Fig. 8.1B). The heads of the infant and toddler (Fig. 8.1C,D) are proportionately larger. The same hands are used in all four photographs in Fig. 8.1. This change in volume occurs pari passu with changes in dermal (skin, connective tissue, and aponeurosis of the scalp) thickness, inversion of relative amounts of diploic and lamellar components of the skull, diminution in volume of cisternal cerebrospinal fluid and increase in cerebral volume, and closure of fontanels and narrowing of the sutures.

Premature Newborn

For all intents and purposes, and with only the rarest exceptions, neurosurgery on the brain of

Figure 8.1. A: Premature newborn. B: Term newborn. C: Infant. D: Toddler. (Reprinted from Raimondi AJ. *Pediatric Neurosurgery—Theoretic Principles/Art of Surgical Techniques.* New York: Springer-Verlag, 1987.)

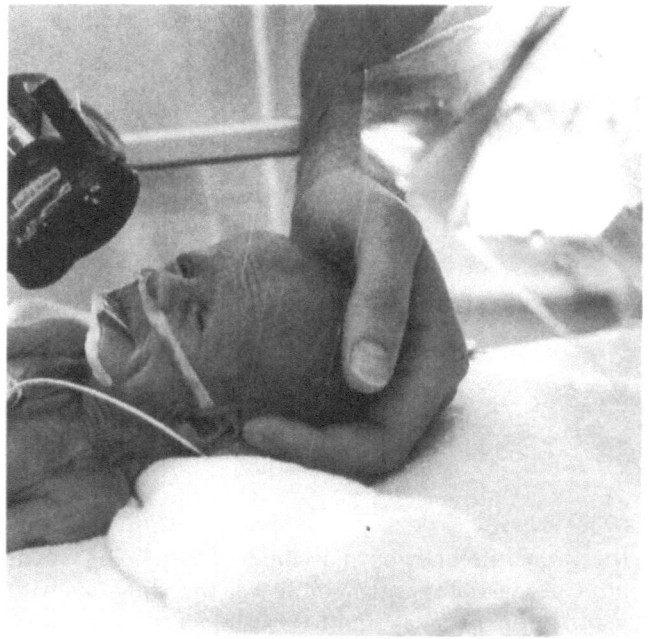

A

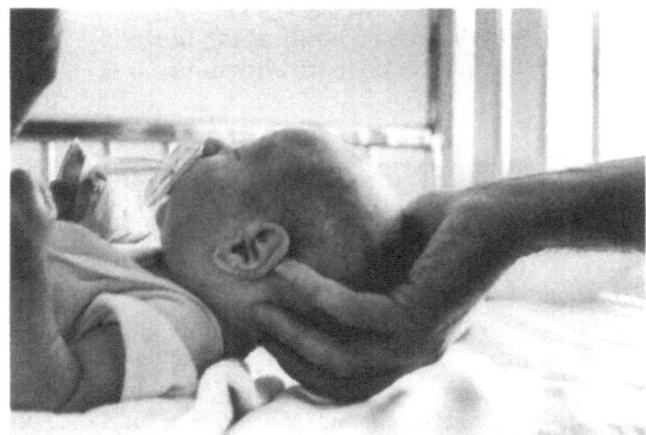

B

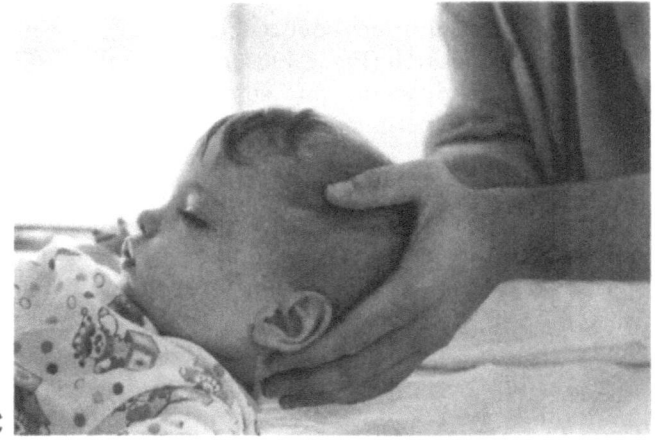

C

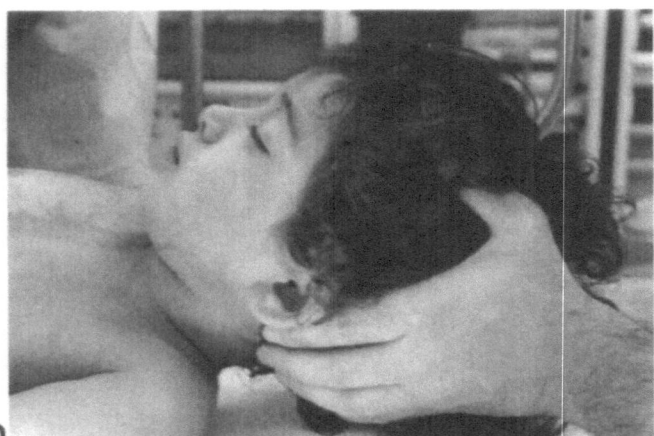

Figure 8.1. (cont.)

the premature newborn is limited to placing an external ventricular drain or inserting a ventriculoperitoneal shunt. Consequently, the supine position, with the head turned to either side, is all that is used in this age category. The exception is the prone position for posterior fossa hematoma secondary to birth injury.

Term Newborn and Infant

The term newborn and the infant can suffer the full range of neurosurgical diseases, so that it may be necessary to operate on children in these age ranges with the patient in the supine, the prone, or the sitting position. Although the sitting position in the newborn is extremely difficult to maintain (he keeps slipping away from the drapes), the infant may be more securely positioned sitting. The need to arrive at the region of the culmen monticuli of the cerebellar vermis, fortunately, does not occur often.

The prone position (Fig. 8.2) is for occipital, craniovertebral junction, and some posterior fossa lesions. It permits optimal exposure of the occipital lobes and craniovertebral junction, but the anatomical structures within the posterior fossa exposure are so located as to permit one to work effectively only in the inferior cerebellar triangle. The position of the surgeon, vis-à-vis posterior fossa contents, makes this obvious (Fig. 8.3). The disadvantages of this position are most notable when performing a suboccipital craniectomy for de-

compressing the foramen magnum in children with the Chiari II malformation. One is never able to work efficiently, either in the superior cerebellar triangle for posterior fossa masses or at the foramen magnum in Chiari II children, with the patient prone. It is also difficult to gain a direct line of vision to the superior cerebellar triangle in the newborn because of the short posteroanterior (clivus-squamous occipital) and the long superoinferior (tentorial opening–foramen magnum) distances. These anatomical characteristics impair significantly the surgeon's ability to visualize the superior aspect of the culmen monticuli by lowering and extending his head.

Toddler

The toddler may be put safely and effectively into either the sitting or lounging positions because his trunk is long enough to sit him up, and his skull, generally speaking, is thick enough to offer purchase to the pins of standard head holders. It is fortunate indeed that this is true, since there is a high incidence of posterior fossa pathology after the second year of life, including such lesions as medulloblastoma, primitive neuroectodermal tumor of the superior cerebellar vermis, arteriovenous malformations of the galenic system, pineal tumors, and arachnoidal cysts of the quadrigeminal and superior cerebral category.

Figure 8.2. A: Access to the cervical spine, the craniovertebral junction, and the occipital lobes may be had with the newborn or infant prone. It is necessary to place pillows or sandbags under the shoulders and to flex the head. The shoulders should be taped in the caudad direction (arrow), distracting the neck, and the head should be taped to the headrest. B: A lateral view showing the degree of flexion of head on neck. Note that the frontal eminences, not the face, nestle into the headrest. C: The surgeon's view of the child's occipital and posterior parietal areas when positioned prone. Again, the pendant position of the head is apparent, not real, a result of the two-dimensional limitations of photography. True perspective may be appreciated by looking at the lateral view in either Fig. 2B or 3. (Reprinted from Raimondi AJ. *Pediatric Neurosurgery—Theoretic Principles/Art of Surgical Techniques*. New York: Springer-Verlag, 1987.)

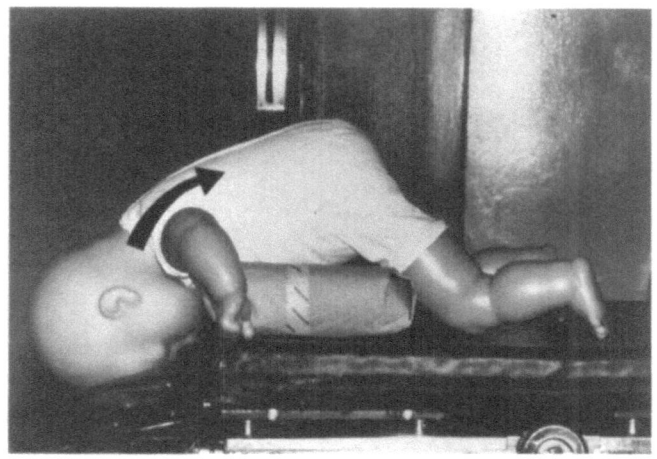

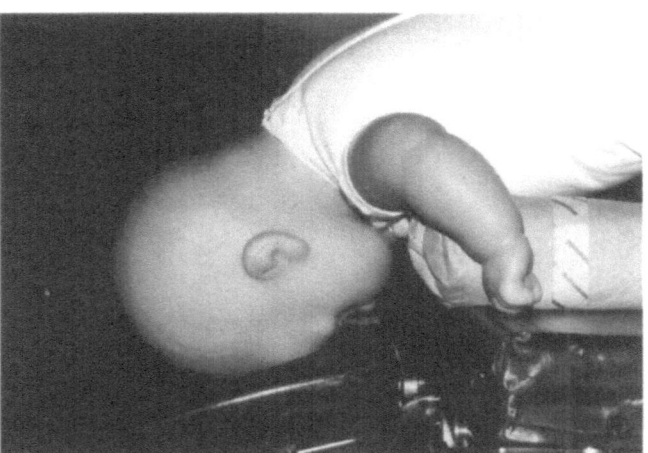

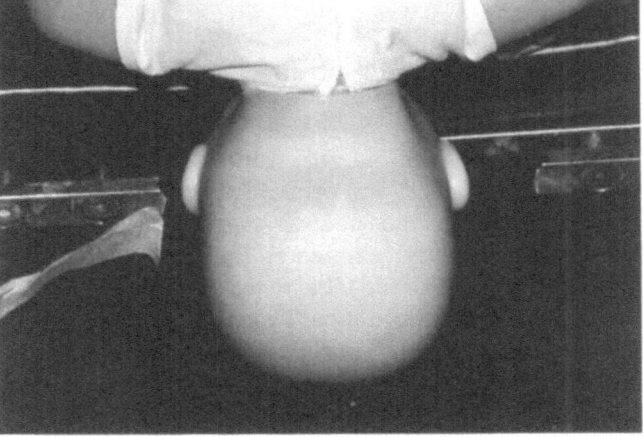

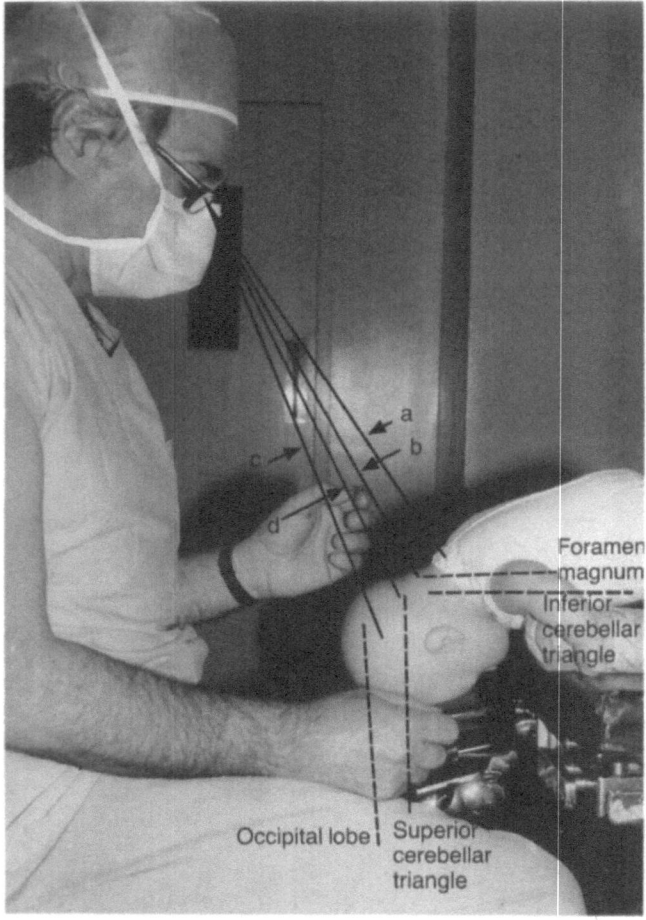

Foramen
magnum
Inferior
cerebellar
triangle

Occipital lobe | Superior
cerebellar
triangle

Figure 8.3. The relative positions of the surgeon and the child's head, with the newborn prone, illustrate (A) an excellent line of vision to the cervical spine; (B) an adequate line of vision to the foramen magnum (except in Chiari II children), and the inferior cerebellar triangle; (C) an unacceptable line of vision to the superior cerebellar triangle because of the ledge of squamous occipital bone and the transverse sinus; (D) a good line of vision to the occipital lobes. (Reprinted from Raimondi AJ. *Pediatric Neurosurgery—Theoretic Principles/Art of Surgical Techniques*. New York: Springer-Verlag, 1987.)

Specific Positions

Supine Position

The supine position is for frontal, frontopterional, parasellar, and orbital lesions. Placing the head in the neutral position, and extending it slightly, eliminates the need for lowering the head of the table when working at the chiasm or optic foramina. Conversely, flexing the head slightly provides more direct visualization of the cerebral convexity along the posterior frontal and anterior parietal regions of the brain. With the head neutral and slightly flexed, the supine position offers immediate access to the convexities and parasagittal areas of the frontoparietal, parietal, and parieto-occipital lobes. Turning the head

to either side (bringing the coronal suture parallel to the sagittal plane of the body), affords access to the convexity of the hemisphere, exposing the frontal, temporal, or occipital poles, and to the floors of the anterior and middle fossae, the tentorium, and the lateral surface of the opticocarotid region. It also puts the child into perfect position for a ventriculoperitoneal shunt, permitting the surgeon to insert the ventricular end into the body of the lateral ventricle through either the occipital horn (and the trigone) or the frontal horn.

Although extension of the head around the axis running through the auditory canals does not embarrass venous drainage, flexion may cause the horizontal rami of the mandibles to compress the internal jugular veins. Distraction of the skull prior to flexion minimizes this

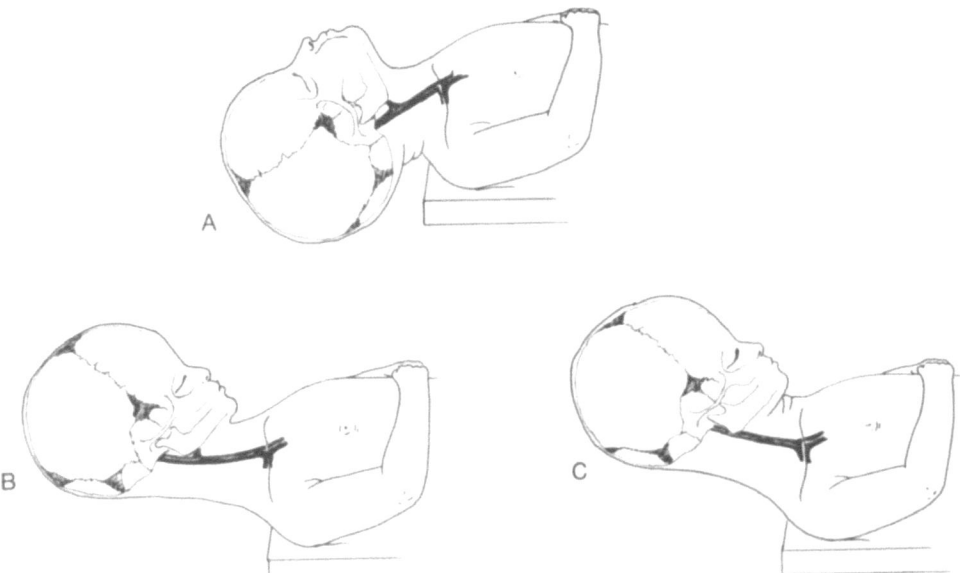

Figure 8.4. The head is drawn schematically, illustrating that, in extension, one need take no particular precautions to avoid compressing the jugular veins by the horizontal rami of the mandible, but that it is necessary to distract the head to avoid this in flexion. A: The head is extended around an axis running through the external auditory canals. B: The head is flexed around the same axis and distracted prior to being secured in position (either onto a headrest or in pins), avoiding jugular vein compression. C: The same as B, but the head has not been distracted, resulting in compression of the vertical ramus and angle of the mandible against the internal jugular vein. Diminished venous return and increased intracranial pressure are the consequences of this compression. (Reprinted from Raimondi AJ. *Pediatric Neurosurgery—Theoretic Principles/Art of Surgical Techniques.* New York: Springer-Verlag, 1987.)

risk of jugular compression of the mandibles (Fig. 8.4).

Prone Position

By placing the child prone with the head in the neutral position, one may expose the lambdoidal sutures (the parieto-occipital region) for immediate access to the occipital lobes. Flexing the head, and distracting it at the craniovertebral junction provides access to the squamous occipital, craniovertebral, and cervicothoracic regions. This position is used for occipital, inferior cerebellar triangle, foramen magnum, and superior cervical cord lesions (Fig. 8.5). When the child is prone, as when he is supine, particular care must be taken to distract the skull from the cervical spine prior to flexing it around the axis that runs through the auditory canals.

The pressure exerted by the weight of the skull tends to jam the mandible against the jugular veins, greatly diminishing cerebral venous drainage. This is worsened by the horseshoe headrest (which must be used in newborn and infants), but somewhat facilitated by the Gardner-Wells head-holder (which may be applied to the toddlers and older children). Whether using the horseshoe or Gardner-Wells head-holders, adequate clearance between the symphysis mentes and the body mat must be provided so that the endotracheal tube is not compressed. If this happens, it may either kink or be forced into one of the main stem bronchi. The weight of the drapes, especially as they become soaked during the procedure, may be enough to cause a decubitus of the chin. One must leave enough room for the anesthesiologist to check and manipulate the endotracheal tube.

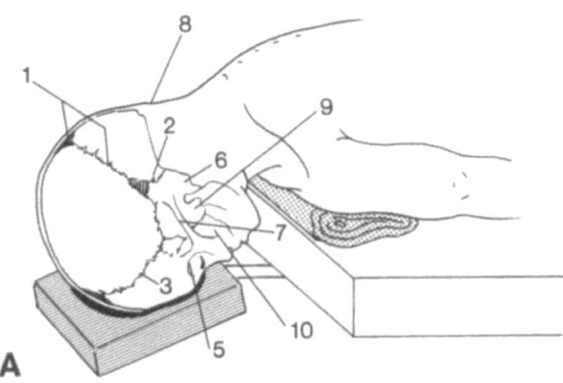

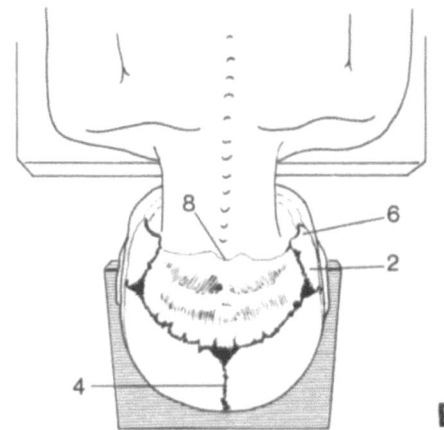

Figure 8.5. The prone position as herein illustrated demonstrates the lambdoidal (1), occipotomastoid (2), coronal (3), sagittal (4), and zygomaticofrontal (5) sutures; and mastoid (6) and the zygomatic arch (7); the rim of the foramen magnum (8), and the squamous temporal (9), and greater wing of the sphenoid (10) bones. (Reprinted from Raimondi AJ. *Pediatric Neurosurgery—Theoretic Principles/Art of Surgical Techniques.* New York: Springer-Verlag, 1987.)

Lounging (Sitting) Position

The "lounging" position is ideal for access to the posterior third ventricle, the superior cerebellar triangle, and the falx-tentorial junction. Irrespective of the physical inconvenience to the surgeon (Fig. 8.6) and the truly negligible risk of air embolism if appropriate anesthesiologic precautions are taken, it is the only safe way to operate lesions in the superior vermis, brachium conjunctivum, superior cerebellar hemispheres, opening of aqueduct into the fourth ventricle, the pineal region, and the great vein of Galen.

The same problems concerning mandibular compression of the jugular veins are encountered, to a much greater extent, when operating on the child in the lounging position as in either the supine or the prone positions. Here, again, the head must be distracted in order to avoid compression of the jugular veins. It must then be flexed around the axis of the auditory canals to provide the surgeon a direct line of vision to the superior portion of the cerebellar vermis and the tentorial opening. Fixing it securely holds it suspended against its own gravitational force. Figure 8.7A shows this with the use of a horseshoe head-holder in an infant, and Fig. 8.7B with the use of the

Gardner-Wells head-holder, which has been scaled down for children, but which has not been designed for the thinner calvarium or relatively more voluminous diploic spaces. The risk of air emboli through the diploë remains very real.

At times one must adapt. It may be necessary to place the head-holder very close to the operative field in order to assure solid purchase, and then to use a jugular vein for a central venous pressure line (essential in either the sitting or lounging positions). Some form of plastic draping may be used to cover the tubing. Such a situation is illustrated in Fig. 8.8, which also cones down on the distracted head, allowing one to appreciate how this separates the rim of the foramen magnum from the arch of C-1. All too often, consequently, because of the very wide range in body and head size of the pediatric population and the standard size of operating tables, the surgeon must improvise in positioning the child, and in securing him firmly in place. Pillows, sandbags, sheets, and so on, are pressed into service, even in the best-equipped pediatric operating rooms. A well-constructed car seat, which can be purchased almost anywhere, serves this purpose well. It may have to be cut, molded, or padded, but it is far superior to anything else avail-

Figure 8.6. The sitting position (A) requires the surgeon to sit or stand in a more tiring and uncomfortable posture than the prone or supine positions (B). (Reprinted from Raimondi AJ. *Pediatric Neurosurgery—Theoretic Principles/Art of Surgical Techniques*. New York: Springer-Verlag, 1987.)

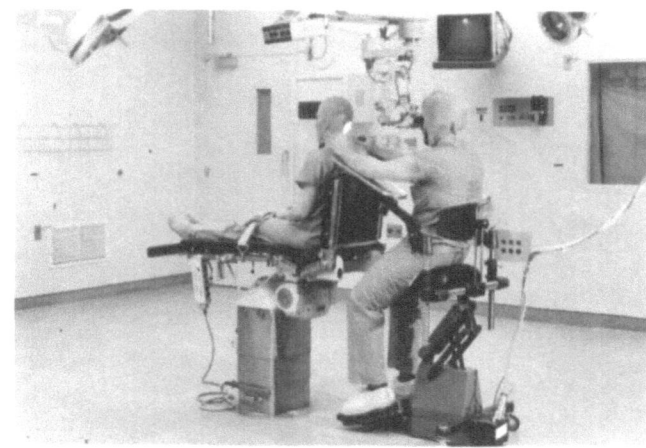

A

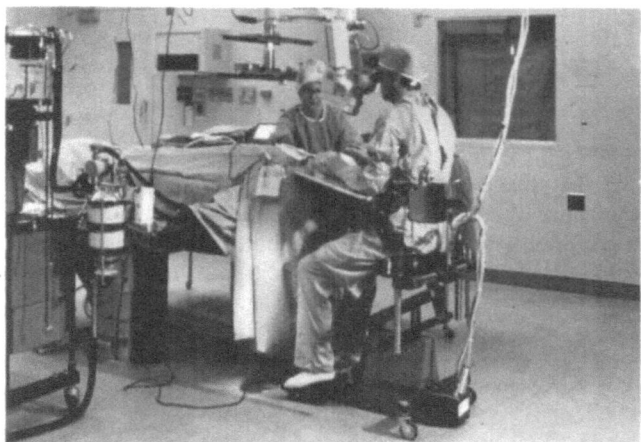

B

able or to any combination of pillows, towels, and sandbags. It is ideal for moving the child onto the operating table, and from it to the cart at the end of the procedure or in the event of an emergency. Most importantly, it facilitates fixing the infant or tiny toddler in position.

All this must be done relatively quickly because the anesthetized child, especially the newborn and infant, loses body heat rapidly.

Positioning of the Child Vis-à-vis the Surgeon's Line of Sight

The single most-important consideration in positioning the child for surgery is not to complicate his already diseased or injured central nervous system. The second most-important consideration is to position the child securely on the operating table so that the surgeon may move him at will, bringing him into a variety of positions throughout the procedure, so as to realize the primary goal of successful positioning: bringing the target area for the specific aspect of surgery being performed at that moment along the surgeon's line of vision. When this is accomplished, the operative exposure is optimal.

If the child is positioned properly, and if the surgeon takes advantage of the full range of motion (body pitch, roll, yaw, and slight elevation or depression of head and/or body), he may work comfortably with elbows relaxed at his side, and with his line of vision extending directly to the target area. This diminishes fatigue in that it allows the surgeon to work with

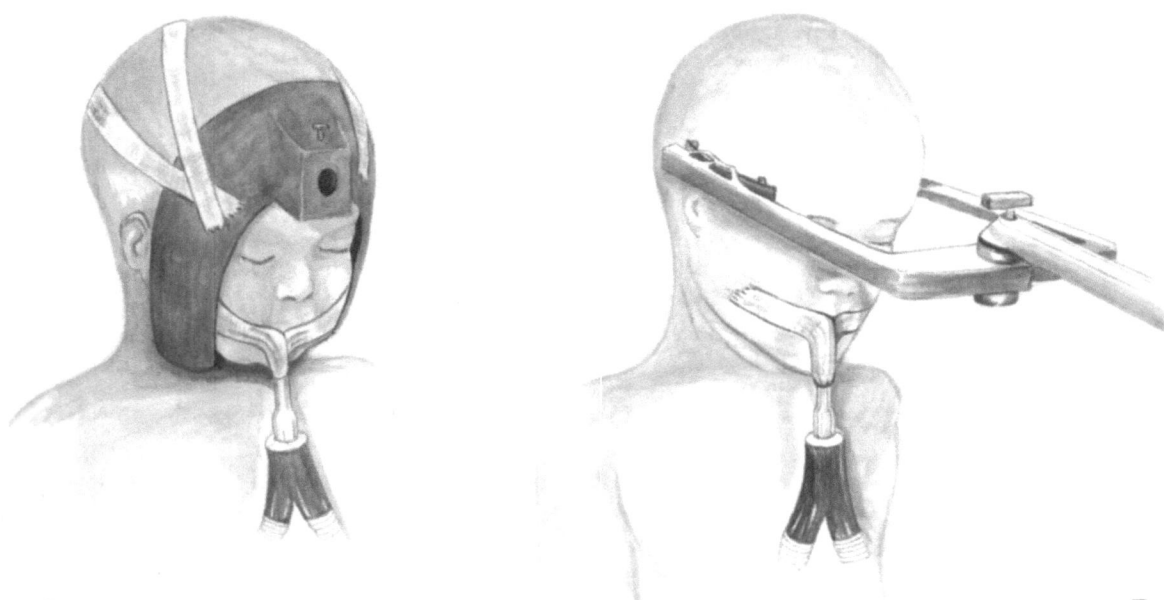

A   **B**

Figure 8.7. Fixation of the head in the lounging position is extremely important. In order to ensure maintenance of craniocervical junction distraction in the infant, one should tape the head to the horseshoe headrest and nestle the chin into the bottom of the headrest (A) or use the Gardner-Wells head-holder on a toddler (B). (Reprinted from Raimondi AJ. *Pediatric Neurosurgery—Theoretic Principles/Art of Surgical Techniques.* New York: Springer-Verlag, 1987.)

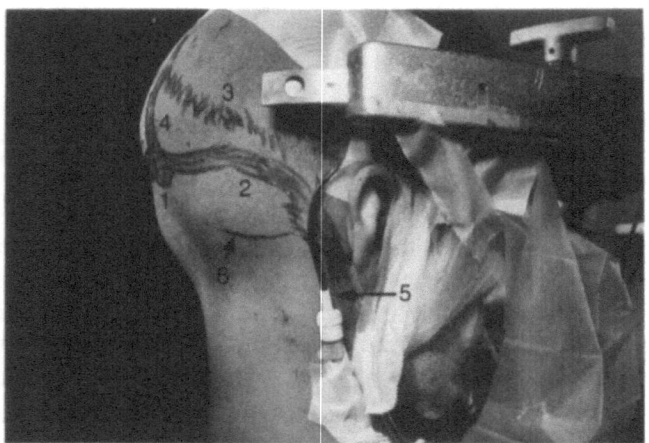

Figure 8.8. After distraction, the head-holder is locked, maintaining head and neck position throughout the operation. In this child, one of the pins had to be set close to the operative field, something which at times is unavoidable, and the tubing for the central venous line had to be brought superiorly and curved around the helix of the ear. The torcular Herophili (1), transverse sinus (2), squamosal suture (3), superior sagittal sinus (4), internal jugular vein (5), and horizontal plane of the squamous occipital bone (6) have been drawn on the scalp to provide orientation. (Reprinted from Raimondi AJ. *Pediatric Neurosurgery—Theoretic Principles/Art of Surgical Techniques.* New York: Springer-Verlag, 1987.)

his body in its natural posture. There should be little need to move about continuously, to use platforms, and to stretch or stoop during the operative procedure.

General Positions

The three basic positions—prone, supine, lounging—refer only to the body, not the head. After the body has been positioned, the anesthesiologist finalizes arrangement of his tubes to assure himself easy access to the face. The head is then positioned on the body, by the surgeon, to permit access to intracranial areas and anatomical structures.

In conceptualizing the operative procedure the surgeon must "visualize" the lesion, or desired anatomical area, within the head for the operation: head extended on a supine body for performing a bifronto-pterional craniotomy to expose the optic chiasm; head distracted and flexed at the craniovertebral junction with the body supine for exposure of the tentorial opening and pineal region; child's body in the lounging position with head distracted on C-1 and slightly flexed, for visualization of lesions in the superior cerebellar triangle; and so on. This overview guarantees correct anatomical orientation. It is used to transmit a holistic concept of positioning, structural anatomy, and surgical technique.

Prone Position

As in the supine position, if the head is kept neutral when the child is prone, the surgeon is obliged to lower it an inordinate (dangerous) distance in order to visualize directly those craniocerebral regions best exposed with the child prone: the occipital bone and the medial surfaces of the occipital lobes, the craniovertebral junction, inferior cerebellar triangle lesions and masses within the inferior portion of the fourth ventricle, and the upper cervical cord. Cisterna magna lesions are also exposed to advantage with the child prone.

The surgeon's best view of the posterior parietal region is with the head in the neutral position. Exposure of the occipital lobes, in-

ferior cerebellar triangle, and of the craniovertebral junction, necessitates lowering considerably the child's head and, thus, increasing intracranial venous pressure. In addition to this, the horizontal portion of the squamous occipital bone presents a visual obstacle, a ledge, separating the surgeon's line of sight from the craniovertebral junction. It puts the surgeon in an undesirable position for exposure and removal of upper cervical cord masses, decompression of the foramen magnum, and cisterna magna lesions extending into the region of the vallecula. If the head is distracted from C-1 and then flexed on it, then the medial surfaces of the occipital lobes, the region of the torcular Herophili and transverse sinuses, the foramen magnum and craniovertebral junction, the cisterna magna and inferior cerebellar triangle, and the superior cervical cord all come into a more direct line of vision and, subsequently, may be operated on more effectively.

It is important to consider in detail the anatomy of posterior fossa lesions when deciding whether to operate with the child in the prone or lounging positions. Factors other than pooling of blood within the posterior fossa warrant consideration if one operates on the prone child. Since the surgeon has no choice but to work standing at the head of the patient, it is impossible for him to position himself so as to have a direct line of vision to the region of the superior cerebellar triangle, the supracerebellar and quadrigeminal cisterns, the pineal gland Fig. 8.9, and the posterior portion of the third ventricle, when the child is prone. Although he may have an adequate line of vision of the inferior portion of the fourth ventricle and the vermis (from the fastigium inferiorly to the pyramis and then anterosuperiorly to the nodulus), he is in no position to deal effectively with superior draining veins going to the transverse sinuses and tentorium. Flexing the head upon the neck at the craniovertebral junction, and the neck on the thorax at the cervicothoracic junction, may increase somewhat the surgeon's visualization of the fourth ventricle and posterior surfaces of the transverse sinuses. It offers only partial visualization of the superior cerebellar triangle and, if pushed

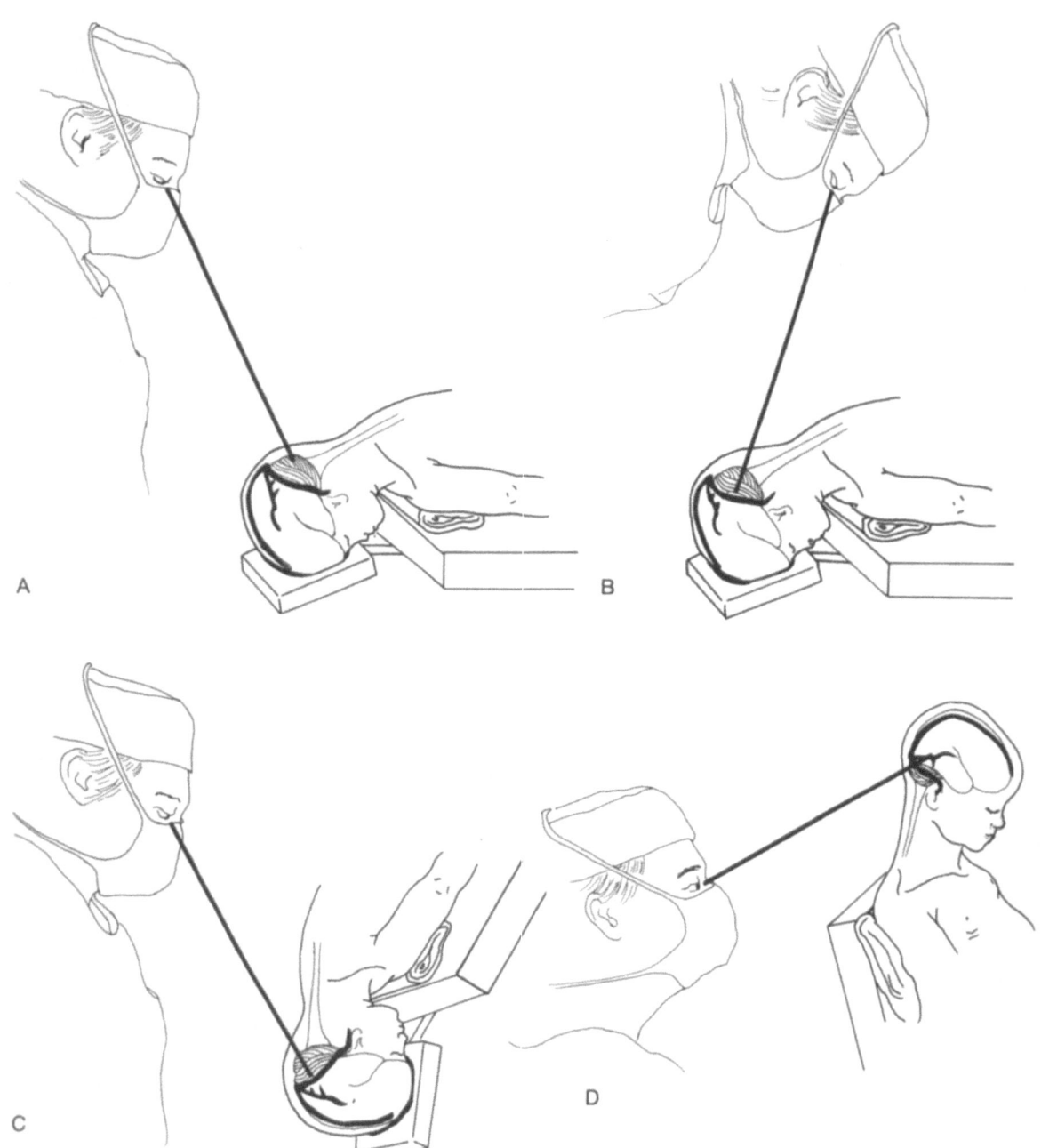

Figure 8.9. With the child prone (A) the surgeon cannot position himself to view the superior cerebellar triangle contents, the superior fourth ventricle, or the aqueduct because he is obliged to work from the head of the patient. In order to obtain a line of vision to the tentorial opening, the surgeon would have to elevate his head and move it caudad (B), or bring the child's head so low as to have him almost in a "headstand" position (C). In order to view completely the structures within the posterior fossa (D), the surgeon should place the child in the lounging position and place himself so that this line of vision is 45° from the horizontal. (Reprinted from Raimondi AJ. *Pediatric Neurosurgery—Theoretic Principles/Art of Surgical Techniques.* New York: Springer-Verlag, 1987.)

to the extreme, increases prohibitively intracerebral venous pressure.

In order to visualize the superior cerebellar veins and the structures within the superior cerebellar triangle, one must place himself so that his line of vision centers along a plane running 45° upward from the horizon. Consequently, the decision to operate on the posterior fossa with the child supine or lounging should not be one of preference of the surgeon, but one predicated entirely upon the location of the lesion that must be dealt with!

In 1974, Meridy and coworkers[1] reported complications during neurosurgery in the prone position in children. They noted an 8% incidence of cardiac arrhythmias, 3% incidence of respiratory complications (one of whom died), 2% incidence of cardiac arrests (two of whom died), and 1.6% incidence of air emboli. They state:

Many anesthetists and neurosurgeons advocate the sitting position for posterior fossa exploration. Such positioning provides an excellent view of the posterior cranial fossa with the operative site situated at the surgeon's eye level. In this position gravity effectively drains spinal fluid and blood from the operative wound. It also facilitates venous return to the heart, relieving intracranial venous stagnation and so controlling venous pressure and ooze, and ultimately brain swelling. . . . Many anesthetists and surgeons are fully aware of the disadvantages of the sitting position. Such pitfalls include the risk of venous air embolism, cardiovascular instability leading to systemic hypotension and diminished cerebral blood flow, the possibility of a patient sliding down the table during the operation and difficulty with temperature control.

Analysis of their results, comparing them to work published by others, especially Michenfelder et al.[2] reveals that there is no difference in the incidence of air emoblism or hypothermia in the two groups; the work reported by Michenfelder et al. studied over 2,000 patients.

The most experienced posterior fossa neurosurgeons[3-8] prefer the lounging position. Bucy[9] states:

For many years I operated in the posterior fossa with the patient lying prone and with the upper part of the body raised so that the long axis formed an angle of approximately 40° with the floor. I am now convinced that the sitting position is superior to this and less hazardous. Most of the risks of this position, principally those of air embolism and of arterial hypotension, can be avoided with care and are more than adequately compensated for by the advantages.

Lounging (Sitting) Position

The head should be distracted and flexed upon the atlas for both midline and lateral suboccipital craniotomies. The height of the table is then set so as to allow the surgeon a direct, horizontal, line of vision for making the skin incision and dissecting the muscle from the skull and atlas, but the setting should allow the table to be elevated when the craniotomy is performed and elevated and tilted forward when opening the dura and entering the superior cerebellar triangle. Also, convenient regulation of the surgeon's height with the operating table, raising it or lowering it, adds a significant amount of security to control of the Hudson brace for either perforator or burr use.

Unfortunately, one often speaks of the "sitting" position when, in fact, practically no neurosurgeon uses the sitting position. Rather, the patient, adult or child, is, in fact, put in the "lounging" position. This diminishes greatly the number of complications previously observed with the patient in the sitting position. These include significant diminution of cerebral blood flow, hypotension, and air emboli. Controlled ventilation has resulted in further diminution of the incidence of air emboli and cardiac arrhythmias, as have the routine insertion of central venous catheters. In fact, Marshall[10] reported that the incidence of air embolism dropped from 15% to 0% when positive/negative ventilation was used. Michenfelder and coworkers[2] reported only a 2% incidence of air emboli in 2,002 neurosurgical procedures performed on patients who were positioned "upright." They also noted a significant difference in air emboli in those patients positioned "upright" for cervical laminectomy and temporal craniectomy (less than 0.1%) when compared to those in the

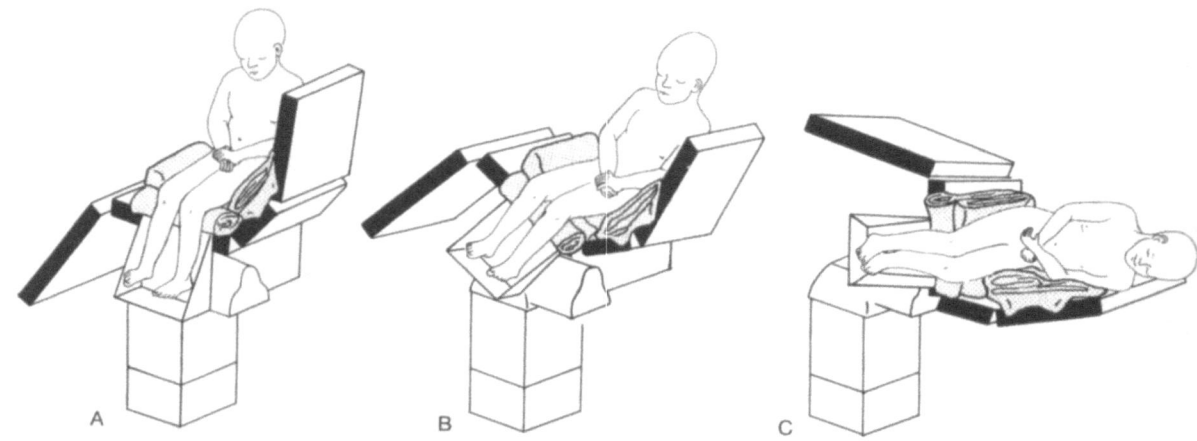

Figure 8.10. The child is positioned sideways (A) with the vertical axis of his body perpendicular to the long axis of the table, so that his arms are resting on the backrest and his legs are extended perpendicular to the table. Then, pushing the table downward (B) brings the child in to the horizontal position (C), without obliging the surgeon to stop his operative procedure. (Reprinted from Raimondi AJ. *Pediatric Neurosurgery—Theoretic Principles/Art of Surgical Techniques.* New York: Springer-Verlag, 1987.)

same position for suboccipital craniotomy (approximately 2%).

When Michenfelder and his associates[11] used the Doppler, they observed that the percentages of "air emboli diagnosed" rose to 6%, although the incidence of clinically significant air emboli did not change. It was Michenfelder et al.'s conclusion, consequently, that the Doppler diagnoses incidences of air embolism that would never become clinically significant complications, that the "threat of air embolism is not sufficient to contraindicate operating the patient in the sitting position." In fact, in his entire series he observed only 53 patients in whom air emoblism was diagnosed. The only death in his series was unrelated to air embolism. Michenfelder's "upright" position is a semireclining (lounging) posture.

An extremely interesting variant of the "sitting" position is one reported by Garcia-Bengochea and coworkers.[12] In brief, it consists of positioning the patient sitting, or preferably, lounging, but seated sideways on the operating table (Fig. 8.10). Lowering of the table in the event of air embolus, or other intraoperative complication necessitating positioning the patient horizontally, may be easily, safely, and immediately carried out.

The lounging position may minimize, not eliminate, the theoretical disadvantages of the "sitting" position. The child is placed horizontal, flexing the elevated calves upon the thighs, and the trunk at the hips, as illustrated in Fig. 8.11. This position is used whenever one wants to sit the child up, whether for a midline or lateral posterior fossa craniotomy. It is easier to place a child, especially an infant, in the lounging position than it is to sit him up, since one need only to distract and flex the head on the neck at C-1, place a pillow or sandbag across the thoracolumbar area, and center a pillow at the popliteal fossae.

Though an upper cervical laminotomy may be performed with the child in the lounging position, it really is not advisable, since it offers no advantages over the prone position. When the child is in the lounging position and the surgeon seated in a mechanical chair, rotation of the operating table around its axis cocks the head forward. This permits better visualization of the superior cerebellar triangle but does put the child into a sitting position (Fig. 8.12). As the child is rotated forward, the surgeon must both elevate his chair and extend his arms.

This position is ideal for occipital and suboccipital craniotomies (whether midline or

Figure 8.11. The table is pitched backward, bringing the knees in the same plane as the shoulders. (Reprinted from Raimondi AJ. *Pediatric Neurosurgery— Theoretic Principles/Art of Surgical Techniques.* New York: Springer-Verlag, 1987.)

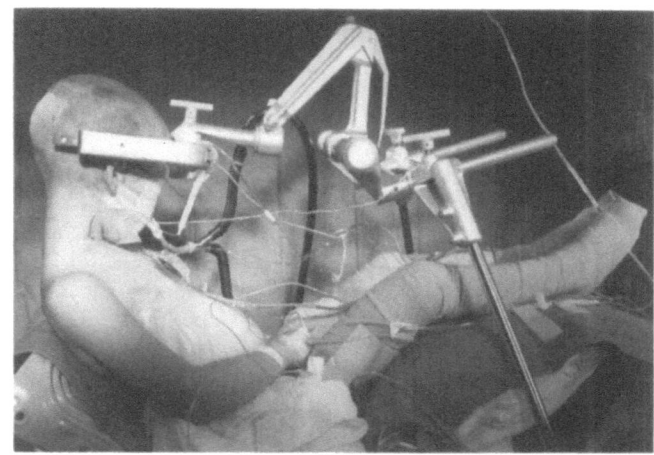

lateral), burr holes (unilateral or bilateral, diagnostic or therapeutic), mid- or lower-cervical laminotomy, and for bilateral ventriculoperitoneal shunts (whether shunting from occipital or frontal horns). It is not recommended for upper cervical laminotomy, even if the surgeon suspects that it may be necessary for him to enter the posterior fossa; the prone position is simpler and permits adequate visualization of the craniovertebral junction. The lounging position is considered feasible for mid- and lower-cervical laminotomy only when one expects to encounter either an arteriovenous malformation of the cervical cord or an intramedullary tumor, which may bleed considerably.

Incisions

Suboccipital Incision

Suboccipital skin flaps may be either medial (midline) or lateral, depending upon whether one must reflect the squamous portion of the occipital bone for a vermis tumor (medial), a cerebellar hemisphere, or a pontocerebellar angle tumor (lateral). The medial incision permits exposure of either the inferior cerebellar triangle (beneath the great horizontal fissue of the cerebellum) or the superior cerebellar triangle (above the great horizontal fissure of the cerebellum). The lateral incision permits a craniotomy, exposing the most lateral portion of the cerebellar hemisphere and the pontocerebellar angle.

Draping

Draping for both the midline and lateral incisions should allow for exposure of the skin for approximately 3 cm to either side of the incision.

Incision

The midline skin incision extends from approximately 1 cm above the inion to C-6. The lateral suboccipital incision extends from just above the lambdoidal suture down to the level of C-5, in a parasagittal plane, midway between the midline and the mastoid process.

Combined Supra- and Infratentorial Incisions

Draping

The draping is for a lateral suboccipital incision beneath the horizontal line of the base of the mastoid, and for an occipital incision above this line.

One of two combined supra- and infratentorial incisions may be used for such rare tumors in childhood as meningioma, acoustic neuro-

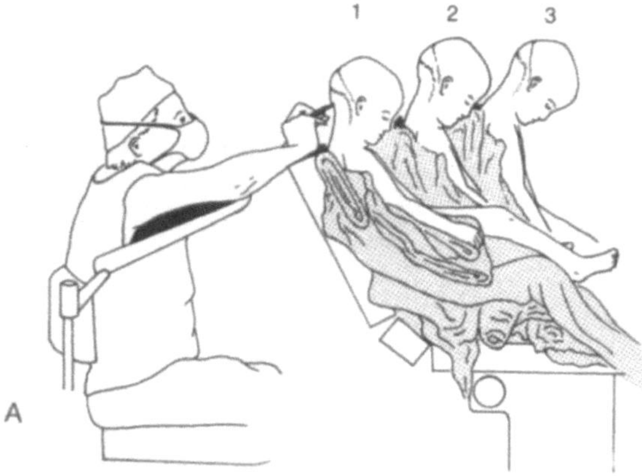

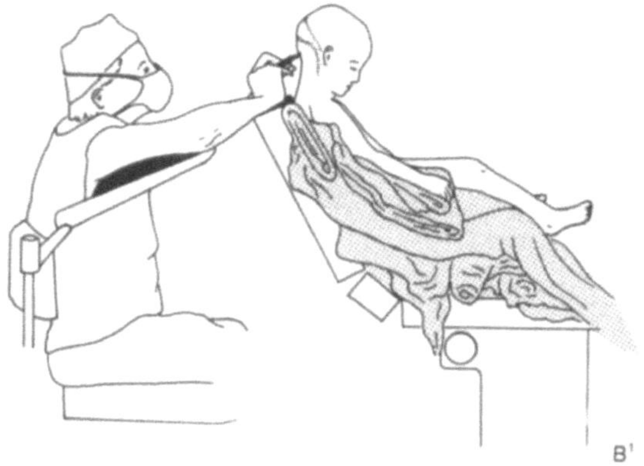

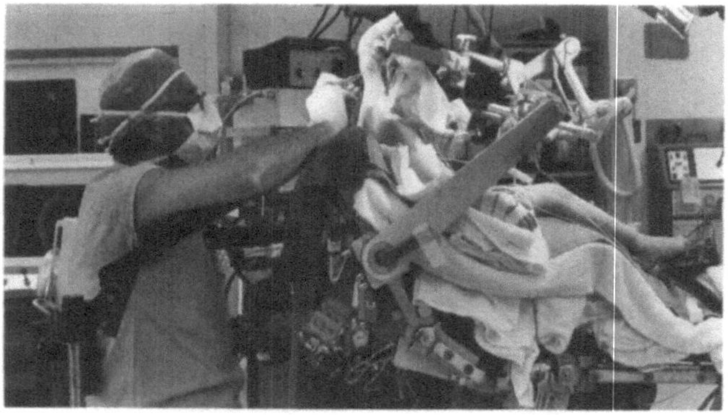

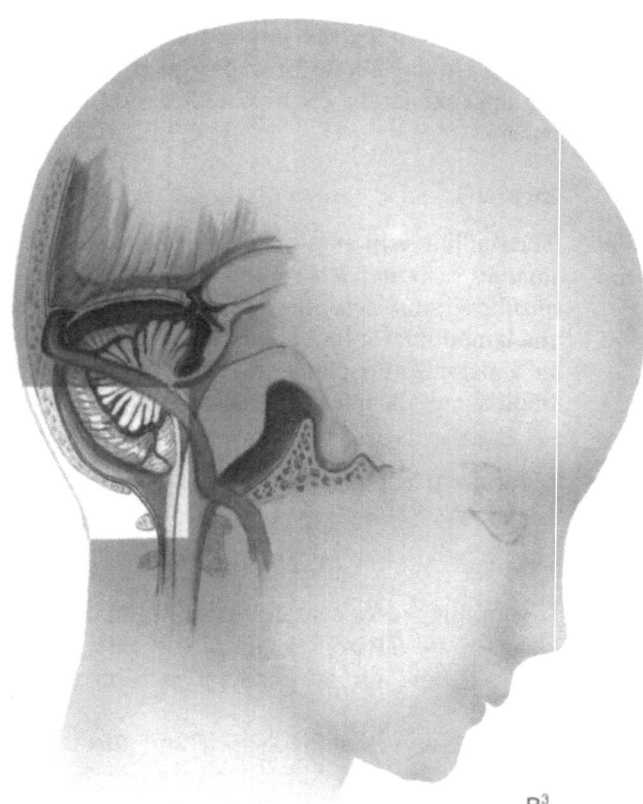

Figure 8.12. A: The surgeon is seated, his arms on a rest, for skin incision, muscle dissection, craniotomy, and inferior cerebellar triangle work (1). Pitching the operating table forward permits access to the IV ventricle and aqueduct (2) and superior cerebellar triangle (3). Notice that, as this is done, the child's head is progressively elevated. B: Photographic and diagrammatic demonstration of relative positions of surgeon, child, and posterior fossa contents for opening and exposure of inferior cerebellar contents. C: As the operating table is rotated forward the surgeon's arms are somewhat extended to permit work within the fourth ventricle. D: Exposure of the superior cerebellar triangle structures and the region of the quadrigeminal cistern necessitate further forward rotation of the child and extension of the surgeon's arms. (Reprinted from Raimondi AJ. *Pediatric Neurosurgery—Theoretic Principles/Art of Surgical Techniques.* New York: Springer-Verlag, 1987.)

Figure 8.12. (cont.)

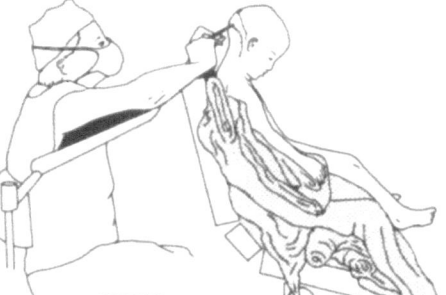

C'

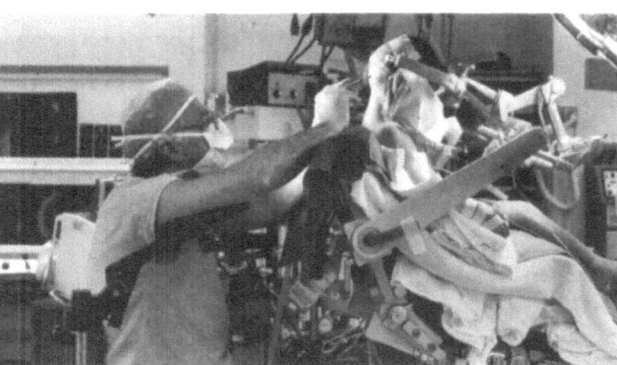

C²

C³

Figure 8.12. (cont.)

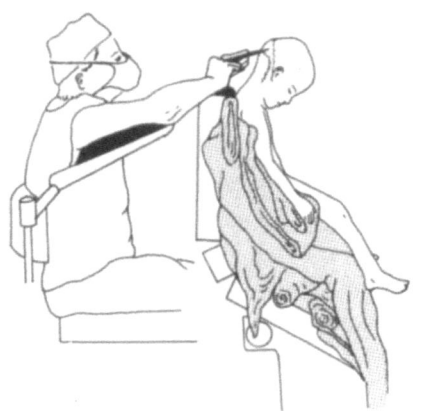

D¹

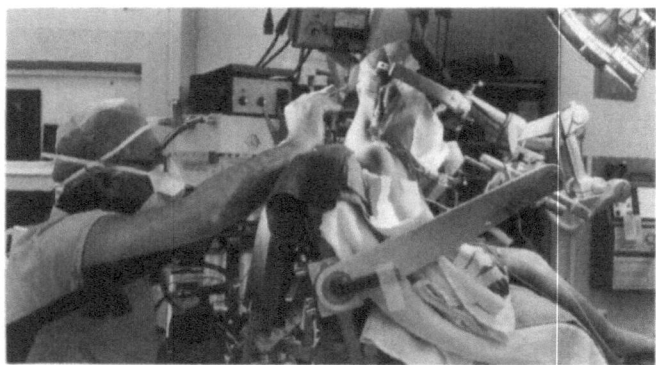

D²

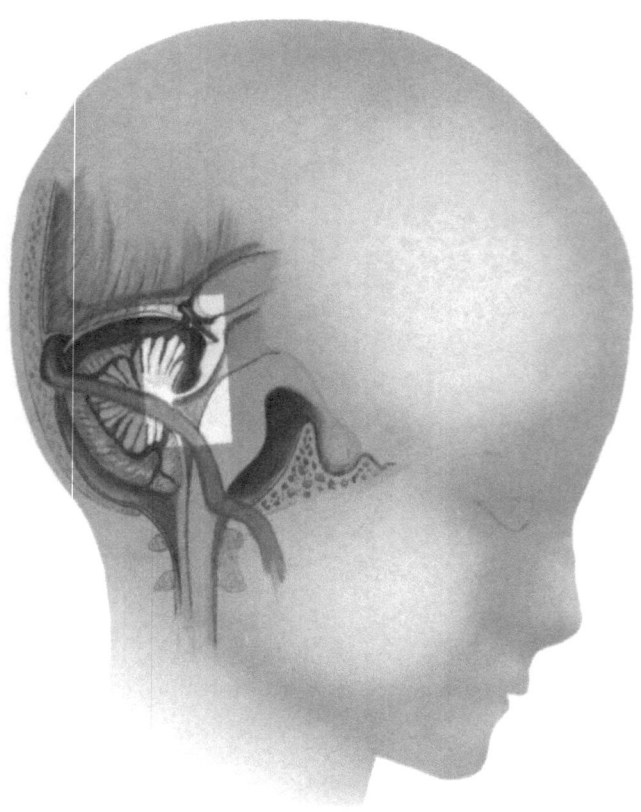

D³

ma, and glomus jugulare, which may grow within the supra- and infratentorial spaces as independent, "dumbbell" tumors growing on either side of the tentorium, or as large extra-parenchymal tumors extending into the supratentorial compartment from the pontocerebellar angle or into the posterior fossa from the rim of the tentorium. The incisions are the following:

1. For lesions involving the tentorium, a question-mark incision can be used, whose vertical limb extends superiorly from approximately the level of C-4 to the inion, and whose curvilinear limb extends anteriorly to the parietal eminence and then inferiorly to over the temporalis muscle. It is not necessary for the vertical limb to be located in the midline. In fact, since tumors that extend into both the supra- and infratentorial compartments either grow from the tentorium or from the pontocerebellar angle, much is in favor of the vertical limb being located midway between the midsagittal plane and the apex of the mastoid bone.
2. Access to glomus jugulare tumors also requires consideration of supra- and infratentorial flaps. However, since the glomus jugulare tumor begins within the temporal bone, it is essential to place the skin incision so as to have access to the mastoid, petrous, squamosal, and styloid portions of the temporal bone. A "sine-wave" incision is used (Fig. 8.13).

Suboccipital Flap

Suboccipital bone flaps may be midline or lateral.

Midline Suboccipital Craniotomy

The midline suboccipital craniotomy may be superior or inferior, depending upon whether the surgeon wishes to expose the superior or inferior cerebellar triangles (Figs. 8.14 and 8.15).

The superior cerebellar triangle has the horizontal fissure of the cerebellum as its base, the culmen monticuli as its apex, and the (inferolateral coursing) superior surfaces of the cerebellar hemispheres as its sides. The apex of the superior cerebellar triangle points upward.

The inferior cerebellar triangle also has the great horizontal fissure as its base, but its apex, the interval between the tips of the two cerebellar tonsils, points downward. The lateral surfaces of the inferior cerebellar triangle consist of the (superolateral coursing) cerebellar hemispheres.

Lesions within the superior triangle are tumors of the culmen monticuli and culmen declive, pineal tumors, and those arteriovenous malformations of the galenic system whose tributaries enter the great vein of Galen posteriorly. Inferior triangle lesions include medulloblastoma, cerebellar hemisphere astrocytoma, ependymoma of the fourth ventricle, foramen magnum tumors, arachnoid cysts of the cisterna magna, and other space-occupying lesions of the inferior vermis or cerebellar hemisphere.

Suboccipital Craniotomy Versus Craniectomy

The suboccipital craniotomy is preferable to the craniectomy! It permits the repositioning of a solid bone flap over the closed dura (Fig. 8.16), giving the child an anatomical reconstruction of the suboccipital area, not entrusting protection of the contents of the posterior fossa to the very thin muscle layers at the base of the skull. It eliminates completely the all-too-common suboccipital bulge observed in children who have had a posterior fossa craniectomy, a bulge holding herniated cerebellum (hence stretched cerebellar peduncles) and cerebrospinal fluid.

The practice of performing a suboccipital craniectomy and not closing the dura should be avoided! Failure to close the dura mater results in herniation of the posterior fossa contents into the dead space beneath the erector capitis and trapezius muscles, with resultant adhesions of cerebellar surface to muscular tissue and prolonged postoperative morbidity. The performance of craniectomy precludes replacement of the bone flap, resulting in the forma-

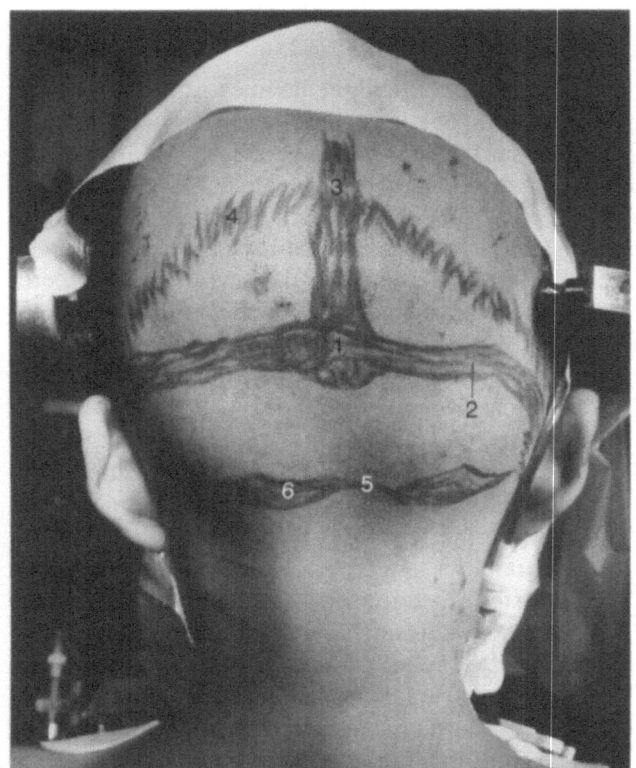

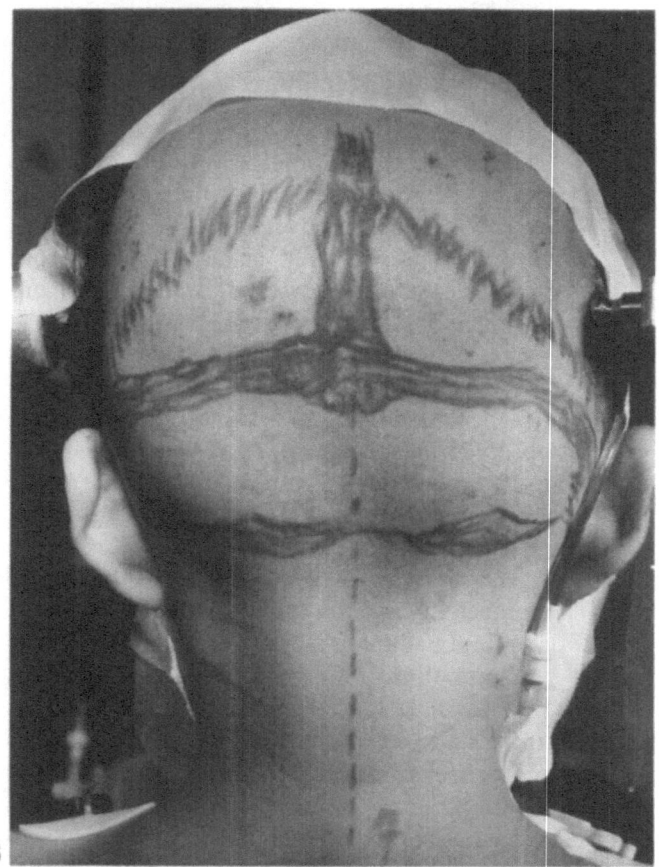

Figure 8.13. A: The significant landmarks for a suboccipital craniotomy have been drawn in. They are the torcular Herophili (1), the transverse sinus (2), the superior sagittal sinus (3), the lambdoidal suture (4), the rim of the foramen magnum (5), and the projection of the occipital condyles (6). Visual conceptualization of these landmarks permits one to plan appropriately for exposure of foramen magnum and inferior and superior cerebellar triangle lesions. B: The skin incision (broken line) has been drawn in. It extends from the inion to the level of C-7. C: The skin incision (black line) is shown in this transparency drawing of the skull and cervical vertebral column, as seen from the surgeon's point of view. The incision's center is at the rim of the foramen magnum (1), its upper extremity at the inion (2), its lower extremity at about C-7 (3). One may envision that retracting it (4), and the underlying erector capitis and cervicis muscles, as far laterally as the digastric grooves (5), exposes the entire squamous occipital bone (6), the bifid spinous process of C-2 (9). The retracted skin and erector capitis muscles are indicated (—o—) as is the retracted skin (–––) inferior to the level of the foramen magnum. It is not necessary to dissect the erector cervicis muscles from C-2, C-3, C-4, etc. D: This oblique transparency drawing permits one to envision the curvilinear course of the skin incision from over the squamous occipital bone, onto ther craniovertebral junction, and then along the supinous processes of the upper cervical vertebrae. The retracted tissue is indicated. The vertebral artery, and the entrance of Batson's plexus into the dural sinuses is at the most lateral exposure of the field (arrows). (Reprinted from Raimondi AJ. *Pediatric Neurosurgery— Theoretic Principles/Art of Surgical Techniques.* New York: Springer-Verlag, 1987.)

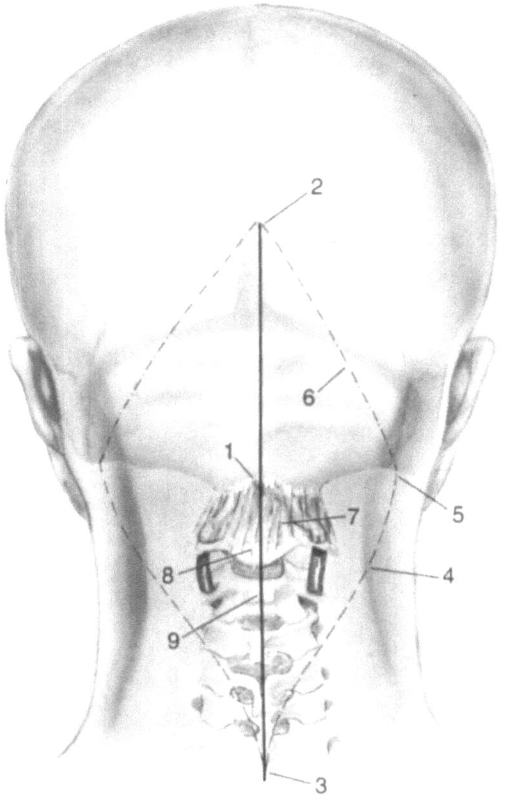

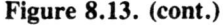
Figure 8.13. (cont.)

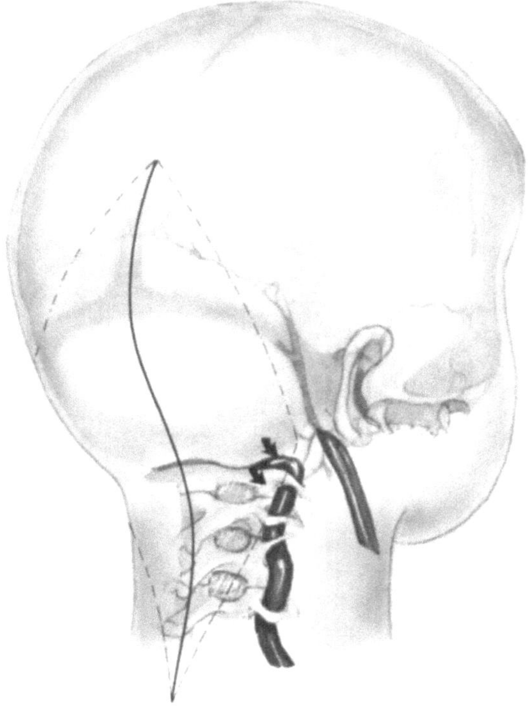

C

D

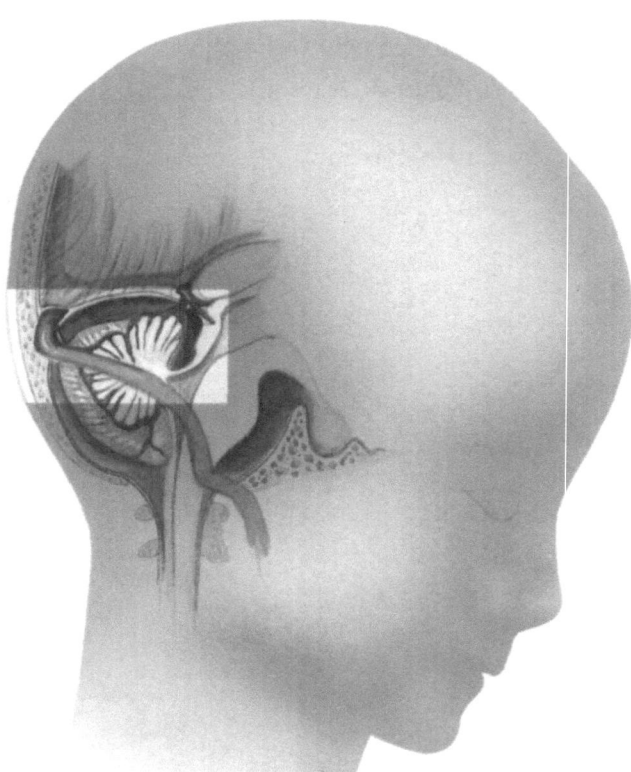

Figure 8.14. Superior cerebellar triangle. (Reprinted from Raimondi AJ. *Pediatric Neurosurgery—Theoretic Principles/Art of Surgical Techniques.* New York: Springer-Verlag, 1987.)

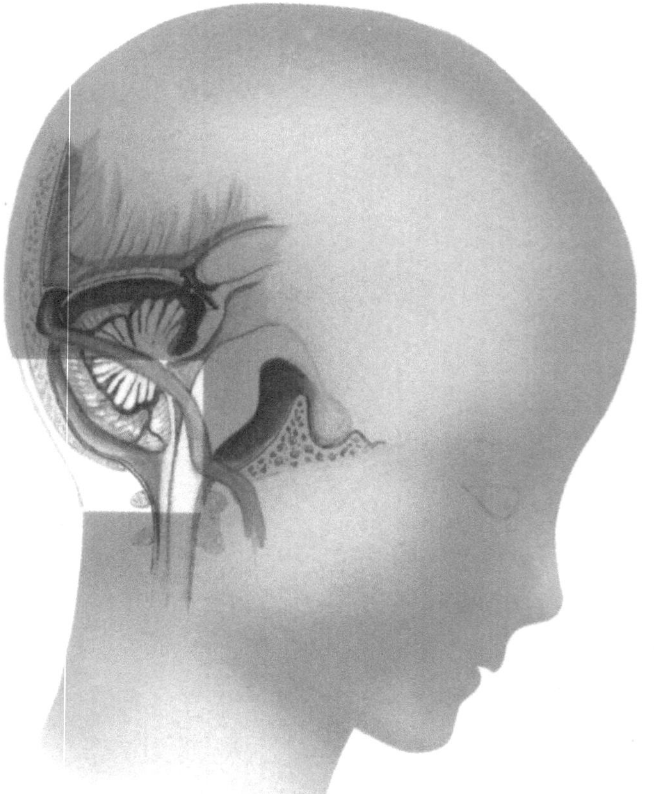

Figure 8.15. Inferior cerebellar triangle. (Reprinted from Raimondi AJ. *Pediatric Neurosurgery—Theoretic Principles/Art of Surgical Techniques.* New York: Springer-Verlag, 1987.)

tion of dense scar tissue between muscle and dura, and in an extremely high incidence of suboccipital bulging. This leaves the child with a weakened area over one of the most vital portions of the human brain. Craniectomy should be performed only when the craniotomy, for technical reasons, proves impossible to perform.

Lateral Suboccipital Craniotomy

The lateral suboccipital craniotomy is used for access to the most lateral portion of the cerebellar hemisphere, the pontocerebellar angle, the clivus, the jugular foramen, the posterior inferior cerebellar artery, and the region of the 9th, 10th, and 11th cranial nerves.

As has already been described, dissection of the soft tissue for exposure of the squamous portion of the occipital bone entails stripping of the periosteum from it (Fig. 8.16). However, this stripping is not complete because it is limited to the highest and lowest nuchal lines, the insertion of the erector capitis and trapezius muscles, respectively. Above and below the highest nuchal line the periosteum may be preserved, but not below it except at the rim of the foramen magnum. In planning either a superior or an inferior midline occipital flap, one must remember that the lambdoidal suture runs well superior to the transverse sinus medially, but that it becomes superimposed on the venous sinuses at the point where the transverse sinus passes into the sigmoid sinus. This is also the area where the parieto-occipital (lambdoidal), occipitomastoid, and parietomastoid sutures meet.

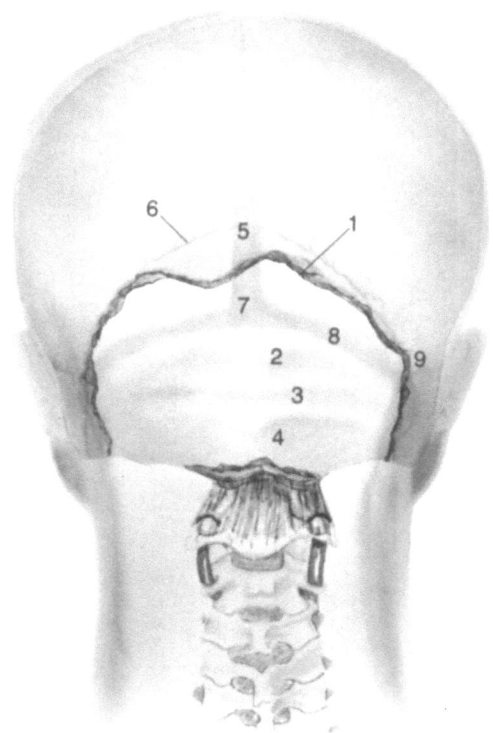

Figure 8.16. Periosteal dissection for suboccipital craniotomy. The periosteal dissection (1) has been brought above the highest nuchal line (2). This drawing shows both the intermediate (3) and lowest (4) nuchal lines. Lambda (5) and the squamosal suture (6) are superior to the torcular Herophili (7) and the transverse sinus (8) medially, but the squamosal suture is at the same level as the sigmoid sinus (9) laterally. (Reprinted from Raimondi AJ. *Pediatric Neurosurgery—Theoretic Principles/Art of Surgical Techniques.* New York: Springer-Verlag, 1987.)

Midline Suboccipital Craniotomies

Inferior Suboccipital Craniotomy

Suboccipital craniotomy for access to the inferior cerebellar triangle (Fig. 8.17) consists of reflecting a triangular bone flap whose base is located beneath the transverse sinus, along the highest nuchal line, and whose (flat) apex is the rim of the foramen magnum. Care should be taken to dissect the periosteum from the outer (posterior) rim of the foramen magnum, but

not to extend the dissection around the rim of the foramen magnum, since use of periosteal elevators in this area may cause damage to the annular sinus, causing profuse venous bleeding or air emboli.

The Gigli saw guide should be passed horizontally from one burr hole to the other, and then the Gigli saw should be used to connect the burr holes with a linear osteotomy. Passage of the saw guide horizontally presents no difficulties, but great care must be taken at the midline, where there is often a spine of occipi-

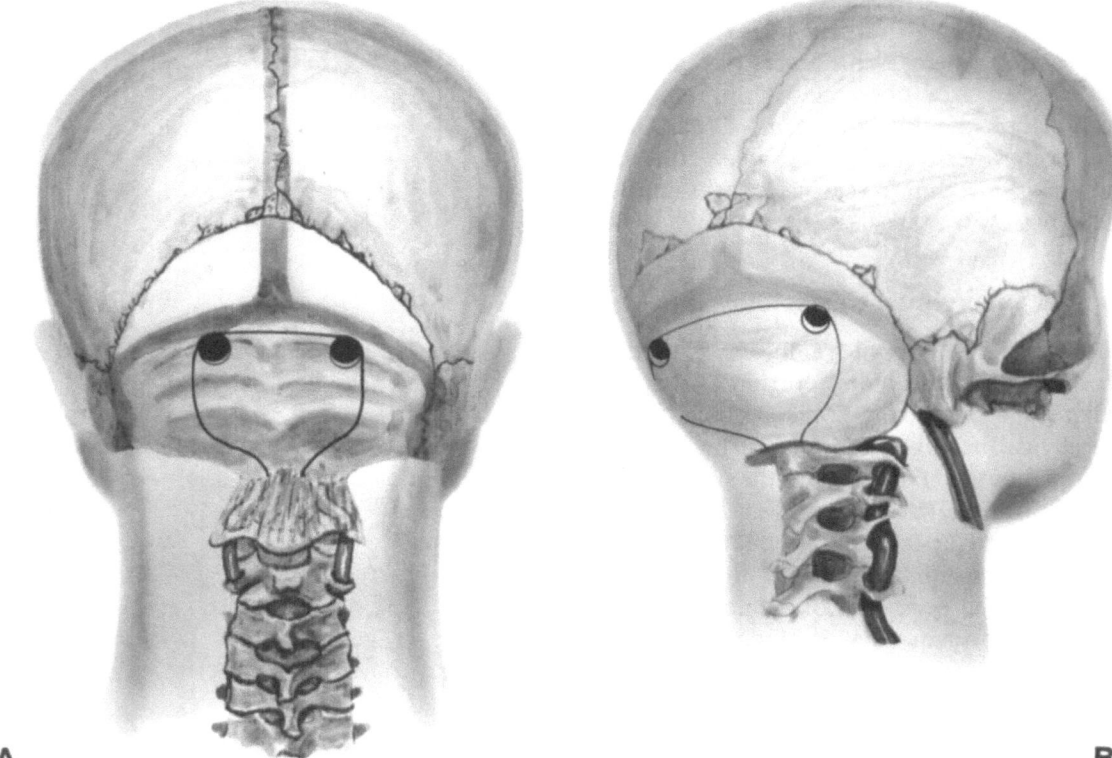

A   **B**

Figure 8.17. A: Inferior suboccipital craniotomy as viewed in a straight posteroanterior line, illustrating the burr holes and osteotomy lines outling the free (squamous) occipital bone flap. B: Inferior suboccipital craniotomy as viewed in a postero-oblique line. (Reprinted from Raimondi AJ. *Pediatric Neurosurgery— Theoretic Principles/Art of Surgical Techniques.* New York: Springer-Verlag, 1987.)

tal bone extending into the dural groove at the fissure between the cerebellar hemispheres. Molding of the tip of the Gigli saw guide, if obstruction is encountered at the midline, and dissecting first from the right and then from the left, always feeling the tip of the guide against bone and dura, eases the guide across the midline into the contralateral burr hole. If it proves to be difficult to pass the guide directly horizontally from one burr hole to the other, the tip should be directed inferiorly toward the rim of the foramen magnum (where the inner occipital spine is least prominent) and then to sweep it superiorly once the tip has crossed the midline.

The saw guide should then be used to dissect the dura from the inner surface of the occipital bone toward the foramen magnum, by advancing it in that direction, remembering that the opening of the posterior rim of the foramen magnum is extraordinarily small (measuring 2.0 cm) and that the lateral surfaces of the foramen magnum consist of thick bony struts that lead to the occipital condyles. Therefore, an attempt to pass the Gigli saw guide directly inferiorly from the burr holes will result in the guide encountering the bony struts along the superior surface of the occipital condyles, and then being deflected medialward.

It is not advisable to attempt to pass the saw guide from a burr hole downward across the rim of the foramen magnum, in the epidural space, since this, too, puts the annular sinus at risk. Rather, the guide should be advanced inferiorly as far as the rim of the foramen magnum, removing it from time to time to measure the length of guide inserted (to be certain that one is at the foramen magnum). No attempt should be made to strip the outer layer of the dura mater from the rim of the foramen magnum; it adheres tenaciously to the rim, the point at which it is continuous with the periosteum. In fact, the outer layer of the dura mater (which is, indeed, the inner periosteum of the skull) is continuous with the periosteum (pericranium) at all foramina of the skull. This dural duplication forms the annular sinus.

A craniotomy is used to connect the lateral surface of each burr hole to the rim of the foramen magnum, but it must not be brought all the way through the bone lest it tear the annular sinus. The triangular, free bone flap is separated from the dura by use of a Penfield No. 3 dissector or an Oldberg periosteal elevator, gradually lowering the base, as the dissection proceeds, until the dural-periosteal transition point at the rim of the foramen magnum is visualized. Now, dura-periosteum may be dissected from the rim of the foramen magnum, within the free flap, under direct visual control, either with a sharp periosteal elevator or by cutting it from the bone with a No. 15 blade. This exposes the point at which the dura mater, atlanto-occipital membrane, and periosteum/pericranium join. This now redundant mass of connective tissue, measuring approximately 3×5 mm, may be dissected from the inner layer of the dura mater as it continues inferiorly over the craniocervical junction. If one wishes a bit more lateral exposure at the rim of the foramen magnum, a rongeur may be used to nibble away 2 or 3 mm of bone, extending the bites toward the occipital condyles.

Superior Suboccipital Craniotomy

The superior suboccipital crnaiotomy (Fig. 8.18) is performed by placing four burr holes in a quadrilateral fashion, the upper two along the highest and the lower two along the lowest nuchal lines. The same precautions as for the inferior suboccipital craniotomy are taken in passage of the Gigli saw guide across the midline. The Gigli saw is recommended for connecting the burr holes to one another, since one will not be crossing the foramen magnum. Once the Gigli saw guide has been passed horizontally across the midline, it may be swept in an arc from the opposite superior to the opposite inferior burr hole in one direction first, then in the opposite direction. This frees all of the dura, and permits safe osteotomies.

Lateral Suboccipital Craniotomy

The lateral suboccipital opening (Fig. 8.19) is placed entirely within the squamous portion of the occipital bone, at its most extreme lateral portion (immediately inferior to the transverse sinus and posteromedial to the jugular bulb).

Consequently, the occipitomastoid suture and the digastric groove are at the anterior edge of the bone flap, and the lambdoidal suture is considerably superior to it. The access it offers to the lateral surface of the cerebellar hemisphere is excellent. It is the only flap that permits one to work effectively in the pontocerebellar angle, the jugular foramen, or along the lateral surface of the medulla oblongata and pons. A craniectomy is neither necessary nor advisable.

Because these flaps are very small, measuring approximately 4×4 cm in surface area, one should use a single burr hole. This is placed in the squamous occipital bone, immediately beneath the point at which the transverse sinus passes into the sigmoid sinus. The linear osteotomy is then performed with a craniotome, since it is not possible to use the Gigli saw properly for such a small flap. Also, the beveling of the squamous occipital bone as it passes from its vertical to its horizontal portions at the base of the skull, thickening remarkably both medially at the inner surface of the occipital condyles and laterally at the mastoid base, renders attempted passage of the Gigli saw guide dangerous.

Medial (Midline) Suboccipital Dural Opening

Medial suboccipital openings (Figs. 8.20, 8.21, and 8.22) permit exposure of either the inferior or superior cerebellar triangles, with the

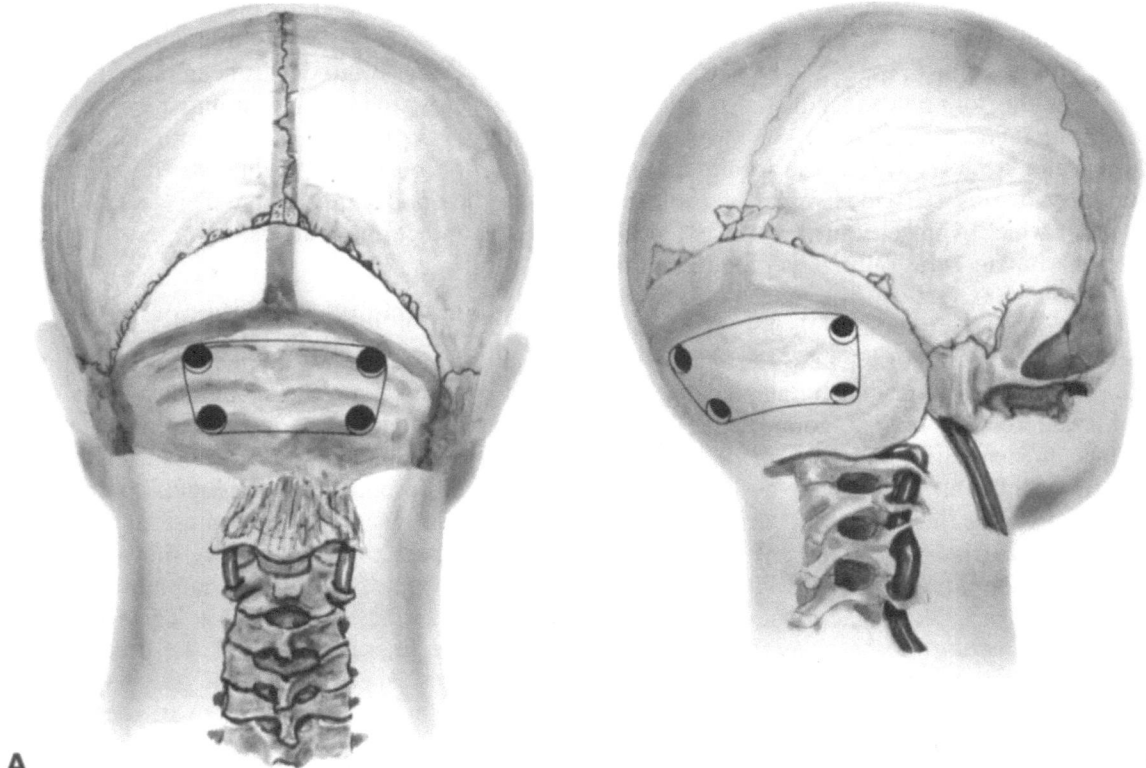

A   **B**

Figure 8.18. A: Superior suboccipital craniotomy as viewed from the straight posteroanterior line. The upper burr holes are inserted along the highest nuchal line, the bottom two along the lowest nuchal line. The middle nuchal line, when present, runs across the center of the free flap. B: Superior suboccipital craniotomy as viewed from a postero-oblique line. (Reprinted from Raimondi AJ. *Pediatric Neurosurgery— Theoretic Principles/Art of Surgical Techniques.* New York: Springer-Verlag, 1987.)

former being used either for inferior vermian/ fourth ventricle lesions or for lesions within the foramen magnum, and the latter for superior vermian and pineal region tumors.

Inferior Cerebellar Triangle Dural Opening

Inferior cerebellar triangle exposure may be used for lesions within the fourth ventricle and inferior cerebellar vermis, or for those extending across the foramen magnum. This distinction (inferior and superior cerebellar triangles) is of value since fourth ventricle and vermian lesions, which are generally very large at the time of surgery, may be removed without opening the dura across the annular sinus and without extending the durotomy into the

atlanto-occipital membrane. Thus, for inferior triangle lesions (within the inferior vermis or fourth ventricle), careful placing of the durotomy incision allows the surgeon to fashion a sling from the inferior portion of the dura. Such a sling serves to suspend the inferior cerebellar hemispheres and tonsils, preventing them from herniating into the operative field, and into avoid potentially damaging traction on the brain stem.

The dura is cut inferomedially from the point of opening (which is best made at approximately the junction of the superior and inferior thirds of the dura exposed by the suboccipital craniotomy). A cut across the midline from right to left, connecting the two inferomedially coursing durotomy incisions, is

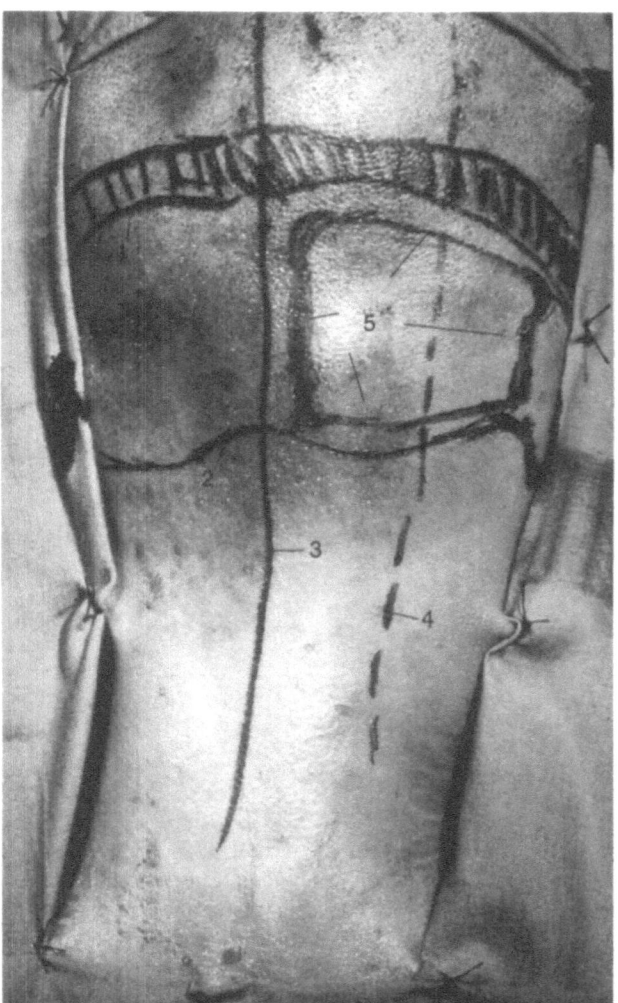

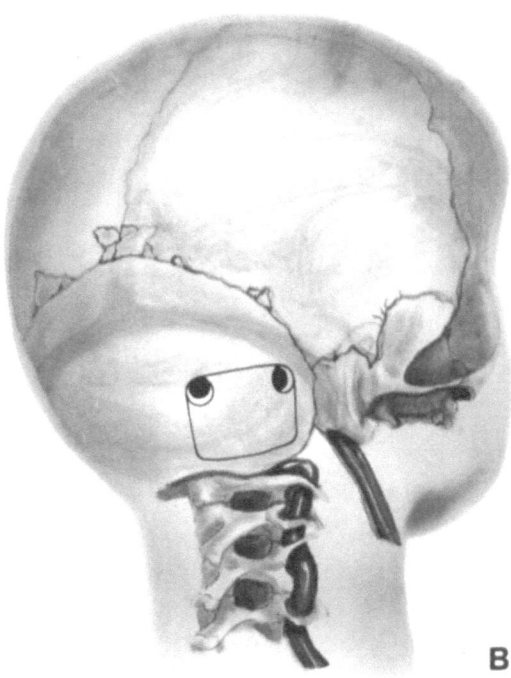

Figure 8.19. A: Lateral suboccipital craniotomy for removal of a solid cerebellar hemisphere astrocytoma. Transverse sinus (1), foramen magnum (2), midline (3), and incision line (4) have been marked off. Subsequent to this, the area for the suboccipital craniotomy (5) was drawn on the skin. B: Lateral suboccipital craniotomy as viewed along a posterior oblique line, showing the flap in relationship to the transverse sinus superiorly, the sigmoid sinus anteriorly, the point at which the squamous occipital bone passes from a vertical to a horizontal structure inferiorly. Note that the flap does not extend to the midline. At times, one may find it advantageous to place two burr holes, as illustrated here. (Reprinted from Raimondi AJ. *Pediatric Neurosurgery—Theoretic Principles/Art of Surgical Techniques.* New York: Springer-Verlag, 1987.)

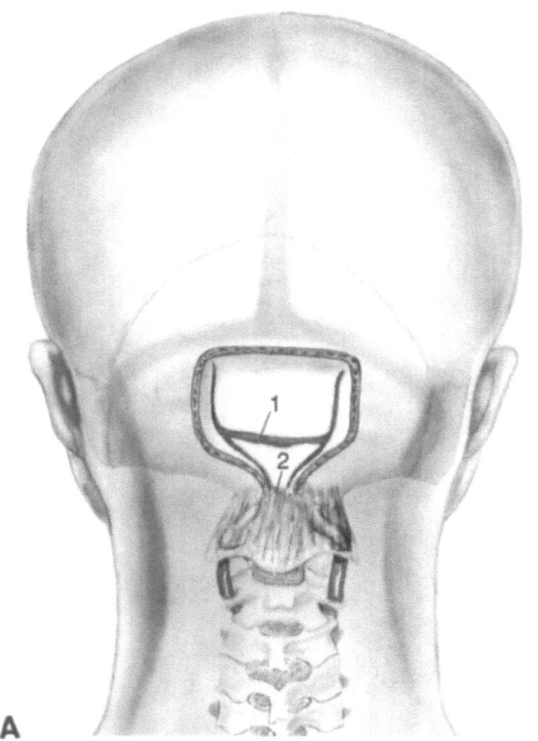

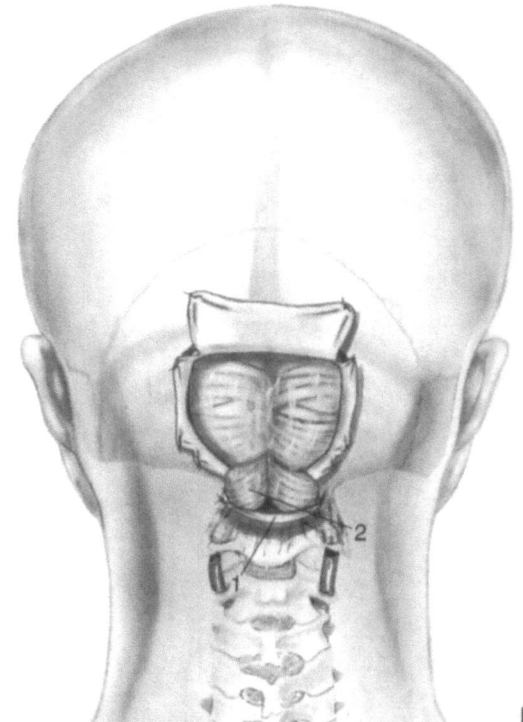

A

B

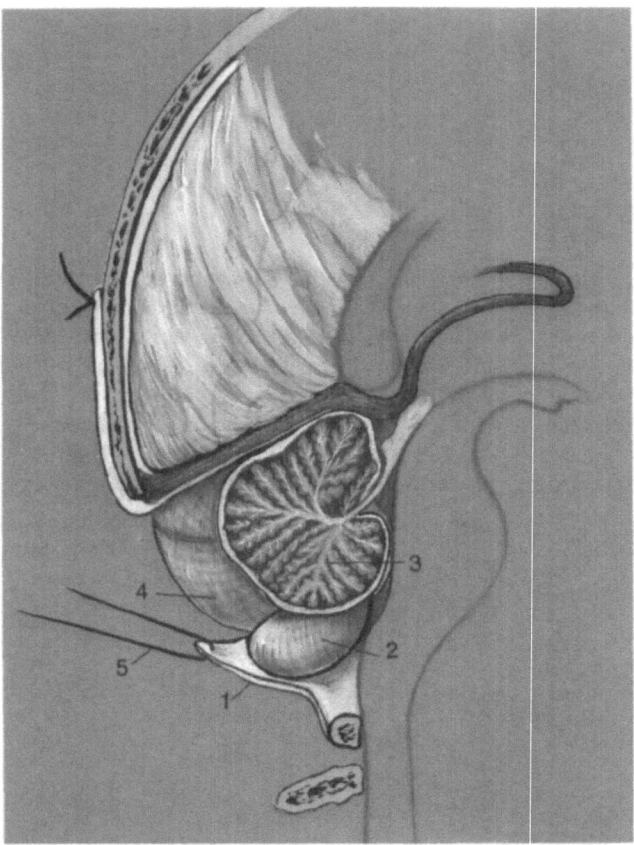

C

Figure 8.20. A: Dural flaps for access to the inferior triangle. The lines of the two U-shaped dural flaps are indicated. They permit opening the dura so as to fashion a sling to suspend the cerebellar tonsils and minimize traction on the cerebellar peduncles. The horizontal dural cut (1) is placed well above the rim of the foramen magnum (2). B: The dura is reflected laterally over each side and superiorly over the base of the triangular laterally over each side and superiorly over the base of the triangular craniotomy. The sling (1) is shown supporting the tonsils (2) in the posterior fossa. This latter point is illustrated to much better advantage in C. C: The sling (1) gives support to the tonsils (2) and, consequently, to the inferior cerebellar vermis (3), and medial portions of the cerebellar hemisphere (4). The ligatures suspending it (5) are sewn to the erector capiti muscle fascia. (Reprinted from Raimondi AJ. *Pediatric Neurosurgery—Theoretic Principles/Art of Surgical Techniques.* New York: Springer-Verlag, 1987.)

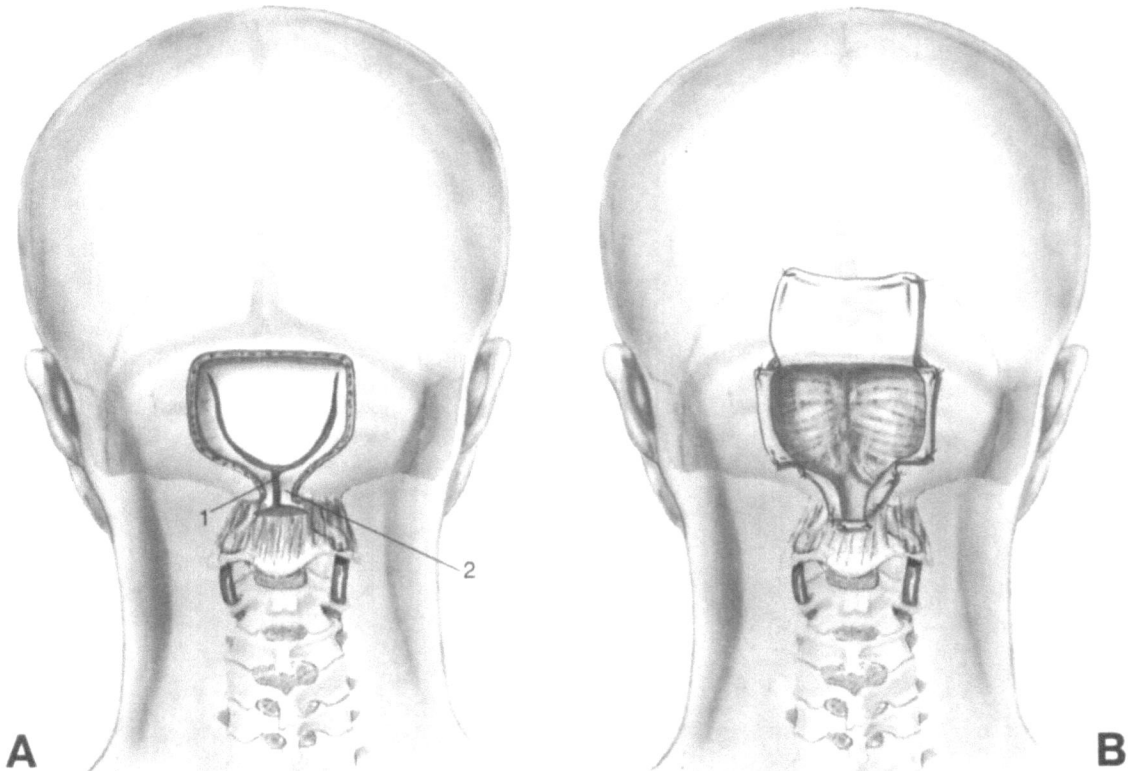

Figure 8.21. A: This is the recommended durotomy for lesions within, or extending into, the foramen magnum. There is a vertical durotomy (1) across the level of the foramen magnum (2). B: The dura is reflected superiorly over the craniotomy edges and inferiorly over the arch of C-1. This exposes completely the tonsils, inferior vermis, and cisterna magnum. (Reprinted from Raimondi AJ. *Pediatric Neurosurgery—Theoretic Principles/Art of Surgical Techniques.* New York: Springer-Verlag, 1987.)

made with tenotomy scissors. The cut across the midline may have to be made with heavier scissors because of the dural reduplication at the annular and cerebellar sinuses. If a dural sinus is encountered it may either be coagulated with the bipolar forceps or clipped. This latter technique is discouraged, since the clips may become dislodged at the time of closure. The result may be bleeding into the posterior fossa, which, unfortunately, may occur without the surgeon being able to identify it. Also, and of more immediate danger, opening the dural sinuses subjects the child to air embolism. Immediate, or incomplete, closure (often the case when clips are used) of these dural sinuses may present continued risk of air embolism throughout the operative procedure.

Opening of the dura over the craniovertebral junction for inferior triangle lesions at the foramen magnum, entails fashioning a U-shaped dural flap, with the convexity pointing inferiorly beginning at the superolateral border on each side of the craniotomy. It should be extended inferomedially to approximately 0.5 cm above the dural fold located just beneath the posterior arch of the foramen magnum bilaterally. Then, a midline durotomy is cut vertically across the foramen magnum, coagulating the annular sinus with a bipolar forceps on either side of the cut. The spinal dura (there is only one layer) is then cut horizontally, first to one side and then to the other, immediately above the arch of C-1. (It is almost never necessary to remove the arch of C-1 in order to gain complete access to the structures within the foramen magnum. In rare circumstances

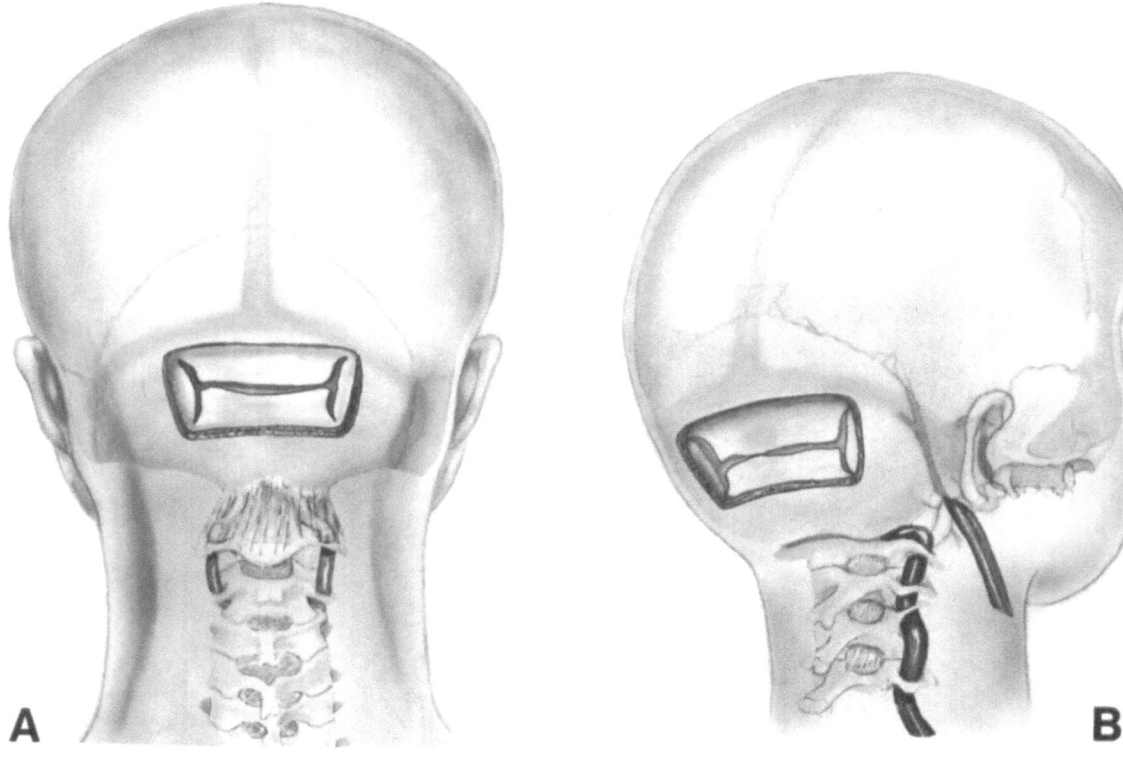

Figure 8.22. The double trapdoor durotomy for access to the superior cerebellar triangle permits the surgeon the option of reflecting only the superior trapdoor, or both. A: The durotomy lines are depicted for complete exposure of the superior cerebellar triangle. B: Postero-oblique perspective of the double trapdoor durotomy. (Reprinted from Raimondi AJ. *Pediatric Neurosurgery—Theoretic Principles/Art of Surgical Techniques.* New York: Springer-Verlag, 1987.)

the tumor does extend beneath the level of C-1, at which time an osteotomy at either lateral extremity of the arch of C-1 allows the surgeon to displace this arch inferiorly and, thus, extend the dural incision almost to the level of C-2). The arch of C-1 may then be anchored back into anatomical position at the end of the procedure.

Superior Cerebellar Triangle Dural Opening

Superior cerebellar triangle exposure and access to the pineal region, through a quadrilateral craniotomy flap, is attained by a double trapdoor durotomy. This permits one to reflect the upper trapdoor superiorly, if the culmen

monticuli and pineal region are the target area(s), and the lower trapdoor inferiorly, if the superior portion of the cerebellar hemispheres is the target area.

Lateral Suboccipital Dural Opening

For access to the lateral cerebellar hemisphere or the pontocerebellar angle (Fig. 8.23), a double trapdoor durotomy with the superior trapdoor being larger than the inferior, is reflected. The advantages of a larger superior segment rest in ease of identification of the superior cerebellar veins and the lateral sinus to which they are tributary.

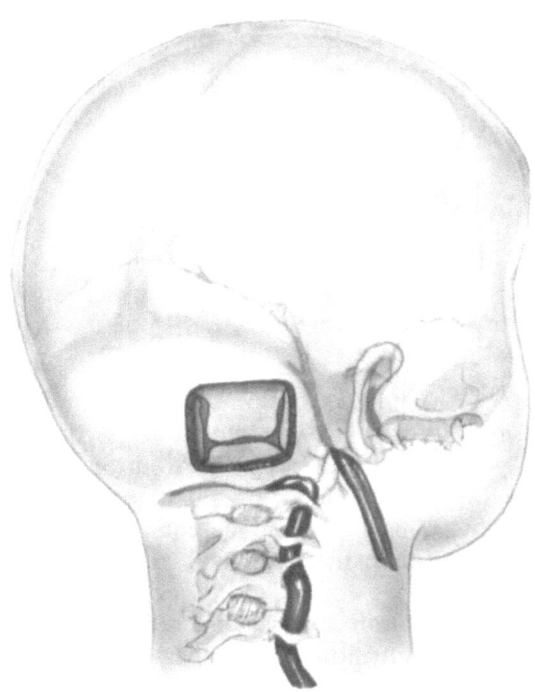

Figure 8.23. This is an asymmetrical double trapdoor durotomy flap. The transverse sinus has not been exposed. (Reprinted from Raimondi AJ. *Pediatric Neurosurgery—Theoretic Principles/Art of Surgical Techniques.* New York: Springer-Verlag, 1987.)

References

1. Meridy HW, Creighton RE, Humphreys RP. Complications during neurosurgery in the prone position in children. *Can Anest Soc J.* 1974; 21:445–453.
2. Michenfelder JD, Martin JT, Altenburg BM, Rehder K, Air embolism during neurosurgery. An evaluation of right atrial catheter for diagnosis and treatment. *JAMA.* 1969;208:1353–1358.
3. Drake CG. Total removal of large acoustic neuromas. A modification of the McKenzie operation with special emphasis on saving the facial nerve. *J Neurosurg.* 1967;26:554–561.
4. Koos WT, Miller MH. *Intracranial Tumors in Infants and Children.* St. Louis: Mosby; 1971: 415.
5. Yasargil CG. *Microsurgery Applied to Neurosurgery.* Stuttgart: Thieme; 1969:230.
6. Kempe LG. *Operative Neurosurgery.* Vol. 2. New York: Springer-Verlag; 1970:81.
7. Symon L. Control of intracranial tension. In operative Neurosurgery. In: Logue, ed. *Neurosurgery.* London: Butterworths, 1971:1.
8. Decker RE, Malis LI: Surgical approaches to midline lesions at the base of the skull: A review. *J Mt. Sinai Hosp.*
9. Bucy PC: Exposure of the posterior or cerebellar fossa. *J Neurosurg.* 24:820–32, 1960.
10. Marshall BM: Air embolus in the neurosurgical anesthesia: Its diagnosis and treatment. *Can Anaesth Soc J.* 12:255–61, 1965.
11. Michenfelder JD, Miller RH, Gronert DA: Evaluation of ultrasonic device (doppler) for the diagnosis of venous air embolism. *Anesthesiology* 32:164–7, 1972.
12. Garcia-Bengoechea F, Munson ES, Freeman JV: The lateral sitting position for neurosurgery. *Anesth-Alag (Cleve)* 55:326–30, 1955.

CHAPTER 9

Surgical Principles and Operative Results

Jean-Francois Hirsch, Elizabeth Hoppe-Hirsch, and Ph. Meyer

Principles in surgery spring from a very simple, obvious, and patent fact: the aim of the surgical procedure is to cure the patient. To reach this goal requires repeated trial and error over the years. Moreover, principles do not remain true forever, but may change with technological advances. For example, at the turn of the century, it was mandatory to operate as fast as possible because long anesthesia was dangerous; speed in surgery is now meaningless since the duration of the anesthetic procedure is no longer a problem. Unfortunately the reasons behind such principles are often progressively forgotten so that their justification is no longer understood. In other cases they may become invalid, but continue to be applied. To understand the present situation a certain knowledge of history is therefore essential. For all these reasons, it may be of some interest to recall what posterior fossa surgery was in the 1950, and what difficulties had to be overcome.

History

Around 1950, when a child was referred to a neurosurgical unit with signs of increased intracranial pressure (ICP), possibly with cerebellar signs, the only available diagnostic tool was Dandy's air ventriculography; the routine clinical use of carotid angiography was in its infancy. In any case, both investigations could only yield one piece of information: the existence of a ventricular dilatation. Sometimes the third ventricle was visualized, but the aqueduct and the fourth ventricle were not seen. Thus at

surgery, the precise localization of the tumor and even its existence were unknown. Within a few years, there was progress, from Sweden, with the development of pneumoencephalography. This technique demonstrating the fourth ventricle, the aqueduct, and the subarachnoid spaces of the posterior fossa gave more information, but was not recommended in cases of acute intracranial hypertension.

Around the same period, the intraventricular injection of Lipiodol replaced air in ventriculography and made it possible to visualize the fourth ventricle. Later, water-soluble contrasts were preferred because they could be resorbed. Vertebral angiography was not always safe and was rarely useful. Isotope scintigraphy became available around 1960 and was the first noninvasive investigation; but it was not considered sufficient for surgical decision.

To summarize the problems during that pre–computed tomography (CT) scan era, investigations were invasive, sometimes dangerous. They could eventually lead to worsening the patient's condition. When multiple investigations were needed, several days were necessary before obtaining diagnosis, during which time abrupt worsening, cerebellar fits, and death due to cerebellar tonsil herniation could occur.

To avoid these dangers, a CSF drainage was inserted. In most cases, it was useful but in some others it was dangerous, being responsible for intratumoral bleeding, upward herniation through the foramen of Pacchioni, or tumoral dissemination.

In 1950 many neurosurgical procedures were still performed under local anesthesia; general anesthesia with tracheal intubation was at its very beginning. Ventilation was controlled manually. Intraoperative monitoring did not exist. It was difficult to compensate blood loss with precision so that neurosurgical procedures in infants and small children were dangerous. Inadequate ventilation was sometimes responsible for an increased ICP.

At surgery, the dura mater was often extremely tense. To reduce the tension, hyperventilation was tried. In most cases, the only way to decrease this tension was to drill a hole and to tap the lateral ventricle. An incision on the cisterna magna could also be efficient, except when the cisterna was squeezed by the tumor. Around 1960 intravenous urea began to be used before being replaced by mannitol.

Once the dura was open, the next step was to determine if there was a tumor and where it was located. It was of course easy when the tumor reached the surface, but often difficult when it did not. When the tumor was on the midline, the policy was to try to see its inferior extremity in the fourth ventricle and to divide the vermis to reach the posterior limit of the lesion. When the tumor was developed in the cerebellar hemisphere, the neurosurgeon, using a blunt needle, pushed into the cerebellum, blindly, was trying to feel some change in the consistency of the hemisphere, which would indicate the localization of the neoplasm. It was obvious that one of the main problems to be solved was how to obtain knowledge of the precise location of the lesion. This was achieved during these past two decades with the development of CT scanning, of magnetic resonance imaging (MRI), and of intraoperative ultrasonography.

Optical magnification was not used; in 1960 the senior author began to operate with binocular magnifying glasses, which was considered unusual. In most cases, tumors were dissected before being debulked so that the retraction exerted on the normal parenchyma was not negligible. Primary debulking was usually contraindicated because it resulted in too much bleeding. In spite of clips, Gelfoam, and monopolar coagulation, which produced lesions beyond the coagulating point, hemostasis was often hard to obtain. Bleeding some-

times occurred in the depth, resulting in abrupt cerebellar swelling, usually fatal.

At the end of the surgical procedure, if the cerebellum was still swollen, the dura was not closed. The consequence was a cerebrospinal fluid (CSF) accumulation beneath the muscles and the skin of the neck. Postoperative follow-up was purely clinical. Monitoring did not exist. Therapy was limited to water and electrolyte equilibration. Intensive care units were not yet individualized.

This rapid description makes it easy to understand that the postoperative mortality rates were by far more elevated that they are now. The mortality rates in the series of medulloblastomas published between 1950 and 1960[1] ranged from 20% to 40%, whereas they now tend toward zero. Neurologic sequelae and postoperative hydrocephalus were frequent. Most malignant tumors were sooner or later fatal. The only tumor that could be cured in children was the cerebellar astrocytoma. Only after 1950 did postoperative radiotherapy delivered to the whole central nervous system make it possible to cure some medulloblastomas.[2]

This short historical review shows that in the 1950s several developments still had not occurred, without which acceptable results could not be achieved. Ways were needed to improve the diagnostic tools, to obtain a more precise localization of the tumor, to shorten the preoperative period to be able to avoid external drainage, to ameliorate the anesthetic procedure and the intraoperative monitoring, to develop intraoperative ultrasonograms to "see" the tumor through the parenchyma, to develop new surgical tools to be able to respect as much as possible the normal nervous tissue surrounding the lesion, and to improve postoperative follow-up.

These difficulties have been progressively overcome. Technological progress has certainly been the major element of evolution with the introduction of bipolar coagulation, of operative microscopes, of ultrasonic aspirators, and of lasers. Two new principles have also been essential. First, the goal of neurosurgery was no longer only to save life, but also to respect function; the problem was not to operate rapidly, but to operate with precision and therefore to use the tools to make it possible. The second principle was that infants and children should be taken care of in pediatric centers, anesthetized by pediatric anesthetists and operated on by pediatric neurosurgeons.

General Principles of Posterior Fossa Surgery

The Preoperative Stage

Because CT scanners are now available to neurologists and general practitioners, the diagnosis of posterior fossa tumor is usually already made when the child is referred to the pediatric neurosurgical unit. In most cases, it is useful to sharpen the preoperative assessment of the patient with an MRI study, which gives an image of the tumor in three planes. Once the diagnosis is made, surgery should be performed as early as possible since any wave of increased intracranial pressure can complete a cerebellar tonsil herniation and induce abrupt and irreversible clinical worsening. Most surgeons have abandoned preoperative shunting or preoperative external drainage. Tumor removal is considered the best treatment of hydrocephalus. In the service of pediatric neurosurgery at *Les Enfants Malades Hospital*, the child is operated on the day following admission. Exceptions to this rule are rare. When the diagnosis is not absolutely definite, when the relationships of the tumor with the brain stem are not clear, or when more information about the vascularity of the tumor is needed, other investigations, such as a vertebral angiography, may have to be performed, leading to a slight postponement of surgery. In developed countries, children are rarely referred very late when repeated vomiting has induced severe denutrition; only in these cases should surgery be delayed after a medical preparation and eventually a CSF shunt.

A preoperative examination is performed by the anesthetist. General principles of preoperative assessment of children should be applied to the "neurosurgical child" with special consideration of his neurological impairment.

The anesthetist should be informed of the surgical position that will be used and the intraoperative complications that could occur. In case of a cardiac murmur detected at auscultation, preoperative echocardiography should be obtained to rule out an intracardiac shunting, which might lead to paradoxical air embolism and contraindicate the use of the sitting position.[3] Laboratory studies are the same as in any preoperative examination. The preoperative visit is the occasion for the anesthetist to evaluate the level of anxiety of the child and to avoid situations that might be threatening.

Premedication should reduce as much as possible the anxiety of the child, who is accompanied to the entrance of the operating theater by his parents or by the nurse who usually takes care of him. We routinely use light oral sedation with benzodiazepines. This premedication is contraindicated in children with an impaired level of consciousness. Shaving of the skull should be performed after induction of general anesthesia.

The validity of prophylactic antibiotherapy is still debated. We use potent drugs active against endogenous and cutaneous organisms. They are started before the surgical incision and discontinued at the end of surgery. Under these conditions, the usefulness of such a policy seems to be proved, at least for long-lasting procedures,[4] and the risk of selecting resistant organisms is minimal.

Anesthesia

The anesthetic management of children with posterior fossa tumors presents specific problems. The first problem is to minimize the risks of acute intracranial hypertension and of aspiration of the gastric content at induction of anesthesia. Therefore a rapid-sequence intravenous induction is preferred. A venous access, which can be facilitated in difficult cases by the adjunction of a light inhalation anesthesia is established; then, short-acting products are administered intravenously. Rapid barbiturates such as thiopental, new hypnotics such as propofol, or rapid-acting narcotics such as fentanyl, and nondepolarizing muscle relaxants are used. Tracheal intubation is then rapidly performed under deep anesthesia with additional topical anesthesia. Mild hyperventilation is instituted. Maintenance of anesthesia can then be conveniently achieved by continuous narcotic infusion and inhalation anesthesia with isoflurane.[5]

Adequate monitoring, insuring adequate ventilation and early detection of intraoperative complications is mandatory. Intraoperative mild hyperventilation prompts the need for continuous monitoring including pulse oximetry and capnography, with serial arterial blood gas analyses. Abrupt cardiovascular reactions resulting in hypertension and bradycardia are well-known signs of alarm; they must be detected early and the surgeon notified. The use of continuous invasive blood pressure and right atrial pressure monitoring is, in our opinion, indicated in all cases.

Positioning the child for the neurosurgical procedure presents certain challenges. Impaired cardiovascular adaptation to positioning puts children at risk of postural hypotension and reduced cerebral perfusion. Excessive hyperflexion of the neck may compromise venous drainage and cause displacement of the endotracheal tube with selective bronchial intubation. Basal thoracic compression could impede lung expansion and lead to hypoventilation with related hypercapnia. All these difficulties, if they occur, must be recognized and remedied while placing the patient in a position that will not be easily modified later on.

Fluid management also represents a difficult challenge. Blood losses are sometimes difficult to evaluate with perfect precision. Inadequate fluid replacement would lead to hypovolemia or increased cerebral edema in case of overhydratation. Adverse cerebral consequences of hyperglycemia are also well known[5] and must be avoided. In practice, baseline requirements are calculated with reference to insensible fluid losses, and diuresis is measured via an indwelling bladder catheter. Fluid replacements are based on hemodynamic conditions and serial measurements of blood hematocrit. A mild hemodilution (hematocrit between 30% and 28%) should be allowed to minimize the risks related to the use of blood products.

Anesthetic management during the surgical procedure should be dedicated to optimization of cerebral perfusion pressure, detection of intraoperative changes, and prevention of specific complications.

Surgery

Surgery is performed with the patient in either the sitting or the prone position. Both positions have their supporters. We have always used the sitting position because bleeding is reduced, blood does not accumulate in the operative cavity, and the upward extension of the tumor toward the incisura tentorii is more easily reached. However, there are two drawbacks. When using the microscope, the surgeon is not in a comfortable operating position, his arms usually being stretched because of the focal length of the objective. The second drawback is more serious: air embolisms are noted in this position in 33% of the children, with related transient cardiovascular complications in 69%.[6] To avoid this complication the surgeon should repeatedly ask the anesthesiologist to perform bilateral jugular vein compression in order to increase the pressure in intracranial veins and to detect those that might be open. This does not represent continuous prevention. Positive end-expiratory pressure (PEEP) proved its inefficacy in preventing venous air embolisms.[7]

A more elegant solution has proven to be effective, at least in children: the use of a G-suit. Since we have used positive lower body pressure generated by military antishock trousers associated with a mild PEEP, we have not observed any detectable air embolism in spite of the fact that continuous capnography represents a reliable tool to detect low amounts of air penetrating in the right atrium and pulmonary circulation.[8] We have now used this technique routinely in more than 75 patients with similar results. However, these two drawbacks lead many neurosurgeons to prefer the prone position. Lateral positions are sometimes use, usually when then brain stem is approached from the side. When using the prone position, the upper chest and hips should be supported on bolsters or special frames so that the mid- and lower thorax and abdomen are free.

Whatever the position, the head is fixed in the Mayfield headrest in children above 3 years of age. When they are younger a horseshoe-shaped headrest is preferred.

Tumors that are located in the vermis or the cerebellar hemispheres are approached on the midline, as well as brain stem tumors that reach the floor of the fourth ventricle. Brain stem tumors that are exophytic on the anterior or the lateral aspect of the pons are reached by infratentorial lateral routes. A subtemporal approach with incision of the tentorium is indicated in brain stem tumors that reach the anterior or the lateral aspect of the cerebral peduncles.

Once the posterior fossa is opened, an intraoperative ultrasonogram should be performed before opening the dura. This investigation is especially useful when the tumor is small, deeply located in the cerebellum, or when it is necessary to recognize the best area to incise a cyst. In most children, however, the tumor is large and is easily found with or without ultrasonogram. Even in these cases, the ultrasonogram is of interest because it allows precise evaluation of the size of the tumor. Ultrasonograms are very useful in reoperations because they limit the size of the new dural incision and reduce the area of the dura that has to be separated from the underlying cerebellum. After incision of the dura, in the sitting position, ultrasonograms can no longer be easily performed; therefore, they cannot be used to check the completeness of the surgical removal.

Surgery can no longer be performed without optical magnification. When the tumor is deep, the equipment must include an operative microscope that allows good vision of the lesion through a small well. When the tumor is large and superficial, magnifying glasses can be used as well. A self retractor and a bipolar coagulator should be available. Ultrasonic aspiration has changed the operative technique because it is now possible to debulk the tumor without too much bleeding and without mobilization of the normal stuctures, especially of the brain stem. When the volume of the lesion is sufficiently reduced, the dissection can be performed without too much retraction of the normal cerebellum.

When the tumor adheres to the brain stem or when it is developed in the brain stem, it is often possible to reach the limit of the tumor and the normal tissue without inducing cardiovascular reactions; to achieve this result, the tumor has to be soft and the intensity of the vibrations of the ultrasonic aspirator reduced. When this is impossible, the CO_2 laser can be used to destroy the last tumoral fragments. However, when there is a cardiovascular reaction, either with the ultrasonic aspirator or with the laser, tumoral removal should be interrupted, at least at the place where the surgical procedure induces these reactions. Because the main danger in posterior fossa surgery is the brain stem and its vessels, the neurosurgeon should be able to visualize its anatomical relations with the lesion all through the surgical procedure.

When the surgical procedure is finished, tight closure of the dura, with or without dural plasty, is mandatory in order to avoid postoperative subcutaneous CSF collections. We systematically insert an external CSF drainage in the lateral ventricle at the end of the operation. This is a good precaution in all cases; it is essential in brain stem surgery because it damps the postoperative waves of increased ICP, which might have disastrous consequences. Around the fourth postoperative day, the bag in which the CSF is collected is progressively elevated. The external drainage is then removed if this can be done without intracranial hypertension. Otherwise a ventriculoperitoneal shunt is inserted. In our series of medulloblastomas, this has been the case in 15% of the children.

After Surgery

The child is positioned in bed in the sitting position if he has been operated on in this position or lying on his back, the head slightly elevated if he has been operated on in another position. The aim is to reduce the venous pressure and to minimize the risk of postoperative bleeding.

The medical treatment includes high-dose dexamethasone and prevention of gastrointestinal complication by the administration of oral sucralfate, which has considerably reduced the risk of stress ulcers. Postoperative per-fusions should balance water and electrolytes losses, a mild plasma hyperosmolarity being tolerated.

In our unit, intubation and controlled ven-tilation under mild sedation with short-acting benzodiazepines and agonist-antagonist narco-tics is maintained for 2 or 3 days after surgery. This practice is debatable after removal of a vermian or hemispheric tumor, but in our opinion it is mandatory when surgery has in-volved the brain stem. Without controlled ven-tilation and sedation in these cases, worsening often occurs on the 2nd or 3rd postoperative day. Sedation and controlled ventilation re-duce the frequency of such worsening and are necessary to overcome its clinical conse-quences once it occurs.

The immediate postoperative follow-up should be clinical and radiological; hemodyna-mic and respiratory variables should always be carefully monitored. Since the use of sedation makes it often difficult to check with precision the state of consciousness of the patient, we always perform a CT scan without and with contrast injection the day after surgery. It re-veals any postoperative bleeding, cerebral col-lapse, or subdural collection. Moreover, per-formed before the postoperative inflammatory reactions, the contrast injection shows if the tumor has been completely removed.

When the postoperative course is normal, without neurological sequelae, and when the tumor is benign, the child is sent home 1 week after surgery. When the tumor is malignant, surgery is followed by chemotherapy and radiotherapy.

Complications sometimes prolong the post-operative course; they include meningitis, coma, and respiratory insufficiency that may require controlled ventilation and eventually tracheostomy, and swallowing difficulties that necessitate feeding the child through a gastric tube and favor the development of pulmonary nosocomial infections. These complications, which may prolong the postoperative course for weeks or months, are particularly dis-astrous in malignant tumors because they post-pone postoperative treatment so that death from tumor recurrence occurs before radio-therapy becomes possible.

Principles of Posterior Fossa Surgery and Postoperative Results in Different Types of Tumor

Posterior fossa tumors in children can be di-vided into four main groups. Three groups are characterized by their cellular pathology: cerebellar astrocytomas, medulloblastomas, and ependymomas. The fourth group is charac-terized by its anatomical location: the brain stem.

Medulloblastomas

Without treatment, all children presenting with a medulloblastoma die within a few months.[9] With surgery alone, the result is the same although it occurs later. When radiotherapy is associated and given only to the posterior fos-sa, survival time is lengthened, showing that the tumor is radiosensitive, but the final evolu-tion is equally bad. As already stated, better outcome in children was obtained when it was realized that these malignancies had a high likelihood of disseminating to the central ner-vous system and that irradiation had to be delivered to the entire neuraxis. Therefore, treatment today associates surgery with-radiotherapy of the whole central nervous system.[2,8,10–12] Chemotherapy is usually given although its usefulness is not yet been com-pletely demonstrated.

There is general agreement as to the approach that should be used: incision of the skin on the midline and resection of the occipi-tal squama and of the posterior arch of the atlas. It is rarely necessary to resect the tuber-osity or the laminae of the axis; in children it is better not to do so in order to avoid the risk of postoperative vertebral instability.[13]

Before opening the dura, intraoperative ultrasonography is useful, but not mandatory; it shows the tumor and its extension and allows its measurement.[11]

It is usually not necessary to tap the lateral ventricle before opening the dura, since mod-ern anesthetic techniques sufficiently reduce ICP. The dura is cut along a Y-shaped incision; the occipital sinus and its branches are ligated or coagulated.

In some cases, the tumor is immediately visible on the midline; sometimes tumoral spots can be seen on the cerebellar hemispheres, indicating subarachnoidal extension of the disease. In most children, however, it is necessary to make a vertical incision of the vermis before being able to see the tumor.

The surgical procedure should always begin with incision of the cisterna magna and the placement of a cotton pad between the two amygdala; this cotton pad should be pushed in the fourth ventricle, unless the tumor is adherent to its floor. This will avoid the diffusion of malignant cells in the subarachnoid spaces. All through the surgical procedure, it will also remain the main anatomical landmark to which the surgeon should go back each time he has difficulty assessing the relationships of the medulloblastoma with the brain stem.

After incision of the vermis, the next step should be to find the superficial limits of the tumor with the cerebellar hemispheres. While initiating this plane of dissection, a vermian branch of the PICA is usually found on both sides; this branch should be coagulated and divided at its point of entry into the medulloblastoma. The upper limits of the tumor with the vermis should also be detected. The tumor is then debulked with the ultrasonic aspirator, the intratumoral blood vessels being progressively coagulated. When the volume of the tumor is sufficiently reduced, the dissection that had been initiated can be continued. The last portion of the tumor to be removed is the part developed on the roof of the fourth ventricle. The tumoral fragment that blocks the aqueduct is easily aspirated. In most patients, it is easy to separate the tumor from the floor and from the edges of the fourth ventricle so that finally total macroscopic removal is obtained. In other children, the medulloblastoma adheres to the floor of the fourth ventricle or even extends within the brain stem. In these cases, it is better to accept subtotal removal rather than to increase the morbidity or the postoperative mortality rate since it is not proven that the risk of recurrence is significantly higher after subtotal than after total removal (when subtotal means "a few cubic millimeters left").

In those rare patients, mainly adolescents or adults, in whom the tumor is located in the cerebellar hemisphere, the surgical procedure is easier since the tumor is not developed against the brain stem.

Progress in anesthesiology and in surgery, bipolar coagulation, ultrasonic aspiration, and optical magnification have progressively decreased the risk of surgery. The postoperative mortality rate, in our series of medulloblastomas reviewed in 1978, was 10.5%[14]; it was 11% in the series of Mealey and Hall.[12] This postoperative rate has further decreased to 6% in our series in 1990.[15] Moreover, in our last 35 children, all operated on with the cavitron, the postoperative mortality rate was nil. Although progress in intensive care has often postponed beyond the first month deaths related to surgery, thus artificially reducing the postoperative mortality rates, it can be concluded that surgical removal of a medulloblastoma is now a benign procedure.

After surgery, the extent of the disease should be assessed. There is now a general agreement that postoperative myelography or MRI study must be performed and that CSF cytology is of some help. A bone marrow study is also advocated. High- and low-risk groups can then be delineated. It is demonstrated that when the tumor is disseminated or when it is only partially removed the prognosis is worse. In these cases, the treatment might be more aggressive.

Surgery, as already stated, has to be followed by radiotherapy of the whole central nervous system (50 Gy on the posterior fossa and 25 to 30 Gy on the hemispheres and the spinal cord). Chemotherapy is now used in most cases associated with radiotherapy. With this treatment the actuarial survival rate at 5 years is 60%, and 53% at 10 years in our series of 120 medulloblastomas.[15] If only the children who complete radiotherapy are taken into account, these survival rates are respectively 73% and 64%. Unfortunately this success is counterbalanced by the behavioral and psychointellectual difficulties of these children after treatment. School problems and difficult social integration are observed in most cases. These difficuties worsen over the years.

Ependymomas

Ependymomas are often recognized before surgery on the CT scan or on the MRI; they are usually isodense before contrast injection, they enhance after injection, and they often extend downward beyond the foramen magnum.

At surgery, the inferior limit of the tumor is often below the foramen magnum and even below C-1. It is mandatory to visualize this inferior limit before beginning to remove the lesion; thus it is sometimes necessary to resect not only the posterior arch of C-1, but also that of C-2. In this case, the risk of postoperative instability is very high in children. This risk is even higher when lower cervical laminae have to be resected.

Usually ependymomas develop in the cisterna magna and seem to be separated from the normal nervous tissue. Once the arachnoid is incised, the downward extension of the ependymoma below the obex can be separated from the medulla and the spinal cord. Further up there is also a separation between the vermis, the cerebellar hemispheres, and the tumor. In most cases, part of the vermis has to be divided on the midline in order to find the superior limit of the tumor; the whole tumor appears as a huge mushroom, the foot of which is implanted on the floor of the fourth ventricle. For this reason, the tumor should be manipulated carefully. Any displacement of the tumor induces a displacement of the brain stem on which it is implanted. Thus cardiovascular reactions sometimes occur at the very beginning of the dissection. Ultrasonic aspirators have simplified this surgery because they make it possible to debulk the tumor or even to remove it without any movement of the brain stem.

The last problem specific to this surgery is to know when to stop. Ependymomas being implanted on the floor of the fourth ventricle, the surgical removal is in most cases only subtotal. Macroscopic total removal was rarely possible in our series. The prognosis was not better in these children probably because total removal was only a fallacious appearance.[16]

Posterior fossa ependymomas sometimes extend to the cerebellopontine angle. In some cases, they seem limited to this region; it is, however, likely that they have a connection with the ependyma of the fourth ventricle, probably at the level of the foramen of Luschka.

The postoperative follow-up of a posterior fossa ependymoma is in no way different from that of a medulloblastoma. The postoperative mortality rate in our whole series is 16%. This rate is reduced to 8% in our last 25 patients, all operated with the cavitron. Postoperative mortality, however, remains higher than in medulloblastomas, very likely because of the brain stem insertion of the tumor. Theoretically a difference should be made between benign ependymomas and malignant ependymomas. Using grading as a means to predict evolution often fails in ependymomas; some children with malignant tumors survive after appropriate treatment, whereas in 10% of the cases benign posterior fossa ependymomas metastasize to the spinal cord.[16] In our series of 75 ependymomas, the 5-year actuarial survival rate is approximately 60% whatever the grade of the tumor. The prognosis of ependymoblastomas which are actually primitive neuroectodermal tumors (PNETs) is, on the contrary, significantly worse. After surgery, radiotherapy in our department is always associated because the tumor is usually subtotally removed and because the predictive value of grading is low. Chemotherapy can also be associated.

Cerebellar Astrocytomas

Cerebellar astrocytomas that develop in the cerebellar hemispheres are in the large majority of cases benign tumors. In our whole series, there were only two grade III cerebellar astrocytomas. Incidentally, these two children were given radiotherapy; their tumors did not recur. Benign cerebellar astrocytomas in the past were called spongioblastoma polare. This term, however, has been a matter of confusion. At present these tumors are recognized by the great majority of authors as piloid astrocytoma. From an oncologic point of view, it is quite clear that the evolution of benign astrocytomas (grades I and II) is different in adults and in children. In children they are actually benign and do not recur if they are totally removed. Total removal is easy in cerebral hemispheric astrocytomas; in our series of supratentorial hemispheric benign astrocytomas, none of those that had been completely removed recurred.[17] Total removal is also possible in cerebellar benign astrocytomas so that recurrence should never be observed; the situation is slightly different in brain stem benign astrocytomas because, in these tumors, surgical removal is in most cases subtotal.

The conclusions that stem from these considerations is that cerebellar astrocytomas should be totally removed; they should not be treated with radiotherapy since they are practically always low-grade tumors; recurrence is not observed in cases of complete surgical removal.

Cerebellar astrocytomas usually exist in the cerebellar hemisphere with or without extension into the vermis. However, the midline location is also possible. In most cases, the tumor is developed on the wall of a cyst. In these cases, the cyst is visualized on CT or MRI; the tumor itself is visualized after contrast injection; the wall of the cyst does not show any contrast enhancement. In these children the tumor should be removed, but not the wall of the cyst, which is made of normal nervous tissue. In other patients part of the cystic wall enhances after contrast injection. At surgery, it is clear that a portion of the cystic wall is invaded and should be removed. Cerebellar astrocytomas occasionally appear as round, solid tumors without any cystic component. The prognosis remains the same, however, at least if the tumor is completely removed.

The posterior fossa cerebellar astrocytoma removal is usually an easy operation. Once the posterior fossa is open, if the tension of the dura is elevated, the cyst can be tapped through the dura before opening, especially when it can be precisely located by an ultrasonogram. After dural incision, the cyst is opened; the lemon-yellow liquid of the cyst is sucked up. Then, depending on its size, the tumor can be dissected and separated from the cystic wall or removed with the ultrasonic aspirator. The operation is slightly more difficult when the tumor invades the cystic wall or

when there is no cyst. Surgery may also be complicated by the adherence of the tumor to the floor of the fourth ventricle. Such adherences are rare. These astrocytomas should be distinguished from those brain stem astrocytomas that develop an exophytic portion.

With modern techniques, the postoperative mortality rate tends toward zero. As already stated total surgical removal is possible and necessary to avoid recurrences. Postoperative radiotherapy should not be given except in these excessively rare malignant cerebellar astrocytomas.

Brain Stem Tumors

A tumor is not usually defined by its anatomical localization. However, this is the case when this localization is more important than the tumor's pathology in the choice of the treatment. This was the case two decades ago for brain stem tumors, which were considered inoperable. It is no longer so since a majority of the benign brain stem tumors are amenable to surgery.[18] In contrast, surgery is useless in malignant brain stem tumors. In our series, all children presenting with a malignant brain stem tumor were dead 36 months after surgery and radiotherapy. The first step is therefore to differentiate before surgery between benign and the malignant tumors. In most children this can be done on the basis of the speed of evolution and on the characteristics of CT scan and MRI. Malignant tumors are diffuse, hypodense, and show no contrast enhancement; in some patients however, an irregular, circular ring of contrast enhancement surrounds the necrotic center of the tumor. Benign tumors, in contrast, are well limited. They are not surrounded by edema. They are sometimes associated with a cyst and often enhance after contrast injection. Stereotactic biopsy, which is advocated by some authors, should be reserved for those cases in which the distinction between benign and malignant tumors cannot be made on the clinical features and radiology.

Benign brain stem tumors are operable either if they show an exophytic portion or if, at least, somewhere they reach the surface of the brain stem. The majority of these tumors are astrocytomas grades I and II.

The surgical route to reach these benign brain stem tumors depends on the anatomical location of their exophytic portion or of the area where they reach the surface of the brain stem, the general principle being to remove the lesion without having to incise the normal brain stem.

When the tumor bulges into the fourth ventricle, the approach is the same midline route as for any other pediatric posterior fossa tumor. If the tumor extends far upward, a vermian incision has to be performed.

For tumors that reach the pons laterally or anteriorly, a lateral route should be preferred. The technique developed in our department[19] is the transpetrosal retrolabyrinthine approach. This route, which preserves auditory function, gives excellent access to the anterolateral aspect of both the pons up to the level of the fifth nerve and the medulla down to the level of the lower cranial nerves. These operations are performed on patients lying in a lateral position. Once the mastoidectomy is performed, the lateral and the sigmoid sinuses are unroofed and the jugular foramen is opened. The approach to the brain stem tumor is made infratentorially after incision of the posterior fossa dura 1 cm below the level of the lateral and the sigmoid sinuses.

The best approach to the peduncular tumors is subtemporal. The temporal lobe is reclined, care being taken not to sever the veins that bind the lobe to the lateral sinus. The tentorium is then divided parallel to the upper edge of the petrous bone, the fourth cranial nerve being respected.

The surgical removal of the tumor is performed with an ultrasonic aspirator. The removal should be total. However, in many children, cardiovascular reactions develop when the limit between tumor and normal brain stem is reached by the surgeon. In such cases, it is better to leave a small portion of the lesion than to risk heavy postoperative complications or even death. In our series of 103 brain stem tumors operated on between 1970 and 1992, there were 75.7% partial and 24.3% subtotal removals before the cavitron became available,

whereas with the cavitron there were 43.9% partial, 36.4% subtotal and 19.7% total removals. The use of this tool has thus clearly improved the quality of removal. The CO_2 laser can also be used to remove some small tumoral remnants. It is of course essential all through the surgical procedure to respect the vessels that course on the surface of the normal brain stem.

The postoperative course of these operations is often stormy. It is in our opinion mandatory to maintain these children under heavy sedation and controlled respiration for several days since worsening often occurs around the third postoperative day. In our series, one third of the children were operated on before and the other two thirds after the use of the ultrasonic aspirator. Before the cavitron era, the postoperative mortality rate was 21.6%, whereas it is 6% now. There were no postoperative deaths among the last 60 patients who were operated on. These results demonstrate that brain stem surgery is feasible.

After surgery, most children present with neurological sequelae, a fact that is not very surprising since all patients show neurological signs before being operated on. However, it should be pointed out that surgery improves or stabilizes the neurological status in 82% of the cases and that worsening is observed in only 18% of the patients.

It is more difficult to demonstrate with our series that surgery is useful in benign tumors of the brain stem since all except eight of our patients received complementary radiotherapy. However, it should be noted that the 5-year actuarial survival rate of these benign brain stem tumors was 91% for total and subtotal removals, whereas it was only 50% for partial removals. It is now our policy not to give complementary radiotherapy, especially in young patients, when removal has been total or subtotal. Children are followed up with repeated MRI studies; radiotherapy is delivered to the brain stem if the tumor recurs after total removal or if there is growth of the tumoral remnant after a subtotal removal.

Other tumors, such as metastases and sarcomas, can develop in the posterior fossa. However, they are very rare in children and do not warrant special comment. Eighth nerve neurinomas are also extremely rare in children; when they occur, they are always associated with other signs of Recklinghausen's disease. They should be removed by surgeons trained in such surgery.

Comparing posterior fossa surgery in children today to the same surgery three or four decades ago, the progress is obvious and impressive. All cerebellar astrocytomas should be cured. Postoperative mortality rates after cerebellar surgery should tend toward zero. About 50% to 60% of the children with medulloblastomas or ependymomas survive 5 years after treatment. Brain stem surgery is feasible and should be proposed each time the tumor is possibly benign. One problem remains unanswered, however—that of malignant brain stem tumors. In spite of many different trials, no efficient treatment is yet available. Malignant brain stem tumors were and remain the darkest chapter of posterior fossa surgery in children.

References

1. Choux M, Lena G. Le médulloblastome. *Neurochirurgie.* 1982;28 (suppl 1):9–229.
2. Paterson E. Medulloblastoma: treatment by irradiation of the whole central nervous system. *Acta Radiol.* 1953;39:323–336.
3. Guggiari M, Lechat P, Garen-Colanne C. Early detection of patent foramen ovale by two-dimensional contrast echocardiography for prevention for paradoxical air embolism. *Anesth Analg.* 1988;67:192–194.
4. Geraghty J, Feelry M. Antibiotic prophylaxis in neurosurgery. *J Neurosurg.* 1984;60:724–726.
5. Cucchiara RF. Anesthesia for patients with increased intracranial pressure. In: *ASA Annual Refresher Course Proceedings.* 1991:432.
6. Cucchiara RF, Bawers B. Air embolism in children undergoing sub-occipital craniotomy. *Anesthesiology.* 1982;57:338–340.
7. Perkins NAK, Bedford RF. Hemodynamic consequences of PEEP in seated neurosurgical patients; implications for parodoxical air embolism. *Anesth Analg.* 1984;63:429–432.
8. Meyer Ph, Jayais P, Quenet G, Barrier G. Prevention of venous air embolism in pediatric neurosurgical procedures by using MAST. *Anesthesiology.* 1990;73(Suppl 6):1100.
9. Cushing H. Experiences with cerebellar medulloblastomas. A critical review. *Acta Pathol Microbiol Scand.* 1930;7:1–86.
10. Lampe, McIntyre. Radiation therapy of medulloblastomas. *Am J Roentgenol.* 1954;71:659–668.
11. Machado HR, Pariente D, Hirsch E, Sauvegrain J, Hirsch JF. L'échographie per-opératoire en neurochirurgie pédiatrique. Expérience sur une série de 40 interventions. *Neurochirurgie.* 1986;32:287–295.
12. Mealey J, Hall PV. Medulloblastoma in children: survival and treatment. *J Neurosurg.* 1977;46:56–64.
13. Penier D, Daussange J, Rigault P, Hirsch JF. Children's cervical spine instability after posterior fossa surgery. *Child's Brain.* 1981;8:77–78.
14. Hirsch JF, Renier D, Pierre-Kahn A, Benveniste L, George B. Les medulloblastomes de l'enfant. Survie et résultats fonctionnels. *Neurochirurgie.* 1978;24:391–397.
15. Hoppe-Hirsch E, Renier D, Lellouch-Tubiana A, Sainte-Rose C, Pierre-Kahn A, Hirsch JF. Medulloblastoma in childhood: progressive intellectual deterioration. *Childs Nerv Syst.* 1990;6:60–65.
16. Pierre-Kahn A, Hirsch JF, Roux FX, Sainte-Rose C. Intracranial ependymomas in childhood. Survival and functional results of 47 cases. *Childs Brain.* 1983;10:145–156.
17. Hirsch JF, Sainte-Rose C, Pierre-Kahn A, Pfister A, Hoppe-Hirsch E. Benign astrocytic and oligodendrocytic tumors of the cerebral hemispheres in children. *J Neurosurg.* 1989;70:568–572.
18. Hirsch JF. Faut-il operer les tumeurs du tronc cerebral de l'enfant? "Les entretiens de Bichat" 1990.
19. Pierre-Kahn A, Perrin A, Hirsch JF. Transpetrosal, translabyrinthic approach for anteriorly extended pontine tumors. Communication to the Paediatric Neurosurgical Section Meeting of the A.A.N.S., Pebble Beach, California, December 1990.

CHAPTER 10

Operative Adjuncts: Laser

Peter W. Ascher

Historical Background

The first successful laser, constructed by Maiman in 1960, soon aroused interest in the industrial and medical communities. Meyer-Schwickerath's work had sensitized ophthalmologists to the possibilities of treatment with light, and it was only a short step to using the ruby laser to produce therapeutic lesions of the retina. The interest of ophthalmologists never waned, and today they use a wide array of lasers.

Laser applications in other medical and surgical specialties had to await the development of the CO_2 laser by Patel and of a light conduction system for the neodynium: yttrium-aluminum-garnet (Nd:YAG) laser by Nath. Laser use then accelerated, and all surgical specialities—except neurosurgery—presented encouraging reports at the First International Congress for Lasers in Surgery and Medicine in Tel Aviv in 1975. There were numerous early attempts to use lasers in neurosurgery. Fox[1] and Lambert and Rossomoff[2] worked with ruby lasers in mice in the early 1960s. Maybe it was their reports of "brain tissue of animals such as mice, cats and dogs driven into cranial openings by ruby laser pulses; hemorrhages; and impacts followed by immediate death or severe neurological damage" that slowed the laser's progress in neurosurgery.

The development of the CO_2 laser and reports by Yahr et al.[3] and Strully and Fiedler spurred Stellar et al.[4] to apply the laser in neurosurgery. Although they recognized the advantages of no-touch cutting, Stellar et al. used the laser only in patients with inoperable glioblastomas of the cerebrum with the goal of vaporizing tumor tissue. Since inoperable cerebral glioblastomas are usually very large and have an extremely abnormal vascular supply, the CO_2 laser had to be used at high-power settings. Applications were limited and very time-consuming. After a few publications and surgical failures, Stellar personally advised prominent neurosurgeons against using lasers at that time. This was the situation when we were first confronted with using lasers for neurosurgery. The idea of no-touch and minimally traumatic cutting convinced us to try the CO_2 laser, but lasers had not yet been adapted to neurosurgical purposes.

The massive probes used in other surgical fields prevented laser applications in neurosurgery. The reasons for this are simple. Once the decision has been made to use an invisible knife, then it would be illogical to surround the device by a material sheath or to decline the potential of aseptic technique by risking contact infection. And it would be especially illogical and defeat the purpose of the new instrument to further narrow the already limited neurosurgical field by again using a material probe.

This problem was solved by using a visible helium-neon pilot laser to accompany the invisible CO_2 laser beam.

A second consideration was the advant of neurologic microsurgery, which led to the requirement that lasers be compatible with conventional operating microscopes. A problem was keeping the focus of the beam narrow at the working distances (25 to 40 cm) used in microsurgery. After this was worked out, the laser was ready for experimental and then clinical use. The first successful neurosurgical procedure with a laser at the Department of Neurosurgery in Graz was performed on July 28, 1976.[5]

At this time the neurosurgical team around Leheta and Goisch[6] and Beck[7] in Munich had begun to test applications of the Nd:YAG laser in neurosurgery. Also, Takizawa[8] had tried to adapt the CO_2 laser for neurosurgical work in the late 1960s. Starting from scratch, he first had to get a laser built at the University of Tokyo. This laser was available for experimental work in 1975–76. But Takizawa's concept was similar to Stellar's in that it envisaged a debulking technique. This meant an a priori limitation of the potential of the CO_2 laser.

In the following years three groups (Graz, Munich, Tokyo) first competed and then cooperated in developing the potential of lasers for neurosurgery. It soon became clear that different problems required different lasers.

Basics of Laser Physics

Laser is an acronym for light amplification by stimulated emission of radiation. The laser was a continuation of the maser.[9] This explains the name but not the phenomenon, and a surgeon should understand the principles of the instruments with which he or she works. Light has both quantum and wave properties, according to which the laser can be explained. A discussion of the laser's quantum properties comprises four aspects: absorption, spontaneous emission, stimulated emission, and inversion.

Absorption

The ground state of an atom is that in which it contains a minimum of energy. Apart from this stationary state there are other defined, higher energy levels. These higher energy states are called stimulated states and are characterized by quantum numbers. At absolute zero, atoms are in their ground state, and this approximately applies at room temperature. An atom in

its ground state cannot release energy, only absorb it. After absorbing energy, it shifts from the ground state (E1) to higher energy states (E2-EN).

Emission

There is only one mechanism of energy absorption, but emission can occur in two ways: spontaneously or after stimulation.

Spontaneous Emission

As the term implies, spontaneous emission takes place without outside influences. The atom reverts from an excited state (EN) to a lower state, until it reaches E1. Therefore, only an excited atom can emit energy.

Stimulated Emission

In stimulated emission an external influence, by means of a corresponding radiation field, prompts the emission of energy. Stimulated emission is the basis of the laser phenomenon. "The emission of an atom system at a higher energy level which is exposed to a radiation field has two components: spontaneous emission, which occurs always, and induced emission, which occurs only in a radiation field."[9]

Inversion

Inversion is required to shift an atom system to a higher energy level. Inversion is present when "a higher energy level is more occupied than a lower level"—i.e., when there is an inversion of occupancy. Inversion requires energy, called the pump energy.[9] There are various methods for producing inversion. A two-tier system cannot produce inversion in the optical range. This requires at least a three-tier system, i.e., from E3 to E1.

The laser effect can also be considered according to the wave properties of light. Normal light results from the spontaneous emission of many atoms and spreads evenly in all directions. Relationships between the timing, direction, and phases of such emissions are random and the resulting light is incoherent.[9] Induced or stimulated emission produces the monochromatic, coherent light that is the basis of the laser phenomenon.

Laser Systems

The three basic types of laser systems are classified according to how the energy required for inversion is produced, or according to the medium. There are gas lasers, solid-body and fluid lasers, and semiconductor lasers.

Gas lasers usually operate continuously, whereas solid-body and fluid lasers operate mainly in pulses. Semiconductor lasers can operate in both modes. Since the amplification depends on the number of excited atoms in the laser medium as well as on the pump energy, solid-body lasers reach a higher amplification than gas lasers, and thus have a higher basal power output.[9] Only a few of the many available laser systems are suited for medical applications. Even fewer lasers are appropriate for surgical use, and only two systems are routinely used in neurosurgery.

The CO$_2$ Laser

This gas laser usually operates continuously but can be switched to a pulsed mode. It is used in all surgical specialties for cutting and vaporization and for coagulation in microsurgery. In the milliwatt range it, like all other lasers, can be used to weld tissue. The CO$_2$ laser is *not* suited for denaturation of protein.

The Neodymium:YAG (Nd:YAG) Laser

This crystal laser operates in a continuous mode. It is used in gastroenterology to coagulate bleeding sites in the gastrointestinal tract and in general surgery to cut parenchymatous organs. In neurosurgery it is the ideal instrument for coagulation and for denaturation of inoperable tumor areas. It has a wide range of endoscopic applications. The Nd:YAG laser can also be used in the milliwatt range to weld tissue. Neither the original 1.06 nm device nor the 1.32 nm version can be used for cutting.

Ruby and argon Lasers have been used occasionally in neurosurgery. Excimer, holmium,

Er:YAG-, KTP-, Dye-, X-ray-, and free-electron lasers are being studied for neurosurgical applications.

Laser Effects on Nervous Tissue

Schalow once permitted us to use the following formula to explain the effects of lasers on nervous tissue to physicians:

Laser light + Nervous tissue = Heat reaction by absorption.

The absorptive properties of the tissue determine the effect of the laser. The diametrically different effects of the CO$_2$ and Nd:YAG lasers result from their different wavelengths.

Different types of applying heat cause different tissue reactions. The CO$_2$ laser is immediately and completely absorbed by the tissue. Its energy is transformed into heat. Up to 55° the laser can weld tissue. Temperatures above 55° produce superficial coagulation and shrinking of the tissue. At temperatures above 100°, a focused beam penetrates directly into the tissue; moving the beam cuts the tissue. A defocused beam (with less energy density) vaporizes superficial tissue. The extent of vaporization depends on the energy density at the surface.

The Nd:YAG laser is poorly absorbed and penetrates into nervous tissue about ten times as far as the CO$_2$ laser. A scattering effect evenly heats a volume of tissue. Human protein is denatured at 70°. Prolonged laser application or increased energy producing higher temperature elicit the so-called popcorn effect. This term refers to explosive changes caused by the vaporization of individual cells. This feared event long hindered the introduction of the laser. Four degrees of tissue reaction can be distinguished according to the temperature produced in the tissue:

First degree (<45°): no effect on healthy nervous tissue.
Second degree (46°–57°): enzymatic changes and slight edema. This is the range in which CO$_2$, argon, and Nd:YAG lasers are used to weld tissue.

Third degree (58°–99°): denaturation and thus destruction of protein. This is where the Nd:YAG laser is used to denature otherwise inaccessible tumor components and highly vascular tumors.

Fourth degree (>100°): vaporization. A focused beam, especially of a CO_2 laser in the superpulsed mode, is used for sharp cutting. Defocused beams cause wide superficial or voluminous vaporization. Temperatures above 100° cause charring of the mineral components of nervous tissue.

This classification was confirmed by histology, electron microscopy, and scanning electron microscopy. These studies showed that the CO_2 laser causes a lesion limited to a radius of 500 nm at most. Tissue more than 0.5 mm away from the laser beam remains completely cold and unaffected. In the superpulsed mode the CO_2 laser causes an even smaller zone of thermal damage.

Material and Methods

Normal human brain tissue was studied under standardized conditions immediately after laser application. Long-term studies of laser lesions stem from autopsies of patients who had undergone laser surgery.

Point lesions were placed in tissue from the temporal or frontal lobe with a CO_2 and with 1.06 nm and 1.32 nm lasers. Energy, time, and focal distance were varied. The tissue surrounding the lesion was removed en bloc. Apart from routine histology, the blocks were also treated with 3% glutaraldehyde, contrasted with osmium tetraoxide (pH 7.4), and embedded in Epon 8. Semithin sections[10] of these blocks were stained with toluidine blue and served to orient subsequent ultrathin (300 Å) sections for electron microscopy. The specimens were studied at magnifications of 10 to 30.000× (Philips EM 200).

For scanning electron microscopy, sections of brain tissue were obtained with the lasers, an electric needle, a Bovy knife, and a cold knife (brain spatula or needle). These specimens were also removed en bloc, prepared, and fixated with critical point drying. After application of gold, the specimens were studied under a scanning electron microscope (SEM, Cambridge Industries, Ltd.).[10]

Results

Irradiation of the cerebral cortex by a focused CO_2 laser (focus diameter 0.2 mm) results in a wedge-shaped incision. The depth of the lesion depends on the duration of irradiation, the energy output, and the mode of the laser [continuous wave (cw) or superpulsed (sp)]. A 1-sec application at 30 watts (W) by a focused laser penetrates 0.8 mm into the tissue.

Three layers can be discerned in the wall of a CO_2 laser incision. The innermost layer shows an irregular, uneven surface of charred particles. Next is a 0.15-mm-thick homogenous zone of coagulation necrosis. The 0.1 to 0.3-mm-thick zone of edema subsides peripherally so that at its edge it resembles only thermal damage of the blood-brain barrier. Magnification of 30.000x shows the extremely heat sensitive mitochondria in this zone to be completely intact.

A focused 1.06 nm Nd:YAG laser produces a completely different lesion. Intact cells can be found at the surface over the center of the lesion, but at a depth of <5.6 mm the tissue looks grossly, as if explosively, damaged. The scattering effect described earlier causes overheating and explosive vaporization of cellular fluid (popcorn effect).

A defocused CO_2 laser beam causes mild edema of the cerebral surface but no deeper damage. A defocused Nd:YAG laser penetrates deep into the tissue with refraction of the beam. This causes homogeneous and sharply demarcated denaturation of the protein. Caution must be exercised so that the temperature of the tissue does not exceed 70°. Histology shows shrinkage and coagulation. Cell structures appear densely packed and vessels are occluded by intimal swelling. Lesions up to 15 mm in diameter can be produced.

Beck and Frank in Munich studied the histologic effects of the 1.32 nm Nd:YAG laser. These studies confirmed that this version of the

Nd:YAG laser represents a compromise between the CO_2 and the conventional 1.06 nm Nd:YAG lasers.

Eggert in Freiburg has reported long-term studies of laser lesions. In animals the extent of the laser lesions continued to develop even hours after the experiment. Sporadic reports of long-term histologic studies of patients who underwent laser surgery showed smooth glial scars and intact nerve cells reaching to the surface of the lesion. This corresponds to long-term computed tomography (CT) findings.

Laser Techniques

There are a number of ways to apply a laser. The first lasers were applied by a pen-like handpiece with an iron focusing device. The advent of pilot lasers improved the handling of the lasers. Today handpieces with an array of lenses and corresponding focal lengths are available. The 125-mm lens has proved most suitable for free-hand use. Special metal mirrors can be used to reflect laser light to regions not accessible by a direct beam.

Normal handpieces and a number of differently shaped or flexible metal applicators are available for Nd:YAG lasers. In contrast to normal handpieces, these instruments have no focusing device. They can be connected to an irrigation system so that the laser beam follows a cooling beam of fluid.[11]

Microadaptors for standard operating microscopes have been available from the onset of the laser era. These permit direct mechanical guidance or electromagnetic guidance via a control panel. Modern adaptors permit focusing and defocusing without altering the plane of observation. Nd:YAG laser light is conducted through optic fibers. Special endoscopes can be used to access intracerebral cavities (ventricles, hemorrhagic, or tumor cysts). Other endoscopes (thoracoscopes) can be used to perform sympathectomies in the thorax. Intra-arterial procedures can be performed with special catheters or arterioscopes with laser light fibers. Special needles and fibers 200 to 400 nm in diameter are used to puncture

herniated intervertebral disks. Sapphire tips for Nd:YAG lasers permit contact with the tissue to be irradiated, vastly expanding the endoscopic applications of the laser.

We are trying to exploit these possibilities for interstitial thermotherapy of inoperable central tumors. The lesion is punctured under CT guidance and a laser probe is introduced. Under continuous magnetic resonance (MR) imaging, the tumor tissue is then denatured from the inside out.

Some authors have advocated using a sapphire-tipped Nd:YAG laser as a glowing knife. We found this technique to entail only disadvantages, and thus do not use it. However, the instrument may be indicated for the treatment of angiomas of the spinal cord and soft tumors in the orbita.

Clinical Results

During the procedures (over 2,000 in 15 years) we have seen advantages and disadvantages of laser neurosurgery. The laser takes twice as long to incise skin as does a scalpel, and laser skin wounds take at least 3 days longer to heal. Similarly, conventional instruments are superior for work on bone. When using a laser the dura has to be protected by a damp strip of gauze because of the varying thickness of the bone and the resulting varying rate of cutting. Also, lasers produce much higher temperatures in bone than in nervous tissue, which contains much water. However, bleeding from the spongiosa can be controlled without wax by coagulation with a CO_2 laser (30 W, defocused, cw). A further indication for using a laser on bone is a meningioma suspected of having infiltrated the skull. Heating the bone denatures organic tumor cell components (CO_2 laser, 30–40 W, defocused, cw). The dura can be incised as quickly with a laser as with a scalpel but a laser causes unwelcome shrinkage.

This section discusses the clinical results of laser neurosurgery for the following lesions:

1. malignant tumors of the cerebral and cerebellar hemispheres,

2. low-grade gliomas of the cerebrum and cerebellum,
3. meningiomas above the cerebral and cerebellar hemispheres and the lateral cranial fossa,
4. brain stem tumors,
5. low-grade astrocytomas but also functionally inoperable (small) malignant tumors,
6. intraventricular tumors,
7. angiomas,
8. cerebellopontine angle tumors.

Malignant Tumors of the Cerebral and Cerebellar Hemispheres

We have operated on about 400 malignant lesions (mainly glioblastomas and metastatic tumors) of the cerebral and cerebellar hemispheres. Lasers are used only in place of conventional instruments during certain phases of the procedures. Three techniques are used, depending on the location and extent of the lesion.

Glioblastomas and metastases limited to the frontal or temporal poles are treated by laser amputation with a margin of healthy tissue. The CO_2 laser is applied with a handpiece containing a 12.5-cm focusing lens. A slightly defocused beam (focus increased from 0.2 mm to 2.0 mm) is used initially at 5 to 10 W. Larger vessels are avoided during cutting with the laser and are either closed incrementally with the laser after further defocusing and simultaneous reduction of the energy (2 to 5 W) or quickly coagulated with bipolar forceps. Dissection is continued with continuous suction to keep the incision dry, and with exposure with nonreflecting brain spatulas. After the amputation the surface of the wound is "sealed" with a defocused beam (5–20 mm focus diameter, 20–30 W, cw).

This procedure does not prevent or postpone recurrences, but postoperative bleeding occurred in only 0.2% of our patients. Postoperative CT studies show surprisingly mild edema and bland healing of the wound within 3 weeks. A hyperdense, 1-mm-thick margin remains visible by CT until the zone of coagulation has been resorbed.

This technique is slightly altered for malignant lesions of the cerebral medulla in nonfunctional regions. A cylinder is cut out of the cortical and medullary tissue with a CO_2 laser. The tumor itself is then dissected as close as possible to its margins and extirpated in the conventional manner with suction, bipolar spatula, and brain gauze. The resulting cavity is then sealed with a defocused CO_2 laser. Radicality must be sacrificed if there is a danger of postoperative functional deficits.

The third technique is used for small malignant tumors in functionally important areas. After adequate exposure and opening of the dura, the tumor, if deep, is located and, if necessary, punctured under ultrasound guidance. The topographically most convenient gyrus is divided over a distance of 2 cm with the laser (CO_2, 5–7 W, cw or sp, slightly defocused) under sight or under the microscope. The gyrus itself is retracted with a specially designed cortex retractor (Aesculap) and dissection continued. The tumor, which is usually highly vascularized, is then vaporized as far as possible under the microscope with a defocused CO_2 laser (5–20 W). Generally, the tumor has been eliminated once the bleeding stops. Radicality is declined for the reasons mentioned above. The resulting cavity is again sealed; this may require metal mirrors to direct the beam to areas of the cavity that cannot be reached directly.

The long-term results of these procedures are the same as those of operations with conventional instruments. Importantly, minimum use of conventional instruments in favor of the laser alleviates the immediate postoperative period. Edema formation is reduced and postoperative bleeding is rare.

Low-Grade Gliomas of the Cerebrum and Cerebellum

The CO_2 laser was used for surgery of the 120 low-grade gliomas shown in Table 10.1. It proved especially suitable for cutting (5–10 W, cw, focused) recurrent astrocytomas with a tough, sometimes rubbery consistency. In these patients the laser was used together with a CUSA. Operating time was markedly reduced. Functionally important vessels must be

Table 10.1. Laser operations of brain stem tumors at the Department of neurosurgery in Graz, July 28, 1976 to July 28, 1987.

Astrocytomas	28
Ependymomas	19
Medulloblastomas	13
Meningiomas	13
Pineal tumors	6
Angiomatous lesions	15
Spongioblastomas	3
Cholesteatomas	1
Papillomas	3
Lipomas	1
Epidermoid cysts	1
Sarcomas	1
Glioblastomas	1
Neurinomas	1
Metastatic tumors	4
Unclassified	3
Total	113

located before excessive laser application. Radicality is aimed for. In isolated cases the CO_2 laser, because of its stronger absorption in edema, can be used for microscopic dissection at the border between the tumor and edema. This involved technique is used for in toto vaporization of single central tumor pegs (15–20 W, cw, defocused to 5–10 mm). As in all tumor procedures, the tumor bed is sealed with the laser. In these patients laser neurosurgery permits radicality more often and with better preservation of healthy tissue than do conventional techniques.

Meningiomas Over Both Cerebral and Cerebellar Hemispheres and the Lateral Cranial Fossa

The technique of extirpating meningiomas depends on the consistency and vascular supply of the tumor. Very hard, partly calcified meningiomas—over both hemispheres as well as at the lateral cranial fossa—are reduced in a piecemeal technique. The CUSA can be used here as well. The laser is used at between 20 and 40 W, focused, and in the cw mode. Otherwise the technique does not differ from that used for conventional tumor surgery. The dura

usually has to be resected and closed with a reconstructive procedure. If it is not clear whether the adjacent bones are involved, the bone is heated at the end of the operation (CO_2 laser, 40 W, defocused, 25–30 mm).

The afferent vessels of vascular meningiomas can be embolized before going after the tumor itself. These vessels usually stem from the external carotid circulation, less often from the internal carotid circulation. The bone is then widely exposed, which usually requires a number of burr holes to avoid tearing the adherent dura. The dura is circumcised with a scalpel and a myrthen leaf. The normal cortex is draped and the tumor preradiated (1.06 nm Nd:YAG laser, 30–40 W, cw, defocused to 10 mm) with continuous cooling of the tumor surface with Ringer's solution. The laser is slowly and repeatedly passed over the area of the tumor. Denaturation can be monitored by the "bleaching effect" (it is important that the laser is not absorbed at the surface) and by the shrinking of the tumor. The duplication of arachnoidea retracts from the healthy tissue, the two layers of the arachnoidea separate, and small bridging vessels can be easily coagulated and divided with bipolar forceps and scissors. During the entire procedure the laser beam must remain directed toward the center of the tumor. Only in this manner can the scattering effect be exploited to denature a maximum of tumor tissue while preserving the adjacent healthy tissue.

This technique can be applied in one of two ways, depending on the size and location of the tumor. If the tumor is small enough, it can be snared and gently exposed. The newly exposed surface of the tumor is irradiated with the laser. The meningioma shrinks under this treatment, and almost delivers itself. The tumor bed, usually intact cortical tissue, is briefly irradiated with a CO_2 laser (5–10 W, strongly defocused to 10–15 mm, cw).

If the tumor cannot be removed by this technique without damaging the cortex, then, after preradiation of the tumor surface, intracapsular compression is performed with suction or the CUSA. The Nd:YAG laser is used again as soon as oozing bleeding develops at a depth of 10 to 15 mm. This technique permits extirpa-

Table 10.2. Operations with the CO_2 laser on tumors of the lower brain stem ($n = 47$).

Histology	Pons	Medulla oblongata	Cerebellum	Cerebellum medulla oblongata	Total
Medulloblastomas	1	5	—	—	15
Astrocytomas	2	3	1	1	—
Spongioblastomas	1	—	—	1	2
Ependymomas	1	—	1	2	11
Papillomas	1	1	—	—	2
Angiomas	3	1	1	—	5
Metastatic tumors	—	—	2	1	3
Unclassified	—	1	1	1	3
Total	10	18	6	13	47

tion of highly vascular meningiomas with a minimum of blood loss.

The rest of the operation is the same for both techniques. The dura is replaced and suspect areas of the calvaria are resected or heated. The soft tissue layers with placement of a subgaleal drain are sutured.

Two special cases need comment. With meningiomas of the falx with invasion (but not occlusion) of the sinus we no longer attempt radicality at all costs in all patients as we did 10 years ago. In older or high-risk patients, after exposing the falx of the invaded sinus the sinus is radiated, thus denaturing tumor tissue in the sinus itself. To avoid a Mantelkantensyndrom, the cortex of the contralateral side can be covered by a blood-soaked patch of brain gauze. The blood flow in the sinus cools and eliminates the danger of thrombosis.

Beck (Munich) has reported a 5-year comparative study of about 80 patients who underwent such subradical surgery with laser radiation and a similar number of patients without laser radiation. Local recurrences developed in 4% and 25%, respectively.

The second special case involves basal and laterobasal meningiomas with invasion of the cranial fossa. Extirpation of the largest part of the tumor is performed as described above. After this debulking, the cranial fossa is worked on under the operating microscope. Usually the CO_2 laser is used (40 W, defocused to 20 mm, cw). The Nd:YAG laser can be used by experienced surgeons to denature residual tumor (30 W, defocused to 10 mm, cw, continuous cooling with saline).

Tumors of the Brain Stem

Brain stem tumors were the first absolute indications for the CO_2 laser, and this is reflected in Tables 10.1 and 10.2. We have operated on a total of 113 brain stem tumors, including 47 of the lower brain stem.

Three of the 47 patients with critically located tumors died within the first 3 postoperative weeks. It must be stated clearly here that the laser surgery cannot cure patients with malignant tumors. But survival was prolonged for an average of 3 years, and preoperative neurologic deficits usually improved.

Brain stem tumors are a domain of the CO_2 laser in combination with the operating microscope. The surgical approach is the same as that for conventional microsurgical operations. Tumors with a volume of <5 cm³ are, if possible, vaporized in toto (15–20 W, defocused to 5–20 mm, cw). Poorly accessible tumors can be radiated by reflecting the laser beam with metal mirrors.

An extracerebral approach to tumors of the cranial fossa is preferred. In the rare cases of highly vascularized tumors the laser-experienced neurosurgeon can use the Nd:YAG laser at high energy in short pulses (80 W, slightly defocused, 0.10 sec) for hemostasis.

Larger ependymomas of the fourth ventricle are reduced conventionally. The laser is used only where the tumor adheres to the surface of the brain stem. This part of the tumor is vaporized in layers with the CO_2 laser (5–10 W, defocused to 5–10 mm, cw) with intermittent irrigation of the surface. Vaporization is continued until the surface shows the same consistency and color as the floor of the fourth ventricle. Tumors directly affecting the pons or the medulla are exposed by dividing the brain stem (CO_2 laser, 5 W, focused, cw or sp) and vaporized, if possible. This procedure illustrates the superiority of the laser most clearly. Even dividing the brain stem causes no vegetative reactions of the patient. The anesthesiologist does not interrupt the procedure as occurs when it is performed with standard instruments. The rest of the operation is the same as that for other microsurgical operations except bipolar forceps are not used.

Surgeons inexperienced with lasers must be warned of the 1.06-nm Nd:YAG laser. The 1.32-nm Nd:YAG laser can be used for short periods only for the coagulation of troublesome bleeding. The laser is used at relatively high power in short pulses (30 w, 0.10 sec, slightly defocused).

Low-Grade Astrocytomas, Functionally Inoperable Tumors

All benign or malignant central brain tumors of a certain size (up to 2 cm of diameter) in patients without neurologic symptoms are indications for interstitial thermotherapy (ITT). ITT has a number of advantages as compared with interstitial brachytherapy. ITT is a simple procedure; the heat reaction of the tumor and surrounding tissue can be monitored directly, and ITT can be performed on all types of tumors. ITT also has the advantages associated with brachytherapy: only local anesthesia is required, sensomotoric function and speech can be evaluated continuously, the procedure can be repeated, and the stereotactic approach permits minimal damage to the surrounding brain tissue.[12]

On the morning of surgery a specially designed plastic coordinate ring is placed on the patient's skull. The coordinates of the center of the tumor and those for an appropriate burr hole are plotted by CT. Trepanation is then carried out under local anesthesia. At the same time the coordinates of the target point and the burr hole are plotted on a phantom. An aiming device is adapted and then transferred to the coordinate ring on the patient's head, the probe is then implanted. Afterward the patient is taken to the MR unit and the laser fiber is introduced to the calculated length under MR control.

The laser is then activated (4 W, 10 min). The first changes in the tumor become apparent on the MR screen after 3 minutes. Further laser applications are adapted according to the size of the lesion and the observed heat reaction. The patient is monitored physiologically during the entire procedure. None of the eight patients to date have reported pain or other sensations. The greatest difficulty is the 10 minutes' motionless fixation of the patient.

Most of our instruments are now MR compatible. Only the aiming device and the fixation of the probe remain to be redesigned. Moving the patient from the CT unit to the operating room and to the MR unit is only a logistic problem.

Intraventricular Tumors

The approach to intraventricular tumors is the same as that for conventional surgery, i.e., transventricular or transcallosal. These approaches are also used for endoscopic procedures. Only the Nd:YAG laser can be used endoscopically. Only for this laser are optical fibers available. Also, CO_2 laser light would be completely absorbed by the cerebrospinal fluid. Operations with an open approach are usually done microsurgically. Of course a transventricular approach permits gentle and dry dissection of a cortical-medullary cylinder with a CO_2 laser and suction. Similarly, dividing the corpus callosum with the CO_2 laser is gentle and technically simple (5–7 W, defocused to 3–5 mm, cw). Small, sharply demarcated tumors can then be vaporized after material has been obtained for a histologic diagnosis (CO_2 laser, defocused to 5–10 mm, cw). Endoscopic procedures are indicated for very small lesions or paraventricular tumors (thalamus). After preradiation (Nd:YAG laser, 20–40 W, cw), small lesions can be morcellated with a microrongeur and removed. Low-grade paraventricular astrocytomas of the thalamus can be left in situ after sufficient radiation to denature the tumor. Serial CT studies showed no remaining tumor in such patients after 2 months. Two patients are alive more than 6 years after the operation. Radiation was applied with a 1.06 nm Nd:YAG laser (30–40 W, cw, with cooling irrigation).

These operations are currently limited to tumors up to 15 to 20 mm in diameter. This is the most the Nd:YAG beam penetrates into the pale brain tissue.

Angiomas

Angiomas are the domain of the Nd:YAG laser. Both the 1.06-nm and the 1.32-nm versions can be used. Arteriovenous malformations (AVMs) are exposed in the conventional manner. If possible, afferent arteries are clipped early on. To close small afferent vessels that can cause annoying bleeding, the lesion is irradiated in the same manner as meningiomas. Care must be taken not to close the larger draining veins early on in the operation.

The second step is microdissection with bipolar forceps and scissors as usual until the edge of the preradiated tissue of the angioma has been reached. The laser is again applied (20–40 W, defocused to 5–10 mm, cw, continuous cooling). This technique usually permits removal of the lesion under adequate exposure with little bleeding.

The 1.32-nm Nd:YAG is preferred for central AVMs or those in sensitive areas of the brain. Its penetration and thus coagulation is limited to 2 to 3 mm. The goal of the operation is always extirpation of the AVM after closure of the circulation.

Cerebellopontine Angle Tumors

In contrast to other authors (Cerullo and Robertson), we do not consider lasers suitable for debulking acousticus neurinomas. There is always a danger of injuring the facial nerve or the inferior cerebellar artery as long as these structures have not been clearly exposed and identified. The CUSA is the instrument of choice for these lesions. The laser was used only to vaporize residual tumor adhering to the nerve or brain stem (CO_2 laser, 10–15 W, single shots, 0.5–1.0 sec, slightly defocused).

Conclusions

One and a half decades after its introduction into neurosurgery the laser has become a widely used instrument. Despite the applications mentioned above, the potential of the laser has only begun to be exploited. New applications will revolutionize medicine. Apart from surgical applications, the diagnostic possibilities of lasers will simplify the treatment of tumor patients. Studies of photochemical and photodynamic laser processes should lead to breakthroughs in the near future. We are studying the use of rare earth elements with the excimer laser. However, lasers will not replace neurosurgeons but will permit good surgeons to perform excellent work. As John Brown said in 1980, "The laser does not make the surgeon, but it makes a good surgeon excellent."

References

1. Fox JI. The use of laser radiation as a surgical light knife. *J Surg Rev*. 1969;9:179–199.
2. Rosomoff HL, Caroll F. Effect of laser on the brain and neoplasm. *Surg Forum*. 1965;16:481.
3. Yahr WZ, Strully KJ, Hurwitt ES. Nonocclusive small arterial anastomosis with a ND:YAG Laser. *Surg Forum*. 1964;15:224.
4. Stellar S, Pollary TG, Bredemaier H. Laser in surgery. In: *Laser Applications in Medicine and Biology*. Vol. II. New York: Plenum Press; 1974:224–293.
5. Heppner F, Ascher PW. Über den Einsatz des Laserskalpells in der Neurochirurgie. *Act a Med Techn*. 1976;24:424–426.
6. Leheta F, Goisch W. Coagulation of blood vessels by argon and Nd:YAG laser radiation. In: *Laser Surgery*, Vol. I. Jerusalem: Acad Lademic Press; 1976:178–185.
7. Beck OJ. The use of the Nd:YAG and CO_2 laser in neurosurgery. *Neurosurg Rev*. 1980;3:261–266.
8. Takizawa T. Comparison between the laser surgical unit and electrosurgical unit. *Neurol Med Surg*. 1977;17:95.

9. Tradowsky K. Laser. Verl. University of Würz-burg, 1975.

10. Ascher PW, Ingolitsch E, Walter G. Unsere mikroskopischen Untersuchungsergebnisse nach Gebrauch des CO2-Lasers am ZNS. In: *Kongreßband*. Wien: Egermann Verl; 1979: 479–482.

11. Ascher PW. Tumors on and in the pons and medulla oblongata. In: Downing EF, Ascher PW, et al., New York: eds. *Lasers in Neuro-surgery*. Springer Verlag; 1985:69–93.

12. Ascher PW. Interstitial thermal therapy of brain tumors with the Nd:YAG laser under real time MRI control. In: Joffe SN, Atsumi K, eds. *Proceedings of Laser Surgery: Advanced Characterization, Therapeutics and Systems, II*. Vol. 1200. SPIE, 1989.

CHAPTER 11

Evoked Potentials in Posterior Fossa Surgical Lesions: Basic Principles and Intraoperative Monitoring

Catherine Fischer and Olivier Bertrand

Human brain stem auditory evoked potentials (BAEPs) recorded from the scalp are a series of potentials corresponding to the sequential activation of peripheral, pontomedullary, pontine, and probably midbrain portions of the auditory pathways.

It is possible with BAEP recording to evaluate the functional condition of the whole cochlear nerve and brain stem. In this way, BAEPs take part in the diagnosis of posterior fossa lesions, particularly brain stem tumors or cerebellopontine angle tumors.

Intraoperative BAEP monitoring consists of recording and interpreting the evoked responses continuously without a time-lag throughout an operation. The monitoring of BAEPs in the operating room raises specific technical problems that will be discussed further on.

The representation of the five successive BAEP waves are usually designated as waves I through V and plotted with the vertex-positive up. The accuracy of neurological diagnosis based on surface-recorded BAEPs comes from an increased accuracy concerning the origin within the brain of each of the waves. During the past 20 years, tremendous effort has been made to determine the origin of the waves. Various approaches have been used in this endeavor. The first experiments have been conducted in animals with intracranial electrodes for comparison with skin electrode recordings.[1,2] More recently, similar surface and intracranial recordings have also been made on humans during neurosurgery.[3,4] Furthermore, information on the origin of the

BAEP waves has been obtained by studying the scalp distribution of the BAEP waves by means of multiple scalp electrode sites and recording arrays.

These studies all agree on the fact that wave I represents the compound action potential of the auditory nerve, probably its distal segment. Wave II would be the complex result of potentials generated in the ipsilateral cochlear nucleus and in the proximal segment of the auditory nerve. Wave III is generated in the pons, most likely in the superior olivary complex, the source being either ipsi- or contralateral. Controversy remains about the precise source of waves IV and V, which are close in time and often fusing in a IV–V complex. With respect to wave IV, human intracranial recordings point to a source in the pons, bilaterally either in the lateral lemniscus or in the inferior colliculus. From the same recordings the origin of wave V could be in the vicinity of the inferior colliculus. Attempts at correlating BAEP recordings with location of lateralized lesions in patients have led to the conclusion that wave V would have mainly contralateral sources. In summary, there is no doubt that wave I is generated by the fibers of the auditory nerve; waves II through V are probably generated by multiple sources.

Evoked Potential Data Acquisition and Processing

An evoked potential (EP) recording device can be functionally divided into two subsystems:

(a) the EP acquisition unit in charge of signal amplification, averaging, and stimulus delivery; and (b) the data processing unit, including storage, filtering, and feature extraction. It should fulfill certain specific criteria for intraoperative monitoring, such as being of reduced size and easily portable on a small cart, and include a high level of automation in data processing to provide in real time reliable data concerning the functional brain status of the patient.

The Acquisition Unit

Recording

The BAEP amplitude, which is of several tenths of a microvolt, is much smaller than the background noise blurring the recorded signal. The noise, part of which is biologically generated, includes spontaneous electroencephalogram (EEG) and muscle activity. Technical factors such as external electrical interference and electromagnetic artifacts produced by the acoustic transducer also contribute to this background noise. By repeating the acoustic stimulus and by averaging the EEG phase-locked to the stimulus, BAEPs can be extracted from noise. Typically, 1,000 to 4,000 sweeps are used to acquire an interpretable response.

Traditionally, BAEPs are recorded differentially between electrodes placed on the vertex (positive input) and on the mastoid process (negative input) on the side of the stimulated ear. Both electrodes record relevant activities and are neither inactive nor true reference electrodes. The lateral electrode mainly records early potentials such as peaks I to III, whereas the vertex electrode mainly records peaks III to V. Sterile hypodermic needle electrodes are generally used, and their impedance should preferably be checked and be lower than 5,000 ohms to avoid large electrical interferences. A ground electrode is placed at the earlobe or mastoid contralateral to the stimulated side, or at the forehead. Both for the patient's safety and to limit powerline artifacts, isolated preamplifiers are preferred. The latter should also quickly recover their base-lines after a voltage saturation occurs. In general, during monopolar coagulation the electrodes need to be disconnected for safe use of the preamplifier, whereas during bipolar coagulation recording is still possible.

Several possibilities are available to reduce the noise level. When recording BAEPs, the bandwidth of the recorded signal is very often reduced to 100 to 1,500 Hz by means of an analog bandpass filter. This efficiently reduces the low-frequency biological and environmental noise in the recordings. With a narrower bandwidth, reducing the noise level even more, greater distortions of the waveforms occur, including significant modifications in latency of the relevant peaks due to a complex phase-shift.[5,6] Artifact-containing sequences, corresponding to large amplitude signals exceeding a fixed threshold, must also be excluded from the averaging process.

An interesting feature of the acquisition unit is the possibility to digitize the signal before the stimulus occurs, i.e., to have a prestimulus period. First, this allows an evaluation of a baseline, free of evoked response. The averaged EP can then be centered around the mean of the prestimulus time samples. Second, it provides an estimation of the residual noise level that can be expected to be still present in the rest of the response, flat baselines corresponding to reliable EPs.

It is also very important to continuously control the spontaneous EEG traces on a display screen, preferably with the same time scale as that of the recorded EP. This allows an easy identification and reduction of the artifacts due to the environment. The quality of the signal can thus be quickly evaluated at any time, and the averaging process can be interrupted when necessary.

Stimulation

Acoustic click stimuli produce well-synchronized BAEPs. Clicks are most commonly used with alternating polarity to reduce phase-locked stimulus artifacts. They are delivered through an inexpensive ear insert transducer, hi-fi "Walkman" style. Because of its reduced size, such an audio transducer is better suited to the operating room environment than a standard earphone.[7] Moreover, it can be securely fixed in the patient's ear. Indeed, there may be audiologically significant differences among individual transducers that could introduce undesirable variability. However, during monitoring sessions relative changes over time have more value than absolute changes compared with statistical norms, the stimulus intensity being kept constant during the entire monitoring session. In any case, a modification of the intensity of the stimulus implies a latency shift of all peaks but with a I–V interpeak latency remaining approximately constant. A masking noise is sent in the contralateral ear to limit the neural response of the opposite auditory pathway due to bone conduction. Since it takes less time to perform a test if the rate of the stimulus is increased, rates of 10 to 15 stimuli per second are usually used when it is important to identify the different peaks accurately. At rates exceeding 20 to 40 stimuli per second, little remains of the early peaks I to III and the response mostly consists of peak V.

The Processing Unit

The role of the processing unit includes the control of the acquisition unit, the process of the EP curves, and the storage and display of the results in a sequential manner. EP processing refers here to digital filtering, artifact rejection, peak detection, and feature extraction, which are generally performed on a microcomputer-based system interfaced to the acquisition unit. Displaying the results as trend curves over hours is also one of the specific aspects of neuromonitoring.

Digital Filtering

When recording EPs, the best technical challenge is to obtain the "best and most clean" waveform with the least number of stimuli. The noise problem becomes acute when testing is conducted in the operating room. A few highly contaminated responses may greatly damage the response even after averaging thousands of sweeps. Applying zero-phase

shift digital filters can significantly improve the signal-to-noise ratio.[8–10] The practical problem then consists of choosing the most optimal bandwidth setting that will eliminate the noise still remaining in the averaged response. Automatic peak detection and comparison of serial records thus becomes possible even with a small number of stimuli.

In general, band-pass digital filters avoid phase-distortion introduced by similar analog filters. They are often based on the widely available fast Fourier transform (FFT) alogrithm to modify the spectrum of the response. Cutoff frequencies are determined empirically on the basis that the narrower the bandwidth is, the lower the residual noise level will be. The problem is to determine the values of the high-pass and low-pass frequencies for which distortion of the evoked response begins, or information is lost. The digital bandwidth setting generally determined by testing the filter on normal subjects is not always adequate for pathological responses. When a component decreases in amplitude or completely disappears, the spectrum of the response becomes wider or shifts toward low frequencies. It is thus very difficult to define a bandwidth that can be securely used for all patients, allowing an effective noise removal. Furthermore, when monitoring EPs, it is difficult to choose an efficient bandwidth during the entire monitoring session.

To overcome the problem of the subjective and arbitrary choice of the cutoff frequencies, automatic procedures have been proposed.[8,11] However, to avoid the drawbacks of a fixed band-pass digital filter, we have developed a filtering algorithm that tends to be both optimal and autoadaptive.[12] After every newly acquired EP, it takes into account modification of the patient's response and, overall, occurrence of large transient noise (Fig. 11.1). It is not the purpose of this presentation to detail the filtering technique, but the reader can refer to Bertrand et al.[13] for more details.

Artifact Rejection

Artifact rejection consists of the elimination, out of the averaging process, of single trial

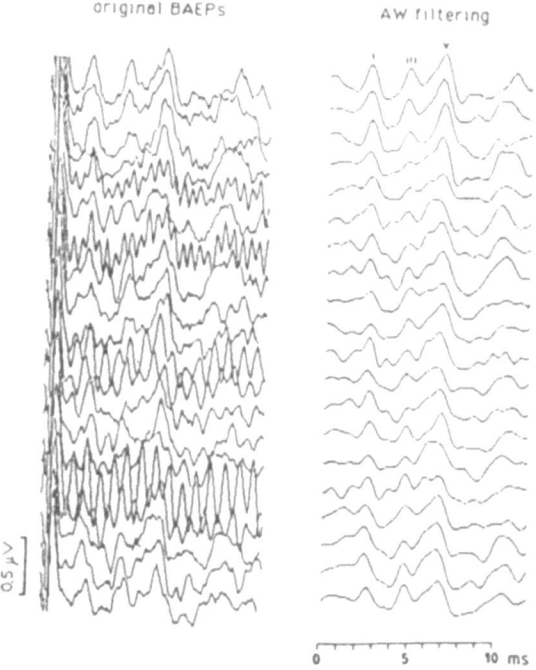

Figure 11.1. Left: Successive BAEPs recorded every minute after 200 stimuli. From time to time, the waveform is contaminated by a periodic noise related to power line interferences. Right: The same BAEPs after adaptative Wiener (AW) filtering. The filter selectively reduces these artifacts, thus leading the clearly interpretable waveforms.

sequences having a large amplitude, exceeding a certain threshold. This is usually done by most of the acquisition units. Nevertheless, large elementary responses at the higher authorized amplitude limit may still distort the averaged EP. Additional stimulations will then be necessary to compensate the effect of such a transient noise. However, the use of the adaptive Wiener filter based on successive subaverages makes it possible to implement more sophisticated algorithms to discard too highly artifacted EPs. After each newly acquired subaveraged response, for instance quickly obtained with 200 stimulations, we may compute a specific criterion allowing us to keep or discard this EP according to the noise level. In this latter case, the adaptive filter is not updated and a new EP acquisition is immediately started. This procedure is repeated until an acceptable response can be recorded. There are various possible criteria to achieve artifact rejection.[14] The energy of the entire current EP, or in a specific frequency band, for instance, can be compared to the energy of the last filtered EP. Thus it seems of great interest for monitoring purposes to acquire EPs as successive small subaverages, followed by the above-mentioned artifact rejection, whether simple or sophisticated digital filtering is used. This avoids the sudden distortion of the moving average, which would become steady again sometime after 10 or more correct successive subaverages.

Feature Extraction

Our main concern in monitoring EPs is to follow, on-line, changes of the response waveform, i.e., the latency and amplitude of waves I, III, and V for BAEPs. Therefore, a computer algorithm that automatically tracks the peak of the waves on the successively filtered curves is necessary. Our method is based on an initial localization manually performed by the operator with a cursor on the computer screen. The latency of the reference peak are stored, and then sequential recording may start. On each new filtered EP, positive or negative peaks are searched within a time window centered on each reference latency. The smoothness of the curves obtained after digital filtering allows a straightforward detection by locating the zero-crossing of the first derivative of the response. This adaptive algorithm allows a continuous tracking of the main waves without being disturbed by some possible aberrant detections.

Once the peaks are identified, clinically relevant parameters can be computed. Peak latencies or interpeak latencies are the most easily derived values. The amplitude difference between a peak and its following trough can then be computed, and provide a baseline-free measurement.

One of the most original characteristics of EP monitoring lies in the elaboration over hours of trend curves of the extracted features. Grand averaged EP waveforms need of course to be compared at different times, but it is also

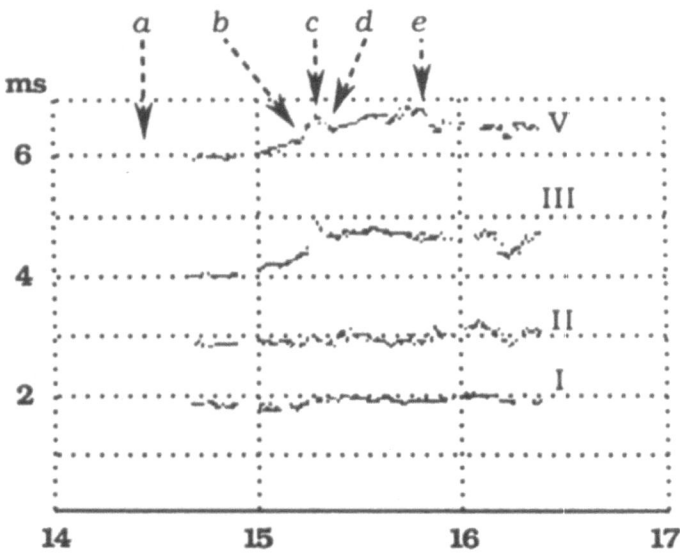

Figure 11.2. Trend curves with automatic detection of wave I, II, III, and V latencies during microvascular decompression of the seventh nerve and cerebellar retraction. Abscissa: time from onset of the operation. Ordinate: wave latencies in milliseconds. a: 14:30—dura open, b: 15:11—retractor on, c: 15:14—warming to the surgeon, d: 15:24—retractor adjusted, e: 15:49—retractor out.

important to extract the relevant information contained in these data, and to present it as a synthesis. The latency values of the detected peaks, as well as their amplitude, are plotted on a graph with the x-axis expressed in minutes or hours, and the y-axis in milliseconds or millivolts. This type of curve provides immediate information on the patient's brain status and his current evolution (Fig. 11.2) A characteristic of neuromonitoring relies on the fact that high-rate sequential recording increases the redundancy of the measured parameters and gives more confidence in the interpretation of response modifications. Significant variations should be assessed by taking into account the variability of the parameters, which could be correctly estimated if a sufficient amount of data is present.

High-level artifact rejection of small, successive subaverages and adaptive digital filtering on a moving average could probably summarize the data processing requirement for EP monitoring. This allows for a fast recording of waveforms reliable enough to alarm or to comfort the neurosurgeon during the different phases of an intervention. Analysis of trend curves of latencies and amplitudes certainly provides meaningful information on the patient's brain status and evolution, in an easily understandable synthesis.

BAEP Abnormalities in Brain Stem Tumors

Since its introduction into clinical practice, BAEP recording has become a routine test for neurologic diagnosis. It has proved to be an objective and sensitive indicator of brain stem impairment. BAEPs are useful to determine the functional state of the brain stem in posterior fossa lesions. For early detection and localization of brain stem tumors, BAEP recordings have nowadays been replaced by magnetic resonance imaging (MRI), which has a much better detecting and localizing value.

Normal BAEP

Normal BAEPs recorded in children above 2 years of age are similar to those recorded in adults (Fig. 11.3). Below 2 years of age, interpeak latencies increase and vary inversely with age.

The principal features used to assess BAEPs are the following:

presence of waves I to V, which should be detected in most normal individuals.
interpeak intervals: The I–V interpeak interval represents the conduction from the eighth nerve to the midbrain. The upper limit for

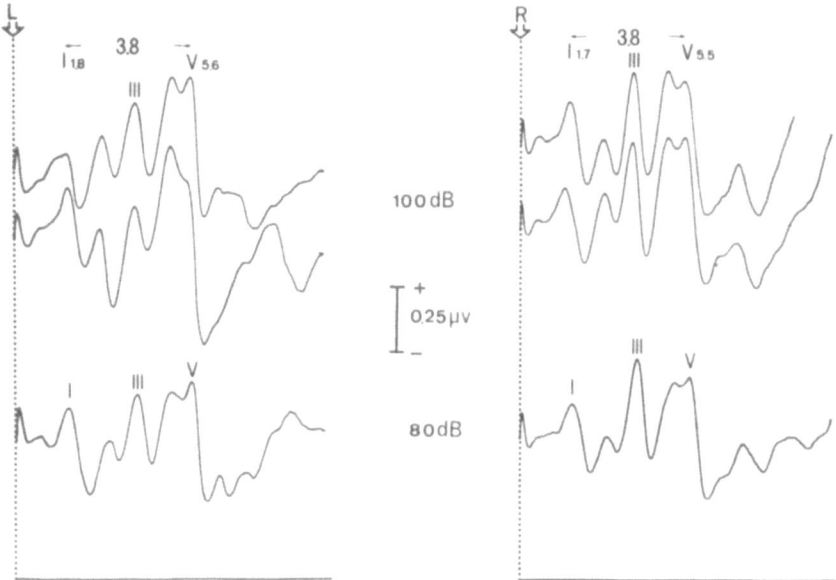

Figure 11.3. A normal brain stem auditory evoked potential (BAEP). Left (L): left ear stimulation. Right (R): right ear stimulation. Stimulation intensity in dBHL. Two normal reproducible traces are superimposerd at 100dB. Waves I and V latencies, and I–V intervals in milliseconds.

normal I–V interval is 4.5 msec, and normal right-left asymmetry for the I–V interpeak interval is not greater than 0.4 msec. The I–III interpeak interval represents the conduction of the eighth nerve into the lower pons. The upper limit for the normal I–III interpeak interval is around 2.5 msec. The III–V interpeak interval represents the conduction from the lower to the upper pons and into midbrain. The upper limit is below 2.4 msec.

I/V amplitude ratio, which should be lower than 1. When it is greater than 2, central impairment decreasing the amplitude of wave V is suspected.

absolute latencies of waves I, II, and V can be of clinical value when there are absent BAEP waves.

BAEP Abnormalities in Brain Stem Tumors

When abnormal in such cases, BAEP recordings show one or several of the typical patterns of retrocochlear impairment.

Criteria for retrocochlear dysfunction are:

1. absence of all waves (unexplained by audiometry),
2. absence of all waves following wave I or III,
3. increase of I–V interpeak interval,
4. abnormal I/V amplitude ratio,
5. interaural I–V interval asymmetry.
   (From American Electroencephalography Society, cited in ref. 15.)

BAEP recordings of patients with brain stem tumors have been reported in the medical literature, most often in very small series.[16–18] Results were similar, with waves I and II being present and normal, and III–V intervals most often bilaterally abnormal.

We have already reported both clinical and electrophysiological data in 30 cases with brain stem surgical lesions.[19] There were 19 men aged from 4 to 54 and 11 women aged from 5 to 60 years. When performed, audiometry was normal in all but one.

BAEP results depended on the level of the lesion in the brain stem:

1. This group includes seven patients with lesions involving the medulla oblongata

(three low-grade astrocytomas, one grade I ependymoma, two hemangioblastomas, one cavernoma). BAEPs were normal in all cases, since in these cases lesions were strictly limited to the medulla and did not cross over the pontobulbar junction.

2. This group includes five patients with lesions involving the medulla oblongata and the pons (two low-grade gliomas, one malignant glioma, one hemangioblastoma, one ganglioglioma). BAEP were abnormal in all cases, bilaterally, whatever the side of the auditory stimulation was. In all cases the I–V interval was delayed, with an abnormal I/V amplitude ratio in one case.

3. This group includes 13 lesions involving the pons and sparing the medulla (five low-grade gliomas, three high-grade gliomas, five vascular malformations). BAEPs were abnormal in all cases. In 12 of the 13 cases abnormalities were bilateral (Fig. 11.4). In two cases all waves following waves I and II were absent. In 10 cases the I–V interval was delayed, even more so with abnormal I/V amplitude ratio. In a single case there was a unilateral obliteration of all the waves; the patient suffered from an angioma with hematoma causing facial palsy and unilateral deafness.

4. In this group there are five lesions involving the midbrain. In three cases BAEPs were normal (two vascular malformations and a small low-grade glioma). In two cases (large malignant tumors) BAEP recording disclosed a slight delay of I–V interval.

BAEP recordings in 30 patients with surgical lesions of the brain stem can be summarized as follows:

wave I was present in all cases but one (patient with a lesion causing unilateral deafness);

when abnormal, BAEP recordings disclosed delays or amplitude abnormalities of waves III to V;

BAEP abnormalities are most often bilateral;

BAEP patterns depend on the topography of the lesion and on its closeness to central auditory pathways.

Intraoperative BAEP Monitoring

Modern neurosurgery tends to take into account methods that improve patient safety during high-risk surgical procedures or that preserve sensory function. By allowing continuous evaluation of the functional condition of the cochlear nerve and brain stem in anes-

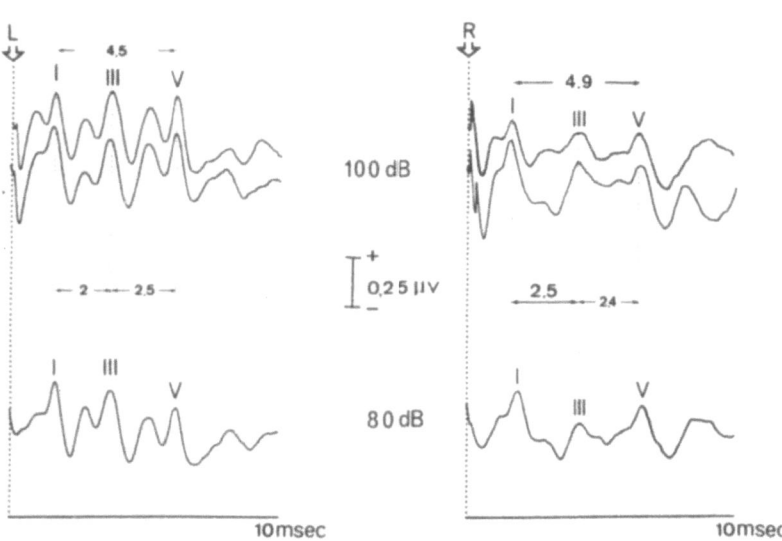

Figure 11.4. Abnormal BAEPs in a case with a pontine lesion. Delay of I–V interval after right (R) ear stimulation. Upper limit of I–V interval after left (L) ear stimulation. Two superimposed traces show the reproducibility of BAEP abnormalities.

thetized patients, intraoperative BAEP monitoring can help attempts at preserving hearing in cerebellopontine angle surgery and can improve patient safety in conditions in which the brain stem is particularly exposed.[20]

Hashimoto et al.[21] published the results of the first intraoperative monitoring in 12 cases with a surgical lesion of the posterior fossa of various etiologies and showed the feasibility of BAEP monitoring during surgery. Subsequenth, Raudzens and Shetter[22] reported their experience of BAEP monitoring of 46 cases of posterior fossa surgery. They concluded that the BAEPs could be routinely recorded in the operating room, and that BAEP monitoring was rather a good predictor of the postoperative hearing condition, and possibly helpful in minimizing nerve damage by alerting the surgeon during surgery. Grundy et al.[23] also reported the results of BAEP monitoring carried out on 54 patients during cerebellopontine angle operations. They suggested that if no modification or even transient or reversible modifications of the BAEPs occurred during surgery, postoperative hearing was preserved. More recently, Schramm et al.,[24] reporting on their initial experience of BAEP monitoring in 31 patients, analyzed the data about significant intraoperative changes. They raised the question, When is it reasonable to react to intraoperative BAEP deterioration?

Monitoring the Functional Condition of the Brain Stem

Information on the functional condition of the brain stem can be helpful during surgery of a tumor or a brain stem hematoma, during posterior circulation surgery, or during removal of large tumors of the posterior fossa. BAEP monitoring can provide reliable information on the functional state of the brain stem. Today intraoperative monitoring is rather time-consuming because it requires the presence of a neurophysiologist all throughout the operation. In the future, thanks to evoked potentials devices including a high level of automation in acquisition and data processing, more and

more surgeons will be able to take advantage of intraoperative monitoring.

BAEP monitoring has been carried out in our department on 16 patients undergoing surgery for a brain stem tumor (14 cases) or a brain stem hematoma (two cases). Eight lesions were completely removed and eight were only biopsied (Fig. 11.5). In all 16 cases BAEPs were altered before operation. In 10 of them there was no deterioration of BAEPs during the operation; for 7 of the 10 patients the postoperative neurological condition was unchanged; the other three worsened. In the case of the other six patients, transient (five cases) or permanent (one case) intraoperative changes were observed. Three of them had uneventful recovery and two of them became worse. It cannot be ascertained whether postoperative worsening was due to surgery or to natural evolution of the lesion. The patient with the permanent changes did not wake up after the operation and died on the 15th day.

Unfortunately, brain stem tumors can greatly disturb the preoperative recording of the BAEPs, thus not allowing efficient monitoring during surgery. The purpose is to survey above all waves III, IV, and V, and the III–V interval, but the preoperative BAEP changes can be such that this is impossible or very difficult.

We have also monitored 12 patients during operation for posterior fossa lesions indirectly compressing the brain stem, or likely to cause brain stem dysfunction during their removal. Five large meningiomas of the cerebellar convexity, four tumors of the cerebellum, one cerebellopontine metastasis, and two Chiari malformations were included in this category. Ten of the 12 patients had very good results. The increase of the I–V interval did not exceed 0.6 msec during the operation. A shift of the I–V interval not exceeding 0.6 msec could be considered as nonsignificant in posterior fossa monitoring. Two patients worsened after surgery. In one of them the I–V interval increased over 1 msec, without any reversibility. In the other case the intraoperative amplitude of wave V very progressively decreased, a phenomenon continuing after surgery. Wave V disappeared on the following day.

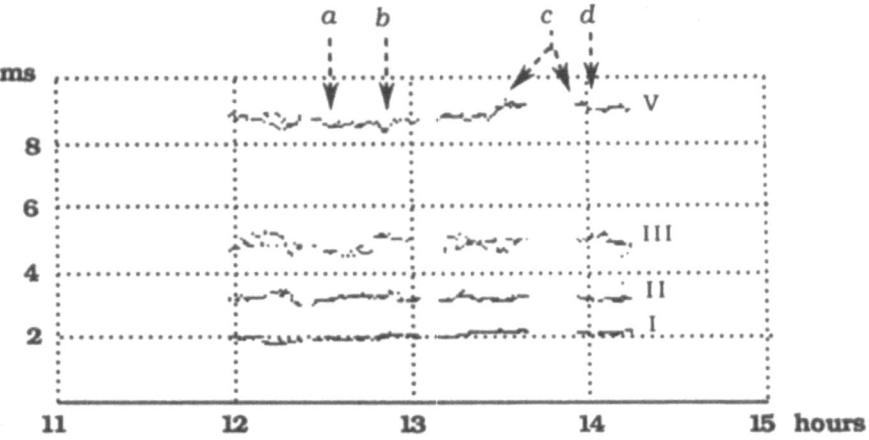

Figure 11.5. Trend curves with automatic detection of wave I, II, III, and V latencies during the biopsy of a brain stem infiltrating tumor. Abscissa: time from onset of the operation. Ordinate: waves latencies in milliseconds. a: dura open (12:32); b: retractor on (12:50); c: biopsy (13:30 to 13:50); d: retractor out (14:03). I–V and III–V intervals are delayed without any significant increase during surgery.

Little et al.[25] have reported BAEP monitoring of 10 patients operated for vascular problems in posterior circulation. There is a correlation of the BAEP abnormalities and the neurological findings before and after operation. They concluded that monitoring BAEPs helps in identifying brain stem dysfunction during posterior circulation surgery.

Monitoring the Auditory Nerve Function

The purpose of BAEP monitoring during surgery of cerebellopontine angle lesions is to prevent damage to the eighth nerve, thus preserving some hearing function. For example, until 1989 our experience of acoustic neuroma surgery dealt with 61 neuromas responsible for incomplete deafness.[26] After surgery 42 of the 61 patients lost hearing function. Thanks to BAEP monitoring we have learned about mechanisms of hearing loss during that kind of operation. Peak V was never present at the end of the operation of the patients who lost hearing function. Some identified mechanisms of BAEP loss and subsequent hearing loss were dura opening, tumor vessel coagulation, cere-

bellum retraction, volume reduction, and tumor removal within the internal auditory canal. After surgery hearing was preserved in 19 of the 61 patients. All of these patients had wave V still present at the end of the operation. Only one-third of the patients who maintained only wave I at the end of the operation preserved some hearing. Preserving peak I does not guarantee postoperative hearing preservation.

Conclusion

The usefulness of monitoring is greater after one has acquired experience in using this neurophysiological technique for given indications such as for acoustic neuroma operations or brain stem tumors operations. Those performing intraoperative monitoring have to learn the significance of the BAEP changes that may be observed during the monitoring period and they have to identify when a change warrants warning the surgeon. BAEPs may change not only because of the surgical procedure, but also because of pharmacologic agents and the patient's temperature.

BAEP monitoring is helpful in attempts to preserve hearing function in cerebellopontine angle operations and in allowing real-time evaluation of the functional state of the brain stem in any posterior fossa surgery. In a general way, it may help improve patient safety during at-risk procedures in the posterior fossa.

References

1. Lev A, Sohmer H. Source of averaged neural responses recorded in animal and human subjects during cochlear audiometry. *Arch Klin Exp Ohr Nase Kehl-Heilk*. 1972;201:79–90.
2. Achor LJ, Starr A. Auditory brainstem responses in the cat. I. Intracranial and extracranial recordings. *Electroencephalogr Clin Neurophysiol*. 1980;48:154–173.
3. Hashimoto I, Ishiyama Y, Yoshimoto T, et al. Brainstem auditory evoked potentials recorded directly from human brainstem and thalamus. *Brain*. 1981;104:841–859.
4. Moller AR, Jannetta PJ. Evoked potentials from the inferior colliculus in man. *Electroencephalogr Clin Neurophysiol*. 1982;78:144–157.
5. Boston JR, Ainslie PJ. Effects of analog and digital filtering on brainstem auditory evoked potentials. *Electroencephalogr Clin Neurophysiol*. 1980;48:361–364.
6. Elton M, Scherg M, Von Cramon D. Effects of high-pass filter frequency and slope on BAEP amplitude, latency and waveform. *Electroencephalogr Clin Neurophysiol*. 1984;57:490–494.
7. Erwin CW, Gulevich SJ. Evaluation of transducers for obtaining intra-operative short latency auditory evoked potentials. *Electroencephalogr Clin Neurophysiol*. 1985;61:194–196.
8. Fridman J, John ER, Bergelson M, et al. Application of digital filtering and automatic peak detection to brainstem auditory evoked potential. *Electroencephalogr Clin Neurophysiol*. 1982;53:405–416.
9. Boston JR. Effect of digital filtering on the waveform and peak parameters of the auditory brainstem response. *J Clin Eng*. 1983;8:79–84.
10. Møller AR. Improving brainstem auditory evoked potential recordings by digital filtering. *Ear Hear*. 1983;4:108–113.
11. Boston JR, Deneault LG, Kronk L, et al. Auto-mated monitoring of brainstem auditory evoked potentials in the operating room. *J Clin Monit*. 1985;1:161–167.
12. Bertrand O, Garcia-Larrea L, Artru F, et al. Brainstem monitoring. I. A system for high-rate BAEP recording and feature extraction. *Electroencephalogr Clin Neurophysiol*. 1987;68:433–445.
13. Bertrand O, Bohorquez J, Pernier J. Technical requirements for evoked potential monitoring in the intensive care unit. In: Rossini PM, Mauguiere F, eds. *New Trends and Advanced Techniques in Clinical Neurophysiology* (EEG J Suppl. 41). Amsterdam: Elsevier; 1990:51–70.
14. Pantev C, Khvoles R. Comparison of the efficiency of various criteria for artefact rejection in the recording of auditory brainstem responses. *Scand Audiol*. 1984;13:103–108.
15. Nuwer MR. *Evoked Potential Monitoring in the Operating Room*. New York: Raven Press; 1986.
16. Rosenhall U, Hedner ML, Bjorkman G. ABR in brain stem lesions. *Scand Audiol*. 1981; 13:117–123.
17. Walser H, Yasargil MG, Curcic M. Auditory brainstem responses in patients with posterior fossa tumors. *Surg Neurol*. 1982;18:405–415.
18. Davis SL, Aminoff MJ, Berg BO. Brain stem auditory evoked potentials in children with brain stem or cerebellar dysfunction. *Arch Neurol*. 1985;42:156–180.
19. Guy G, Jan M, Guegan Y. Les lésions chirurgicales du tronc cérébral. *Neurochirurgie*. 1989; 35(suppl 1):20–24.
20. Fischer C. Brainstem auditory evoked potential (BAEP) monitoring in posterior fossa surgery. In: Desmedt JE, ed. *Neuromonitoring in Surgery*. Amsterdam: Elsevier; 1989;191–207.
21. Hashimoto I, Ishiyama Y, Totsuka O, et al. Monitoring brainstem function during posterior fossa surgery with brainstem auditory evoked potentials In: Barber C, ed. *Evoked Potentials*. Baltimore: University Park Press; 1980:377–390.
22. Raudzens PA, Shetter AG. Intraoperative monitoring of brainstem auditory evoked potentials. *J Neurosurg*. 1982;57:341–348.
23. Grundy BL, Jannetta PJ, Procopio PT, et al. Intraoperative monitoring of brainstem auditory evoked potentials. *J Neurosurg*. 1982;57:674–681.
24. Schramm J, Mokrusch T, Fahlbusch R, et al. Detailed analysis of intraoperative changes

monitoring brain stem acoustic evoked potentials. *Neurosurgery*. 1988;22:694–702.

25. Little JR, Lesser RP, Lueders H, et al. Brainstem auditory evoked potentials in posterior circulation surgery. *Neurosurgery*. 1983;12:496–502.

26. Fischer C, Fischer G. Intraoperative brainstem auditory evoked potential (BAEP) monitoring in acoustic neuroma surgery. In: Schramm J, Møller AR, eds. *Intraoperative Neurophysiological Monitoring*. Berlin: Springer; 1991:187–192.

CHAPTER 12

Chemotherapy of Childhood Posterior Fossa Tumors

Roger J. Packer, H. Stacy Nicholson, and Janis Ryan

Introduction

Chemotherapy has been utilized for patients with brain tumors for the past five decades.[1] Primarily stemming from poor results obtained in adults with malignant gliomas, chemotherapy has been considered an ineffective adjunct to the care of newly diagnosed patients or a last gasp for patients with recurrent disease.[2,3] However, over the past 10 years, results from well-performed trials in children with recurrent brain tumors and, even more recently, in patients with newly diagnosed tumors have shown that chemotherapy has a definite role in the management of primary childhood central nervous system tumors.[4–31] As the rates of survival slowly increase for children with brain tumors, the frequency and degree of treatment-related sequelae become more apparent.[32,33] Radiation therapy, although the cornerstone of postsurgical treatment for most malignant and some benign childhood brain tumors, has been implicated as the major, if not sole, reason for most adverse effects of treatment.[32–35]

Chemotherapy has been proposed as an alternative or adjunct to radiation therapy to potentially reduce (or obviate in selected cases) the amount of radiation therapy needed and resultant sequelae.[22,23,36–38] The obvious drawback to this approach is that if chemotherapy is not as effective as radiotherapy, more children will die of their disease. In addition, the long-term safety of various chemotherapies on the developing nervous system has not been conclusively demonstrated. Despite these potential problems, there is now evidence that chemotherapy is of benefit for some forms of childhood primary central nervous system tumors. The most compelling data come from studies of patients with newly diagnosed medulloblastoma, where chemotherapy is used in an adjuvant fashion with surgery and radiotherapy.[18–22,25,26] For other childhood posterior fossa tumors such as ependymomas, brain stem gliomas, and cerebellar gliomas, evidence for the benefit of chemotherapy is either less impressive or completely lacking.[2,39] However, since survival and the quality of survival are far from optimal for most of these other childhood posterior fossa tumors, further investigations with chemotherapeutic agents seem warranted.

General Chemotherapeutic Principles

In the most simplistic terms, by the time a child shows clinical signs of a primary central nervous system tumor, the intracranial mass has reached a size of at least 0.5 cm or a tumor burden of at least 10^9 cells.[1] Treatment is aimed at reducing this tumor burden and can be conceptualized in a log-kill manner. For any specific treatment, a percentage of tumor cells will be destroyed. Aggressive surgery, although possibly removing the majority of visible tumor, is unlikely to reduce the tumor bulk by more than one log-kill (10^8 cells). Radiation therapy, when effective, usually results in approximately 2 more log-kills, leaving the patient with re-

Table 12.1. Efficacy of chemotherapy.

Delivery–pharmacologic distribution
    Physiochemical drug properties
    Pharmacokinetic drug properties
    Permeabilities of capillaries
    Surface area of capillaries
    Blood flow to tumor
    Drug concentration
    Drug circulation time
    ? Brain-adjacent to tumor content
Tumor sensitivity
    Drug effects
    Spontaneous mutation rate of tumor
    Tumor mitotic activity
Tumor burden
Normal tissue tolerance
    Toxicity to brain
    Toxicity to other organs

sidual of 10^6 cells. It is believed that the body's own immune mechanisms may be able to control a reduced tumor burden, in the 10^3 to 10^4 range. Thus, for chemotherapy to be useful it would need to cause at least an additional 2 log-kill. In the future, it may be possible to augment the patient's immune response so that a greater number of tumor cells are controlled by the body's immune mechanisms.

Although this construct is logical, the chemotherapy of brain tumors is much more complex (Table 12.1). Probably more than in any other region of the body, the accessibility of the tumor to the chemotherapeutic agent is most limited in the brain. The amount of drug that reaches a brain tumor is determined by both the physiochemical and pharmacokinetic properties of the drug and the intrinsic properties of the brain tumor.[2,40] The amount of drug that can cross the capillary wall (the blood-brain barrier) or the blood-tumor barrier is dependent on the permeability of the capillaries to that drug, the surface area of the capillaries available for drug exchange, the blood flow to the tumor, the concentration of drug in the plasma, and the length of time that the drug circulates through the capillaries.[40]

The significance of the blood-brain barrier as it affects the utility of chemotherapeutic agents is far from clear.[2,3,40] There is no question that

the barrier, which usually protects the brain from certain biomolecules that can upset its function, restricts the delivery of anticancer agents. However, for many childhood brain tumors, especially the medulloblastoma, the majority of the tumor has a relatively poor blood-brain barrier (as can be seen by how readily the tumors enhance after the intravenous infusion of contrast agents). Compounding this problem, however, is the distribution of drug to the brain adjacent to the tumor.[2] Malignant cells can migrate from the center of a necrotic tumor (which has a disrupted blood-brain barrier) to the periphery of the normal brain adjacent to the tumor. These tumor cells theoretically are the most viable and have the greatest capacity for proliferation. However, because of the relatively intact blood-brain barrier in this adjacent area, this region may be the most inaccessible to treatment.[3] The properties that influence and enhance the tansport of drugs into the central nervous system include low molecular weight, high lipid solubility, and the lack of significant plasma protein binding.[40]

Concern over the effect of the blood-brain barrier, especially for nonlipophilic drugs, has led to the use of various agents to disrupt the barrier.[3] The efficacy of these approaches to deliver more drug to the regions adjacent to brain has been greatly debated. In addition, all such approaches can have the unwanted effect of delivering the chemotherapeutic agents in high concentration to normal regions of the brain. For drugs such as cisplatin and CCNU, delivery of the drugs to the brain after barrier disruption may result in increased neurologic morbidity.[41]

Another means to enhance delivery of chemotherapeutic agents is to change the route of delivery. Although most agents are still given intravenously or orally, the pharmacokinetic properties of the drug might suggest that an intrathecal or intra-arterial infusion may be more efficacious. On theoretic grounds, those tumors that lie near the subarachnoid space are more amenable to direct intracerebrospinal fluid instillation.[2] However, since these drugs tend to penetrate only a small distance within the tumor, such an approach is of little benefit for patients with bulk disease. The intrathecal approach also carries with it increased risk for neurotoxicity, especially in patients with posterior fossa tumors and altered flow of cerebrospinal fluid.

Intra-arterial therapy has not been utilized widely in pediatric protocols. In theory, intra-arterial administration achieves locally higher drug concentrations for a given amount of systemic exposure. Those drugs with high capillary permeability, a high extraction fraction, and rapid metabolism or excretion, such as the nitrosoureas, are delivered in as high as a fivefold greater concentration and a tenfold greater peak level, after arterial as compared to intravenous delivery.[3] There is some evidence of increased efficacy but with increased neurotoxicity in adult trials.[2,3] Moreover, the basilar blood supply of almost all posterior fossa tumors limits the utility of this approach. Another approach to maximize the benefit of chemotherapy is the utilization of drugs prior to radiotherapy.[18-21] Conventionally, chemotherapeutic agents have been used after the completion of radiotherapy. There is some evidence that radiation therapy, at least transiently, causes microvascular changes, decreases the delivery of drug to the tumor, and possibly makes it less effective.

The underlying premise of the use of any chemotherapeutic agent is that the tumor is sensitive to the drug utilized.[2,28] In principle, chemotherapeutic agents are considered to be either cell-cycle specific or cell-cycle nonspecific. Since some brain tumors have a relatively slow turnover rate, drugs that are given over a longer duration of time or are not dependent on reaching the tumor at a phase of active cellular proliferation, should have an advantage. However, in practice, this distinction has not been of great utility in childhood brain tumors. The agents that have been shown to be effective in the treatment of childhood brain tumors have been identified, by and large, from trial and error approaches. The use of laboratory-based screening tests has been disappointing in determining the efficacy of an agent in an individual patient. Newer animal models, especially the establishment of human tumor cell lines growing in vivo in athymic mice, hold great promise for the rational selection of chemotherapeutic agents. For years, such research has been limited in medulloblastoma by the lack of available human cell lines. However, the recent development of more cell lines has overcome this obstacle.[28]

Other factors that impact on the efficacy of any chemotherapeutic agent are the cellular mechanisms that exist to reverse drug-induced damage.[2] A general oncologic principle is the greater the tumor burden, the less effective the chemotherapeutic agent. The large bulk of some central nervous system tumors combined with their inaccessibility to significant debulking procedures (such as an intrinsic brain stem tumor), is one reason why therapy may be of borderline efficacy. Another is the ability of tumor cells to become resistant to therapy.

In 1979, Goldie and Coldman[42] proposed a mathematical model that related the curability of a malignancy to the appearance of resistant cell lines. They proposed that control of a neoplasm was the function of various factors, including the tumor's spontaneous mutation rate toward resistance. An outgrowth of this construct is that the probability of the tumor being resistant to multiple agents administered simultaneously would be less than the probability of it being resistant to agents used individually. One possible reason for the greater efficacy of chemotherapy in pediatric trials is the use of multiple chemotherapeutic agents. This use of multiple agents may decrease the ability of the tumor to mutate and develop pleiotropic multiple-drug resistance. In addition, if drugs are given over a relatively short period of time, myelosuppression should be less, as damage to the hematopoietic precursor cells is dependent on duration as well as dose of exposure.

A multiagent approach is presently being utilized in most childhood adjuvant chemotherapy trials. Whether this approach is best is yet unproven. The introduction of hematologic growth factors and the application of bone marrow transplantation techniques also may enhance the efficacy of chemotherapy by allowing higher peak doses or greater concentrations of drugs to be given over time, partially obviating the tumor's natural tendency to develop resistance.

Medulloblastoma/Primitive Neuroectodermal Tumor

Medulloblastoma/primitive neuroectodermal tumor (MB/PNET) constitutes approximately 40% of all posterior fossa tumors and is the most common malignant childhood brain tumor.[43] These small cell tumors frequently display histological heterogeneity and their multiclonal nature may partially explain why multiagent chemotherapy has seemed to be more effective than single agent therapy. More is known about the clinical course and response to chemotherapy for medulloblastoma than for any other childhood brain tumor.

Survival figures for patients with medulloblastoma were quite disappointing until recently. Less than one-third of patients diagnosed in the 1950s or 1960s were alive and free of disease 5 years after treatment.[43] Due to several factors, including earlier diagnosis, safer anesthesia, advances in surgical techniques, improved postoperative care, and the more effective use of radiotherapy, disease-free survival rates of up to 50% 5 years after diagnosis are now being reported.[43–45] The introduction of prophylactic radiation therapy to the entire neuraxis at the time of diagnosis is probably the single most important factor leading to these improved "long-term" survival figures.[43,44]

Over the past decade, the usefulness of staging studies has been demonstrated for MB/PNET and these parameters have become the backbone of ongoing treatment trials. Two large prospective randomized treatment trials for children with MB/PNET were undertaken in the 1970s by the Children's Cancer Study Group and the International Society of Pediatric Oncology. Both of these trials concluded that children with medulloblastoma could be stratified into risk groups based on factors such as the degree of surgical resection, size of the tumor at the time of diagnosis, the extent of tumor dissemination at diagnosis, and the age of the patient (Table 12.2).[25,26,46,47] In addition, large single institution retrospective reviews also suggested that these variables were of prognostic importance.[47]

In the Children's Cancer Study Group study,

Table 12.2. Factors portending "poorer" outcome for children with PNET/MB.

Disseminated disease
? Larger tumor
? Subtotal resection
Younger age at diagnosis (? less than 4)
Brain stem involvement

children with localized disease at diagnosis had a nearly 60% 5-year event-free survival, compared with 36% for those with evidence of dissemination.[25] Factors suggesting poor outcome tended to cluster in an individual patient and the independent significance of any one factor has been difficult to prove. The only parameter that has reproducibly been associated with poorer outcome in all studies has been tumor dissemination at diagnosis.[25,46–48] The rate of dissemination at diagnosis has been reported between 15% and 50%, with series weighted toward younger patients (under age 5 at diagnosis) reporting the highest incidence of dissemination.[46,48]

One factor that has been especially difficult to analyze and conceptualize has been age. In almost every large series to date, younger children, especially those younger than 3 years of age at diagnosis, have a lower survival rate.[25,43,46] The significance of age as a predictive factor is confounded by the greater likelihood for younger patients to have disseminated disease at diagnosis and the possibility that these patients receive less aggressive treatment because of their young age.[25,43,46] It is also conceivable that there are inherent differences in the biology of the tumor.

In most retrospective series, aggressive tumor resection at diagnosis has been related to a better outcome. However, in the randomized multi-institutional trials this association was not found when other factors, such as age and tumor dissemination at diagnosis, were taken into account.[25,26] Blurring the situation even further are results from the recent study jointly undertaken by the International Society for Pediatric Oncology and the German Society for Pediatric Oncology. Between 1984 and 1988, 369 patients with MB/PNET were treated in a randomized trial. No prognostic influence of tumor stage or metastasis at the time of diagnosis was found.[49]

Despite these latter findings, the two largest cooperative childhood cancer groups in the United States, the Children's Cancer Study Group and the Pediatric Oncology Group, have adopted a postoperative staging system based on the extent of surgical resection (rather than on the preoperative size of the primary tumor), extent of disease dissemination, presence of brain stem involvement, and age.[50] The stratification systems are not just of academic interest, since in both earlier cooperative trials there was evidence that children with "poor risk" parameters benefited from the addition of chemotherapy, whereas children with "average risk" lesions did not.[25,26] In most centers, cerebrospinal fluid cytological analysis, myelography, and/or spinal magnetic resonance imaging (MRI) with gadolinium, and postoperative neuroimaging of the surgical site [with either computed tomography (CT) or MRI] are standard postoperative investigations (Table 12.2). These factors are taken into account when deciding whether to add chemotherapy to radiotherapy in the postoperative period. If the prognostic significance of these factors is reaffirmed in future studies, they must be taken into account in evaluating the efficacy of any chemotherapeutic regimen. On the other hand, if these parameters are not confirmed to be of prognostic significance, they may be used incorrectly to deny patients needed adjuvant therapy.

Efficacy of Chemotherapy in Recurrent MB/PNET

Medulloblastoma/primitive neuroectodermal tumors are well vascularized lesions and have a high growth fraction. In vitro and in vivo studies of human MB/PNET have demonstrated responsiveness of the tumor to a variety of different chemotherapeutic agents. The recent development of multiple MB/PNET cell lines and improved in vitro models of MB/PNET tumor growth should allow for an even better selection of agents.[28] Clinical evidence for the response of medulloblastoma to chemotherapy has been most clearly substantiated by analysis of patients treated at the time of disease recurrence, and more recently by preradiation therapy trials in which therapy is given after surgery, but before radiotherapy.

Various chemotherapeutic agents, used singly, have been shown to be at least partially effective in children with relapsed MB/PNET (Table 12.3).[6,7,9,12–16,51–57] The earlier studies,

Table 12.3. Objective[a] response of recurrent MB/PNET to chemotherapy: single agent trials.

Author	Therapy	Response/evaluable patients	Median duration of response (months)
Rosen et al. (1977)	Methotrexate	5/7	9
Allen and Helson (1981)	Cyclophosphamide	8/8	5.5
Sexaur et al. (1985)	Cisplatin	4/10	6[b]
Diez et al. (1985)	Cisplatin	0/6	—
Walker and Allen (1988)	Cisplatin	10/14	8
Bertolone et al. (1989)	Cisplatin	3/12	3
Allen et al. (1987)	Carboplatin	6/14	10.5
Gaynon et al. (1990)	Carboplatin	6/19	7.5
van Eys et al. (1987)	Procarbazine	0/1	—
Allen et al. (1987)	PCNU	1/5	—
Friedman et al. (1989)	Melphalan	3/12	3
Chastagner et al. (1989)	Ifosfamide	3/20	NR[c]
Heideman et al. (1989)	Thiotepa	2/5	5.5
Ettinger et al. (1990)	Diaziquone	1/15	NR

[a] Radiographic complete and partial (>50%) responses only.
[b] Reported for complete responses only.
[c] NR: not reported.

done in the pre–CT/MRI era, involved only a small number of patients and described clinical responses without objective radiographic evidence of shrinkage.[12] Drugs said to be effective in such trials included vincristine, BCNU, procarbazine, methotrexate, and cyclophosphamide.[12,13,16,30,58] In this pre-CT era, combination therapy was also utilized. The multiagent approach with procarbazine, CCNU, vincristine, and prednisone demonstrated clinical benefit in greater than 40% of patients at the time of relapse and became the adjuvant arm for the multicentered, randomized studies performed in the late 1970s.[4]

With the introduction of CT scanning in the mid-1970s, responses to chemotherapy could be more convincingly demonstrated. High-dose intravenous methotrexate was shown to result in a 50% or greater reduction in tumor size in five of seven children with recurrent MB/PNET; responses in three of the five children lasted for more than 9 months.[13] The value of methotrexate, especially in the postradiation period, is limited by the risk of associated leukoencephalopathy.[35,41] High-dose intravenous cyclophosphamide was reported by Allen and Helson[16] to result in objective evidence of tumor shrinkage in eight of eight children with recurrent primitive neuroectodermal tumors. Toxicity in this trial was significant and the responses were relatively transient, lasting for less than 6 months in most patients. A major limitation of the drug was that at high doses the cyclophosphamide caused significant bone marrow suppression and multiple doses could not be given.

Multiple independent studies have shown that cisplatinum is an effective agent for children with recurrent MB/PNET.[6,14,15] Objective responses, defined as greater than 50% reduction in tumor size on neuroimaging studies with associated clinical improvement, have been seen in as many as 75% of children treated with *cis*-platinum for recurrent MB/PNET.[14] Although some children treated with cisplatin alone have had relatively long-term responses, most have relapsed within 1 year of initiation of therapy.[6,14,15] Cisplatin's use is also limited by cumulative renal toxicity and irreversible sensorineural hearing loss.

The sensorineural hearing loss seems to be potentiated when the drug is used after radiotherapy.[59]

For these reasons, a variety of different platinum derivatives have been evaluated in an attempt to find one that was as efficacious but less toxic. Carboplatin is the most widely tested drug and in one study demonstrated response in 6 of 14 patients with MB/PNET.[7] Over one-half of those responding were able to maintain their response for greater than 10 months. However, others have not found as high a response rate. Gaynon and coworkers,[9] for the Children's Cancer Study Group, were able to demonstrate an objective response in 6 of 19 children with primitive neuroectodermal tumors and an even lower response rate was found in the Pediatric Oncology Group trial. The use of prior cisplatin did not affect the rate of response in initial trials with carboplatin; however, in the Children's Cancer Study Group (CCSG) trial, patients who had received prior cisplatin were less likely to respond to the carboplatin.[9] The carboplatin did demonstrate significantly less ototoxicity and nephrotoxicity.

The results of these and other single-agent treatment approaches in patients with recurrent disease suggest that chemotherapy could affect the growth of medulloblastoma, but when used in a single-agent fashion at the time of relapse rarely resulted in long-term disease control or cure. This understanding and the above-mentioned concept outlined by Goldie and Coldman[42] (which suggests that a tumor is more likely to be sensitive to multiple agents administered simultaneously) led to the use of multiple agents at the time of relapse (Table 12.4).[8,10,11,17,18,60,61]

The most complex application of rapid sequence, multiagent chemotherapy has been the use of eight different drugs over a 24-hour period (the so-called eight-drugs-in-one-day therapy approach).[18] In patients with MB/PNET, the eight drugs utilized included vincristine, CCNU, cisplatin, hydroxyurea, prednisone, cyclophosphamide, cytosine arabinoside, and procarbazine hydrochloride. Initial results with this combination were encouraging and toxicity was tolerable.[62] In one study, six

Table 12.4. Objective responses of recurrent MB/PNET to chemotherapy: multiple agent trials.

Author	Therapy	Response/evaluable patients	Median duration of response (months)
Cangir et al. (1984)	MOPP[a]	4/9	9
	OPP[b]	3/12	11
van Eys et al. (1988)	MOPP	4/19	NR
Pendergrass et al. (1989)	8-in-1[c]	9/11	NR
Kovnar et al. (1989)	Cisplatin/VP-16	8/14	NR
Mulne (1989)	VP-16/cyclophosphamide[d]	1/10	21+
Lefkowitz et al. (1990)	Cisplatin/vincristine/CCNU	4/6	24
Castello et al. (1990)	Carboplatin/VP-16	5/6	5.2

[a] MOPP: nitrogen mustard, vincristine, procarbazine, prednisone.
[b] OPP: vincristine, procarbazine, prednisone.
[c] 8-in-1: vincristine, hydroxyurea, procarbazine, CCNU, cisplatin, cytosine-arabinosid, methylprednisolone, and cyclophosphamide or dacarbazine.
[d] Oral VP-16/cyclophosphamide.

of nine children treated at the time of recurrence had an objective response to treatment.[18] However, in comparison with other single-agent and multiagent trials, it is unclear whether this approach is any more effective. As early as 1979, Duffner and coworkers[31] reported response to the combination of vincristine, BCNU, methotrexate, and dexamethasone in five of five children with recurrent medulloblastoma. Two of these patients had a long-standing response lasting greater than 30 months. The potential long-term effects (especially leukoencephalopathy) with this regimen, have limited its use. The combination of CCNU, vincristine, and cisplatin showed objective efficacy in four of six patients with recurrent disease.[11] Survival in this series was somewhat better than that reported in single-agent trials as median time to progression was 18.5 months; but once again all patients ultimately relapsed.

During the 1980s, trials began in patients with newly diagnosed medulloblastoma/primitive neuroectodermal tumor utilizing chemotherapy before radiation.[18–22,63] Potential benefits of preradiation chemotherapy include the following: (a) some agents may be effective when used early in disease, whereas the same drugs used after the patient has been treated with other agents (including radiotherapy) may have no benefit; (b) side effects may be less intense because of the lack of previous organ

toxicity, allowing drugs to be used at higher doses; (c) microvascular changes produced by previous radiotherapy, which potentially could limit drug delivery to the tumor site, may be avoided; (d) there may be increased synergy with later radiotherapy; and (e) some drugs, such as methotrexate and cisplatin, are potentially less neurotoxic if used prior to radiotherapy.[64] This preradiation approach has been termed a "neoadjuvant" approach (Table 12.5).

Trials with the eight-drugs-in-one-day regimen and the combination of cisplatin and vincristine have shown efficacy.[18,21] Since many of the patients entered on these preradiation studies have had no residual disease postoperatively, evaluation for objective response is often impossible. In those children with residual disease, both the eight-drugs-in-one-day therapy approach and the cisplatin/vincristine combination have shown an approximately 50% response rate. A major potential drawback of this type of therapy is the delay of radiotherapy, still the best proven form of treatment for medulloblastoma/primitive neuroectodermal tumor. To date, preradiation therapy has not been shown to improve survival for patients, although in the series reported by Kretschmar and colleagues,[21] 11 of 15 children treated with preradiation vincristine and cisplatin were alive a median of 25 months after the completion of treatment.

Table 12.5. Objective[a] response of newly diagnosed MB/PNET to chemotherapy.

Author	Therapy	Response/evaluable patients	Median duration of response (months)
Pendergrass et al. (1987)	8-in-1[b]	16/25	NR[c]
	Methotrexate	1/1	57+[d]
Allen et al. (1988)	Vincristine/cisplatin	5/13	NR
Kretschmar et al. (1989)	MOP[e]	2/4	NR
Kuhl et al. (1989)	HIT '88/89[f]	7/15	NR
Kovnar et al. (1990)	Cisplatin/VP-16	7/8	20[d]
Strauss et al. (1991)	Cisplatin/VP-16	2/3	14

[a] Radiographic complete and partial (>50%) responses only.
[b] 8-in-1: vincristine, hydroxyurea, procarbazine, CCNU, cisplatin, cytosine-arabinoside, methylprednisolone, and cyclophosphamide or dacarbazine.
[c] NR: not reported.
[d] Disease-free survival with irradiation.
[e] MOP: nitrogen mustard, vincristine, procarbazine.
[f] HIT '88/89: procarbazine, ifosfamide, VP-16, methotrexate, cisplatin, cytarabin.

Adjuvant Trials in MB/PNET

Two large, independent, multi-institutional randomized trials were undertaken in the mid-1970s to determine the benefits of chemotherapy when used after radiation therapy for children with MB/PNET.[25,26] In both studies, patients were randomized to receive either radiation therapy alone (3,600 cGy craniospinal plus local boost; total tumor dose of 5,400 to 5,600 cGy) or identical radiation therapy plus vincristine therapy during radiation and postradiation cycles of CCNU and vincristine. For the children in the CCSG trial, prednisone was given for the first 14 days of each postradiation chemotherapy cycle.[25] Although flawed by today's standards because of the unavailability of CT scanning in some institutions and incomplete postoperative staging of other patients for residual primary site disease, these studies did, for the first time, demonstrate a benefit of the addition of chemotherapy for some children with MB/PNET.

In the International Society of Paediatric Oncology (SIOP) trial, children with brain stem involvement at diagnosis, treated with radiation and chemotherapy, had a significantly higher 5-year event-free survival (64%) than children treated with radiation therapy alone (36%).[26] For children treated on the CCSG protocol, the estimated 5-year event-free survival was 60% for patients treated with radiation therapy and chemotherapy and 50% for patients treated with radiation therapy alone, a difference that is not statistically significant.[25] Patients with higher T-stages (an evaluation of the amount of disease present at the primary tumor site at the time of diagnosis) alone did not statistically differ in survival. The 5-year event-free survival for children without metastasis was 50% as compared with 36% for children with metastasis ($p < .003$). In the 30 patients with the most extensive tumors, both large primary sites and metastatic disease, event-free survival was markedly better in the group receiving chemotherapy (48% versus 0%, $p = .0006$). Overall survival was also significantly prolonged by chemotherapy for patients with more locally extensive lesions.

Although the information garnered from the two prospective randomized trials is the most compelling to date, information from other smaller trials also suggests the possible benefit of chemotherapy when used in an adjuvant fashion. McIntosh and colleagues[24] reported that 81% of 21 children with MB/PNET treated with cyclophosphamide and vincristine after radiotherapy were alive and free of disease at a median of 6 years afte diagnosis. In this trial, the cyclophosphamide was used at a low dose and treatment was carried on for 2 years. Toxicity of treatment was minimal. Unfortunately, it is unclear what selection criteria were used to enter patients in this study. In addition, no information was given concerning the extent of disease at time of diagnosis or the extent of surgical resection in these patients. Comparing outcome in this study to results obtained in the randomized trials is essentially impossible.

In 1983, a study was begun at Children's Hospital of Philadelphia that essentially built on the results of the randomized trials.[29] Since CCNU and vincristine seemed to be of benefit in an adjuvant fashion for patients with "poor risk" disease, and cisplatin was showing benefit for patients at the time of recurrence, it was decided to couple the CCNU/vincristine approach with cisplatin. In this study, all patients were stratified at the time of diagnosis. Only those patients with "poor risk" disease (subtotal resection, brain stem involvement, and/or metastatic disease at diagnosis) were treated with adjuvant chemotherapy. The other children seen over this period of time received treatment with radiation therapy alone.

In the first 3 years of the Children's Hospital of Philadelphia study, the doses of radiation therapy employed were identical to those utilized in the Children's Cancer Study Group trial. However, when increasing information became available concerning the detrimental effects of craniospinal radiation in young children, the dose of craniospinal radiation was lowered for patients with nondisseminated disease. For this reason, some patients in the Children's Hospital of Philadelphia trial received lower doses of craniospinal irradiation (1,800 to 2,400 cGy) than patients in the previously described randomized trials. Thirty of the first 34 children with "poor risk" MB/PNET treated on this trial remain alive and free of disease, at a median of greater than 4 years from diagnosis.[29] Outcome in patients in this single-arm trial was compared with historical controls matched for similar risk criteria who had received identical radiation. Survival for children receiving the cis-platinum regimen was statistically better than for those treated with radiation alone or with radiation plus chemotherapy with CCNU and vincristine ($p < .001$). There are obvious problems with a single arm study using historical controls, but this and other studies strongly suggest that chemotherapy improves the short-term survival for children with poor-risk MB/PNET when compared with outcome after radiotherapy alone.

Presently, other trials are under way evaluating other chemotherapeutic regimens. The Children's Cancer Study Group is completing a randomized study comparing radiation therapy coupled with CCNU and vincristine to radiation therapy and pre- and postradiotherapy eight-drugs-in-one-day therapy. Other institutions are applying preradiation chemotherapy protocols utilizing cisplatin and other agents, in an attempt to improve survival. In the largest pre- and postradiation therapy trial reported to date, no benefit was seen for the addition of chemotherapy.[49] This trial, undertaken jointly by the International Society of Pediatric Oncology and the German Society for Pediatric Oncology, evaluated 339 patients. On staging studies, 137 patients were considered to have poor-risk disease as defined by a microscopically incomplete tumor resection or metastasis at diagnosis. All poor-risk patients received conventional doses of radiation to brain and spine followed by maintenance chemotherapy with six cycles of CCNU and vincristine. One-half of the poor-risk patients received preradiation therapy with procarbazine, vincristine, and methotrexate. Patients considered to have average risk disease had a second randomization as one-half of those patients received a reduced dose of brain and spine radiation. Relapse-free survival for the group as a whole was 63% at a median follow-up of 42 months. There was no difference in survival between those children who received preradiation chemotherapy as compared to those who did not.[49]

In summary, results to date in adjuvant treatment trials for children with MB/PNET strongly suggest that some patients benefit from the addition of chemotherapy. Presently, primarily children with poor-risk MB/PNET are being entered on trials evaluating chemotherapy. Recently reported survival figures, however, suggest that patients with so-called poor-risk PNET treated with chemotherapy may survive at a rate equal to or higher than patients with average risk disease treated with radiation therapy alone.[29] It is thus unclear whether average-risk patients (who have probably still no better than a 60% to 70% rate of 5-year disease-free survival) should be excluded from adjuvant drug therapy.

In addition, radiation-induced sequelae are quite common in children with MB/PNET.[34,35] As will be discussed later, the sequelae seem most severe in the very young child. However, patients of all ages are at risk for developing long-term intellectual and endocrinologic sequelae. Another possible role for chemotherapy is as an adjunct allowing for reduction in the dose of radiation needed. In the International Society of Pediatric Oncology trial undertaken in the late 1970s, younger children treated with a slightly reduced dose of whole brain radiotherapy (3,000 cGy) and adjuvant chemotherapy fared as well as patients treated with higher doses of radiation therapy.[46] There are trials presently under way evaluating the safety and benefit of the use of adjuvant chemotherapy, either used prior to or after radiotherapy and a somewhat reduced dose of craniospinal irradiation.

The Use of Chemotherapy in the Very Young Child with MB/PNET

Another potentially important role for chemotherapy in children with MB/PNET is its use in very young children. Children under the age of 7, especially those less than 4 years of age at the time of diagnosis, are extremely sensitive to the intellectual effects of whole-brain radiotherapy.[32,34,35] After conventional treatment with 3,600 cGy of radiation therapy, children between 18 months and 36 months of age have been documented to show progressive decline in intelligence with overall intelligence quotients falling 30 to 40 points from preirradiation values.[32] In addition, almost all children who are less than 7 years of age at the time of initial treatment will require special education classroom settings after completion of radiotherapy.[32] Since MB/PNET is a chemo-

sensitive tumor and present conventional means of treatment are so potentially damaging, there has been a great deal of interest in using chemotherapy in an attempt to at least delay, if not obviate, the need for radiotherapy in the very young child (Fig. 12.1).

The greatest longitudinal experience of this approach is that of workers at M. D. Anderson Hospital in Houston, Texas who have used MOPP chemotherapy (mechlorethamine hydrochloride, vincristine, procarbazine, and prednisone) for infants with malignant tumors, including medulloblastoma.[65] Eight of 18 children with MB/PNET who have been treated with the MOPP regimen are reported to be in complete remission without ever receiving radiotherapy. Patients in this trial have been followed for 6 to 150 months (median 73 months).

More recently, the Pediatric Oncology Group has reported on the use of cisplatin, high-dose cyclophosphamide, etoposide, and vincristine for children younger than 3 years of age with a variety of malignant tumors including MB/PNET.[66] In this study, children were treated for 12 months or until they reached 36 months of age. Unlike the study performed at M. D. Anderson, all patients, regardless of disease state were given full doses of radiotherapy when they reached 36 months of age or after the completion of 12 months of treatment. In the Pediatric Oncology Group Study, this included patients who had no residual disease at the time of completion of chemotherapy. The majority of patients with no residual disease at the onset of treatment were able to complete chemotherapy and begin radiation therapy.

Approximately 50% of patients with residual postoperative disease developed progressive disease prior to 36 months of age and had to begin radiotherapy. After radiotherapy, some of these patients experienced a durable response to irradiation. Other trials are presently ongoing, trying to determine which chemotherapeutic regimen is best in very young children with PNET/MB. An extremely important issue is these chemotherapy-only trials is whether radiotherapy has to be given in patients without objective residual disease at the completion of chemotherapy.

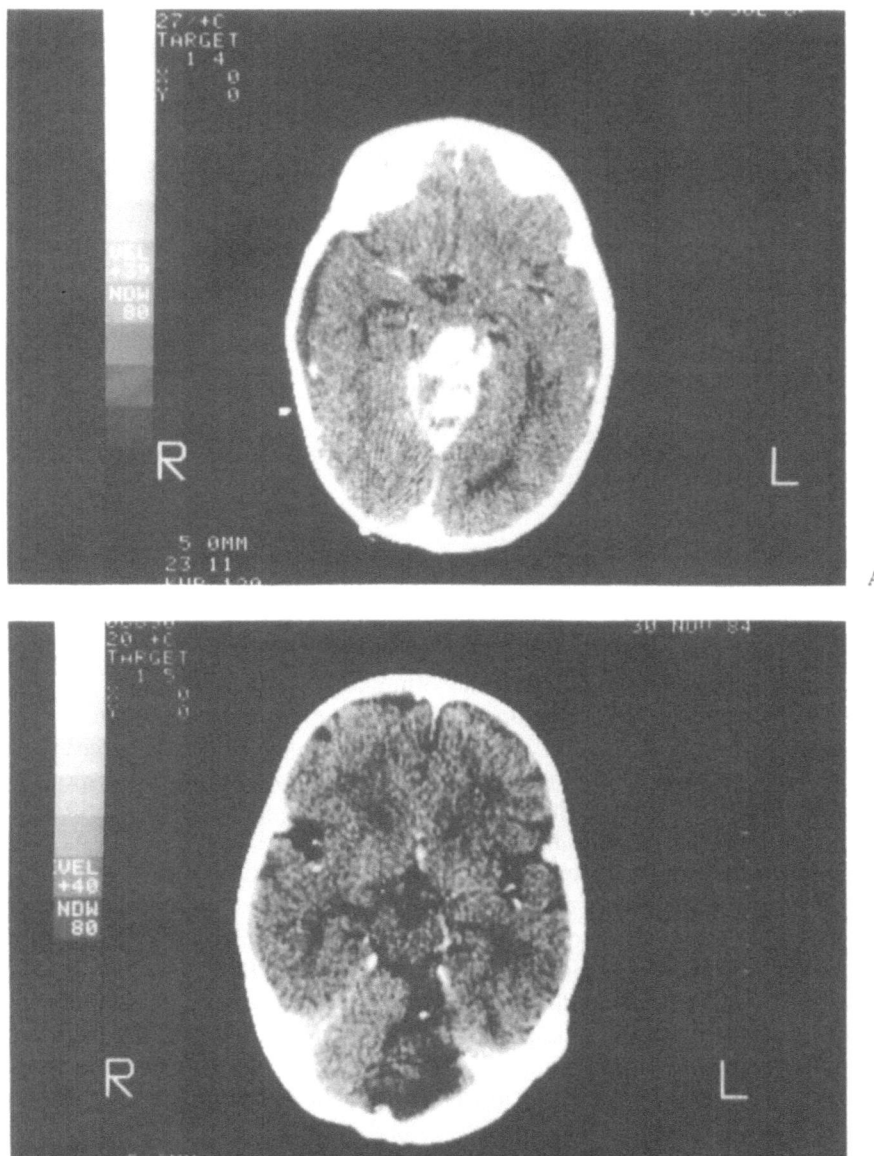

Figure 12.1. A: Postsurgery-enhanced CT of a child with a posterior fossa PNET/MB. B: Enhanced CT of same child after one course of CCNU, VCR, and CPDD.

Ependymoma

Between 5% and 10% of primary CNS tumors of childhood are ependymomas.[67] In children, 90% of ependymomas are intracranial; spinal ependymomas occur more frequently in adolescents and adults. Two-thirds of intracranial ependymomas are in the posterior fossa, and one-third are supratentorial.[68,69] These tumors usually spread by local invasion, with distant subarachnoid spread occurring in approximately 10% of cases.[67] Ependymomas generally convey an unfavorable prognosis with an overall 5-year survival of approximately 40%. When relapses occur, they are overwhelmingly initially local; 20 of 21 relapses

Table 12.6. Selected drug trials in recurrent ependymomas.

Trial	Drug	Objective response*/number in trial
Kahn et al. (1982)	CPDD	3/6
Sexauer et al. (1983)	CPDD	2/15
Walker and Allen (1988)	CPDD	1/2
Gaynon et al. (1990)	Carboplatin	3/14
Ragab et al. (1986)	PCNU	0/10
Seiler (1980)	VM-26/CCNU	2/2
Chastagner et al. (1989)	Ifosfamide	2/8
Ettinger et al. (1985)	AZQ	0/12
Cangir et al. (1984)	MOPP/OPP	2/20

* Greater than 50% objective response in tumor bulk.
CPDD: cisplatin.
MOPP: mechlorethamine hydrochloride, vincristine, procarbazine, prednisone.
OPP: vincristine, procarbazine, prednisone.

(95%) in one series were local, although all patients were not fully staged at relapse.[70]

The utility of separating ependymomas histologically into high-grade (malignant) or low-grade (benign) tumors has been questioned. Most Series have not reported a major difference in survival between histologic subtype, as long as ependymoblastoma are not included. The impact of treatment on outcome has been difficult to discern. In contrast to earlier reports suggesting that the degree of surgical resection does not affect outcome, recent studies have shown that patients have a better survival after "gross-total" resection. The addition of adjuvant radiotherapy has positively impacted survival, although it is unclear if this holds true for patients with total resections. Reported survival rates have ranged from 20% to 70% at 5 years. Most commonly, ependymomas are treated with between 5,000 and 5,500 cGy of local irradiation. Routine craniospinal irradiation in ependymoma remains controversial but has been recommended for high-grade posterior fossa tumors. Recommendations for treatment of low-grade lesions most commonly include local radiotherapy with wide margins.[1]

Chemotherapy in Recurrent Ependymoma

One of the more active agents against recurrent ependymomas has been cisplatin (CDDP) (Table 12.6). One study of recurrent brain tumors utilized 60 mg/m^2 of CDDP in-travenously every 3 to 4 weeks.[5] Six evaluable children with recurrent ependymomas were included and received between one and nine courses of therapy. Of these, two (33%) had complete responses after eight and nine courses lasting 10 and 41 months, respectively. One patient had a partial response after three courses lasting 3 months, and one patient had stabilization of disease for 11 months (while receiving seven courses).

A subsequent multicenter trial in the Pediatric Oncology Group (POG) utilizing the same regimen of CDDP included 15 evaluable children with recurrent ependymoma.[15] Of these, three patients had complete responses (20%), two after two courses and the third after nine courses of therapy; the duration of response was between 3 and 15 months. Four patients had stabilization of disease (27%). However, all had to be removed from therapy 3 to 6 months after beginning CDDP for either ototoxicity or nephrotoxicity. Thus, although 47% of patients experienced some benefit, significant toxicity occurred.

Other investigators have reported the use of 120 mg/m^2 of CDDP as a single dose every 3 to 4 weeks.[71] Two patients with recurrent ependymoma were included in this trial and one (50%) had a partial response lasting more than 7 months.

A Children's Cancer Study Group phase I trial of carboplatin included five patients with ependymoma.[72] Although phase I trials are not conducted primarily to detect activity against specific tumors, one patient with recurrent ependymoma had stabilization of disease for 10 months at a dose of 560 mg/m². The follow-up phase II trial utilizing carboplatin at a dose of 560 mg/m² intravenously every 3 to 4 weeks included 14 evaluable patients with recurrent ependymoma.[75] A greater than 50% decrease in tumor size was seen in three patients (21%), and two additional patients had stabilization of disease; thus 5 of 14 (36%) patients with recurrent ependymoma in this study benefited from carboplatin.

In a combined adult and pediatric series utilizing CCNU for recurrent brain tumors, one 16-year-old boy with recurrent ependymoma was treated with 130 mg/m² of CCNU. Although two of four courses had reduced doses of CCNU, this patient was alive and in remission 11 months after beginning treatment.[74]

Another nitrosourea, PCNU, induced a partial response in the only ependymoma patient included in a phase II trial utilizing between 100 and 125 mg/m² of PCNU.[53] Another phase II trial of PCNU carried out by the Pediatric Oncology Group failed to show a response in 10 patients with recurrent ependymoma.[75] Thus, PCNU does not appear to be a very active agent in ependymoma.

A phase II study of VM-26 and CCNU in recurrent or inoperable, newly diagnosed brain tumors included two patients with ependymoma.[76] Both patients had partial responses lasting 8 and more than 14 months; the doses utilized on this regimen were VM-26 120 mg/m² and CCNU 120 mg/m² (with decreasing doses of CCNU on subsequent courses) every 4 weeks. VM-26 alone has been reported to have induced a partial response in a 16-year-old boy with ependymoma recurring after radiation therapy and CCNU.[77]

Ifosfamide as a single agent at a dose of 3 g/m²/d for 2 days has been studied in patients with recurrent ependymoma.[78] Of eight evaluable patients, two (25%) showed a partial response, and four (50%) had stabilization of their disease. A phase II study of AZQ at 9 mg/m²/d for 5 days conducted by the Children's Cancer Study Group in children with recurrent brain tumors included 12 patients with epen-

dymoma, of whom eight had had sufficient follow-up to be evaluable.[79] Two (25%) had stabilization of disease, but no patients had shrinkage of their tumor on AZQ. Other drugs have also been used. A phase II study of high-dose methotrexate with citrovorum rescue in recurrent brain tumors included one patient with ependymoma who had clinical improvement and survived for 7 months.[80] One adolescent male with recurrent ependymoma had a dramatic response to multiple courses of intrathecal methotrexate (0.25 mg/kg/dose) but died 2 years later of leukoencephalopathy.[81]

A Pediatric Oncology Group protocol in which patients with recurrent brain tumors were randomized to either MOPP or OPP chemotherapy included 10 patients with ependymoma.[17] One patient responded in each arm of the study. Both regimens were less active in patients with ependymoma than in those patients with medulloblastoma or astrocytoma. Intracarotid combination chemotherapy with BCNU, CDDP, and VM-26 has been studied in adult patients,[82] including two patients with ependymoma. Both responded to therapy, but one had only 11 weeks of follow-up, and the other recurred at 35 weeks.

Adjuvant Chemotherapy in Ependymoma

To date, there have been few studies of adjuvant chemotherapy in children with ependymoma. A Children's Cancer Study Group trial that randomized children to radiation only versus radiation followed by adjuvant chemotherapy with vincristine, CCNU, and prednisone showed no benefit for the chemotherapy arm as compared to radiation alone.[70] In this trial, 14 patients were treated with radiotherapy only, and 22 patients were treated on the radiotherapy plus chemotherapy arm. The radiotherapy arm had a 45% 5-year disease-free survival, and the chemotherapy arm had a 37% 5-year disease-free survival.

Chemotherapy in Infants with Ependymoma

As discussed in the section on MB/PNET, there is an interest in delaying or deleting radiotherapy for infants and young children with brain tumors. Two infants with ependymoma were treated on an infant protocol utilizing CDDP at a dose of 20 mg/m²/d and VP-16 at a dose of 75 mg/m²/d for 5 days.[22] One of the infants had a complete response lasting 11 months and the other had a partial response lasting 18 months.

The M. D. Anderson Hospital has treated a number of infants with brain tumors with the MOPP regimen.[83] This trial included three patients with either ependymoma or mixed ependymoma/astrocytoma, all of whom had a complete response. However, all three relapsed between 6 and 15 months after diagnosis. Subsequently, one patient was salvaged and remained alive 33 months after diagnosis.

Summary

It would seem that ependymomas may respond to chemotherapy, but overall responses are infrequent and transient. The platinum derivatives have been the most widely used, but still result in only a 20% to 30% objective response rate. Given the less than optimal outcome in children with ependymomas, there remains interest in using adjuvant chemotherapy. However, it is unclear what criteria should be used to select patients (for example, only those with partial resection) or which drugs should be used.

Brain Stem Gliomas

Brain stem tumors account for between 10% and 20% of all childhood CNS tumors with peak incidence occurring between the ages of 5 and 8 years. This group of tumors encompasses a wide variety of histologic grades of malignancy, and almost half occur in the pons. Neuraxis dissemination is uncommon, but can occur premorbidly.[34] If the rate of local control can be increased, such dissemination may become a more important issue.

The role of surgery in brain stem tumors is limited, and the majority of patients can be diagnosed with MRI and do not require histologic confirmation of their diagnosis. Surgery is probably best reserved for those patients with more focal or localized lesions (i.e., cer-vicomedullary junction), as histology may act as a guide to the aggressivity of treatment undertaken.

Radiation is routinely used in patients with brain stem tumors and represents the only therapy that currently offers at least transient benefit to these patients. However, patients with diffuse lesions or malignant gliomas rarely survive after radiotherapy, reported survival ranging between 0% and 20% at 3 years.

Chemotherapy in Recurrent Brain Stem Tumors (Table 12.7)

In their phase II study of cisplatin at 120 mg/m² in recurrent pediatric brain tumors, Walker and Allen[71] reported one partial response in six (17%) patients with recurrent brain stem tumors. However, this response lasted only 4 months. In the Pediatric Oncology Group phase II study of cisplatin (60 mg/m²/d for 2 days) no patient with a brain stem tumor responded to therapy.[15]

Five patients with recurrent brain stem tumors were treated on the Children's Cancer Study Group phase I study of carboplatin.[72] Two of these patients (40%) had stabilization of their disease; one period of stabilization lasted for 6 months following treatment with 350 mg/m² and one lasted for 4 months following treatment with 420 mg/m². No patient had shrinkage of tumor in this study.

In the Children's Cancer Study Group phase II study of carboplatin utilizing 560 mg/m², three of 14 (21%) patients with recurrent brain stem tumors showed greater than a 50% decrease in their tumor size.[73] These partial responses lasted more than 14 months. In addition, one patient had stabilization of disease lasting more than 6 months.

Zeltzer et al.[84] have reported the encouraging response of one patient on this regimen who was diagnosed at 15 months of age with a low-grade brain stem glioma. She had a dramatic partial response to carboplatin and at publication remained without enlargement of her residual tumor 14 months after completing therapy and 39 months after diagnosis.

The phase II study of CCNU previously discussed included a 13-year-old boy with a

Table 12.7. Selected drug trials in children with recurrent brainstem gliomas.

Trial	Drug	Objective response/ Number in trial
Walker and Allen (1988)	CPDD	1/6
Gaynon et al. (1990)	Carboplatin	3/4
Seiler (1980)	VM-26 and CCNU	2/4
Allen et al. (1987)	PCNU	3/17
Chastagner et al. (1989)	Ifosfamide	0/3
Miser et al. (1989)	VP-16 and ifosfamide	1/18
Rodriguez et al. (1988)	5-FU, CCNU, hydroxyurea, and 6-mercaptopurine	3/14

brain stem tumor who had progressed after radiotherapy.[74] He responded to therapy and, at publication, continued to improve 8 months after beginning CCNU. In the Swiss Pediatric Oncology Group study of VM-26 and CCNU, four children with brain stem tumors were treated[76]: one had a complete response lasting more than 32 months and one had a partial response lasing more than 12 months. Thus, two of four (50%) patients with brain stem tumors responded to this regimen. Allen et al.[53] reported that 3 of 17 (18%) patients with recurrent brain stem tumors had partial responses to PCNU; two additional patients had stabilization of disease. Although 29% of patients with brain stem tumors responded or had stabilization, the authors concluded that PNU did not offer any benefit over other nitrosoureas.

None of the three patients with recurrent brain stem tumors treated on the phase II trial of ifosfamide had a response.[78] In the Children's Cancer Study Group phase II study of VP-16 and ifosfamide,[85] only one of eight (13%) evaluable patients with brain stem tumors had a partial response; one additional patient had stabilization of disease for more than 7 months. Other agents that have not shown efficacy in brain stem tumors include high-dose methotrexate and AZQ.[79,80]

Thirteen patients with recurrent brain stem tumors were treated at the University of California at San Francisco with the combination of 5-fluorouracil, CCNU, hydroxyurea, and 6-mercaptopurine.[86] Of these, four (31%) had partial responses, but three subsequently progressed within 12 weeks. A total of nine patients (69%) had a partial response or stabilization of disease, but the median time to

progression was only 25 weeks (range 6 to 98 weeks), suggesting that this regimen was not beneficial to patients with recurrent brain stem tumors.

Adjuvant Chemotherapy in Brain Stem Gliomas

Adjuvant trials in children with brain stem gliomas have been disappointing. In a CCSG trial, the use of postradiotherapy CCNU, vincristine, and prednisone did not improve survival, as compared to treatment with radiotherapy alone.[39] Similarly, the use of preirradiation 5-fluorouracil and CCNU followed by hydroxyurea and mesonidazole during radiotherapy did not show any clear benefit.[87]

Summary

The response of brain stem gliomas to chemotherapy has been quite disappointing. Although occasional responses are seen, most are very transient. Outcome in patients with diffuse or malignant lesions is extremely poor, as few patients survive with present means of treatment. New approaches are desperately needed and work to identify useful agents or combinations of agents continues. One approach is to treat patients with promising agents prior to radiotherapy, since the tumor may be more sensitive to the drug if given prior to radiotherapy. How well these often critically ill patients will tolerate this approach or the extra fluids needed is unknown. Such therapy also delays the use of radiotherapy—the only known effective (albeit primarily transient) treatment.

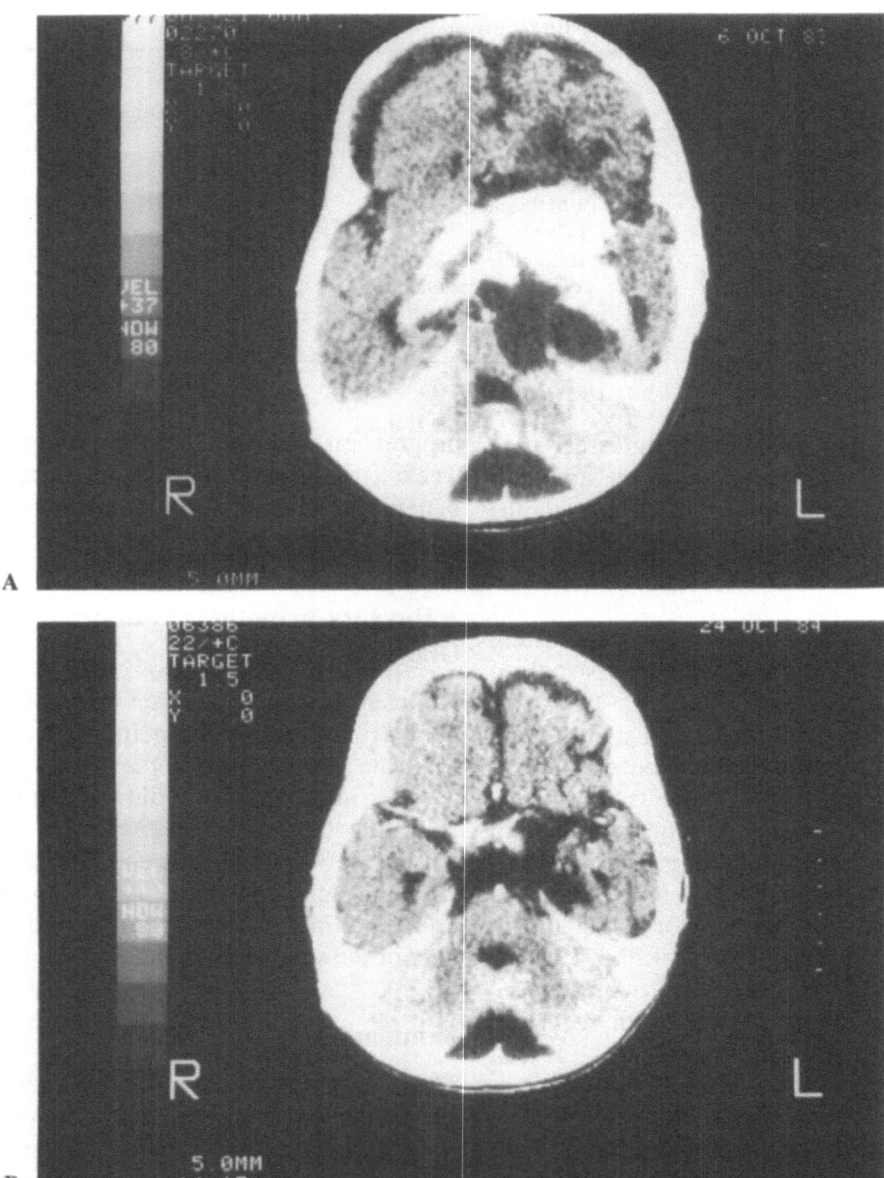

Figure 12.2. A: Postsurgery-enhanced CT of a child with a chiasmatic low-grade glioma. B: Enhanced CT of same child after one course of chemotherapy (actinomycin D and vincristine).

Cerebellar Gliomas

Cerebellar astrocytomas, the most common form of which in children are pilocytic astrocytomas, are primarily surgical lesions. Even at times of recurrence, second surgical resections can be curative. Partially resected low-grade lesions can at times be treated with radiother-apy, with some evidence of prolonged survival. Fewer patients with low-grade tumors have received chemotherapy. Occasionally patients with recurrent low-grade tumor in other sites in the nervous system have had long-lasting responses to treatment with chemotherapy, with drugs such as CCNU and vincristine or the eight-drugs-in-one-day regimen[88] (Fig. 12.2).

A subgroup of children with cerebellar gliomas will have histologically more aggressive tumors.[89,90] These have been classified by different names, including the Gilles-B or "diffuse" cerebellar gliomas. They tend to be less accessible to complete resections and outcome is much poorer than in cerebellar pilocytic astrocytomas, with survival rates after treatment being in the 30% to 40% range. The role of either chemotherapy at the time of recurrence or in an adjuvant fashion for "diffuse" tumors is unclear. One study suggests that the use of vincristine during radiotherapy, and vincristine, CCNU, and prednisone after radiotherapy, increases the 5-year rate of disease-free survival for children with cortical malignant gliomas to 40%, as compared with 10% after treatment with identical radiotherapy alone.[91] Until there is further information, one potential approach is to treat children with these "diffuse" cerebellar gliomas with radiotherapy and the same drug regimen found of benefit in the cortical malignant glioma trial.

References

1. Heideman RL, Packer RJ, Albright LA, Freeman CR, Rorke LB. Tumors of the central nervous system. In: *Principles and Practice of Pediatric Oncology*. Philadelphia: JB Lippincott; 1989:505–553.
2. Levin VA. Chemotherapy of primary brain tumors. *Neurol Clin*. 1985;3:855–866.
3. Dropoho EJ, Mahaley MS. Chemotherapy for malignant gliomas in adults. In: Thomas GT, ed. *Neuro-Oncology: Primary Malignant Brain Tumors*. London: Arnold; 1990:222–241.
4. Crafts DC, Levin VA, Edwards MS, et al. Chemotherapy of recurrent medulloblastoma with combined procarbazine, CCNU, and vincristine. *Neurosurg*. 1978;49:589–592.
5. Kahn AB, D'Souza BJ, Wharam MD, et al. Cisplatin therapy in recurrent childhood brain tumors. *Cancer Treat Rep*. 1982;66:2013–2020.
6. Bertolone SJ, Baum ES, Krivet W, Hammond GD. A phase II study of cisplatin therapy in recurrent childhood brain tumors: A report from the Children's Cancer Study Group. *Neurooncol*. 1989;7:5–11.
7. Allen JC, Walker R, Luks E, et al. Carboplatin and recurrent childhood brain tumors. *J Clin Oncol*. 1987;5:459–463.
8. Castello MA, Clerico A, Deb G, et al. High-dose carboplatin in combination with etoposide (JET regimen) for childhood brain tumors. *Am J Pediatr Hematol Oncol*. 1990;12:297–300.
9. Gaynon PS, Ettinger LJ, Baum ES, et al. Carboplatin in childhood brain tumors: A Children's Cancer Study Group Phase II Trial. *Cancer*. 1990;66:2465–2469.
10. van Eys J, Baram TZ, Cangir A, et al. Salvage chemotherapy for recurrent primary brain tumors in children. *J Pediatr*. 1988;113:601–606.
11. Lefkowitz IB, Packer RJ, Siegel KR, et al. Results of treatment of children with recurrent medulloblastoma/primitive neuroectodermal tumor with lomustine, cisplatin, and vincristine. *Cancer*. 1990;65:412–417.
12. Ward HWC. Central nervous system tumors of childhood treated with CCNU, vincristine and radiation. *Med Pediatr Oncol*. 1978;4:315–320.
13. Rosen G, Ghavimi F, Nirenberg A, et al. High-dose methotrexate with citrovorum factor resuce for the treatment of central nervous system tumors in children. *Cancer Treat Rep*. 1977; 61:681–690.
14. Walker RW, Allen JC. Cisplatin in the treatment of recurrent childhood primary brain tumors. *J Clin Oncol*. 1988;6:62–66.
15. Sexauer CL, Khan A, Burger PC, et al. Cisplatin in recurrent pediatric brain tumors: A POG phase II study. *Cancer*. 1985;56:1497–1501.
16. Allen JC, Helson L. High-dose cyclophosphamide chemotherapy for recurrent CNS tumors in children. *J Neurosurg*. 1981;55:749–756.
17. Cangir A, Ragab AH, Steuber P, et al. Combination chemotherapy with vincristine (NSC-67574), procarbazine (NSC-77213), prednisone (NSC-10023) with or without nitrogen mustard (NSC-762) (MOPP vs OPP) in children with recurrent brain tumors. *Med Pediatr Oncol*. 1984;12:1–3.
18. Pendergrass TW, Milstein JM, Geyer JR, et al. Eight drugs in one day chemotherapy for brain tumors: Experience in 107 children and rationale for preradiation chemotherapy. *J Clin Oncol*. 1987;5:1221–1231.
19. Allen JC, Walker R, Rosen G. Preradiation high-dose intravenous methotrexate with leucovorin rescue for untreated primary childhood brain tumors. *J Clin Oncol*. 1988;6:649–653.
20. Kovnar EH, Kellie SJ, Horowitz ME, et al. Preirradiation cisplatin and etoposide in the treatment of high-risk medulloblastoma and other malignant embryonal tumors of the cen-

tral nervous system: A phase II study. *J Clin Oncol.* 1990;8:330–336.

21. Kretschmar CS, Tarbell NJ, Kupsky W, et al. Preirradiation chemotherapy for infants and children with medulloblastoma: a preliminary report. *J Neurosurg.* 1989;71:820–825.

22. Strauss LC, Killmond TM, Carson BS, et al. Efficacy of postoperative chemotherapy using cisplatin plus etoposide in young children with brain tumors. *Med Pediatr Oncol.* 1990;19:16–21.

23. Packer RJ, Siegel KR, Sutton LN, et al. Efficacy of combination chemotherapy with cisplatinum (CPDD), lomustine (CCNU), and vincristine (VCR) in children with primitive neuroectodermal tumors—medulloblastoma (PNET-MB) of childhood. *Ann Neurol.* 1985; 18:394–400.

24. McIntosh S, Chen M, Sartain PA, et al. Adjuvant chemotherapy for medulloblastoma. *Cancer.* 1985;56:1316–1319.

25. Evans AE, Jenkin DT, Spasto R, et al. The treatment of medulloblastoma: Results of a prospective randomized trial of radiation therapy with and without CCNU, vincristine and prednisone. *J Neurosurg.* 1990;72:572–582.

26. Tait DM, Thornton-Jones H, Bloom HJG, et al. Adjuvant chemotherapy for medulloblastoma: the first multi-centre control trial of the International Society of Paediatric Oncology (SIOP I). *Eur J Cancer.* 1990;26:464–469.

27. Tamura M, Ono N, Kurihara H, et al. Adjunctive treatment for recurrent childhood ependymoma of the IVth ventricle: chemotherapy with CDDP and MCNU. *Childs Nerv Syst.* 1990; 6:186–189.

28. Friedman HS, Schold SC. Rational approaches to the chemotherapy of medulloblastoma. *Neurol Clin.* 1985;3:843–853.

29. Packer RJ, Sutton LN, Goldwein JW, et al. Improved survival with the use of adjuvant chemotherapy in the treatment of medulloblastoma. *J Neurosurg.* 1991;74:433–440.

30. Lassman LP, Pearce GE, Banna M, et al. Vincristine sulphate in the treatment of metastases from cerebellar medulloblastoma. *J Neurosurg.* 1969;30:42–49.

31. Duffner PK, Cohen ME, Thomas PRM, et al. Combination chemotherapy in recurrent medulloblastoma. *Cancer.* 1979;43:41–45.

32. Packer RJ, Sutton LN, Atkins TA, et al: A prospective study of cognitive deficits in children receiving whole brain radiotherapy: 2 year results. *J Neurosurg.* 1988;70:707–713.

33. Duffner PK, Cohen ME, Thomas PRM, Lansky SB. The long-term effects of cranial irradiation in the central nervous system. *Cancer.* 1985; 56:1841–1847.

34. Gamis AS, Neglia JP, Robison LL. Neuropsychological sequelae of radiotherapy. In: Plowman PN, McElwain TJ, Meadows AT, eds. *Complications of cancer management.* Oxford: Butterworth; 1991:348–360.

35. Packer RJ, Atkins T, Littman P, et al. Neurologic and neuropsychologic sequelae in survivors of childhood brain tumors. *Proc Int Soc Pediatr Oncol.* 1983;15:71.

36. Horowitz ME, Mulhearn RK, Kun LE, et al. Brain tumors in the very young child: Postoperative chemotherapy in combined-modality treatment. *Cancer.* 1988;61:428–434.

37. Duffner PK, Cohen ME. Treatment of brain tumors in babies and very young children. *Pediatr Neurosci.* 1986;12:304–310.

38. Levin VA, Rodriguez LA, Edwards MSB, et al. Treatment of medulloblastoma with procarbazine, hydroxyurea and reduced radiation doses to whole brain and spine. *J Neurosurg.* 1988; 68:383–387.

39. Jenkin RDT, Boesel C, Ertel I, et al. Brainstem tumors in childhood: A prospective randomized trial of irradiation with and without adjuvant CCNU, VCR and prednisone. A report of the Children's Cancer Study Group. *J Neurosurg.* 1987;66:227–233.

40. Groothius DR, Blasberg RG. Rational brain tumor chemotherapy: The interaction of drug and tumor. *Neurol Clin.* 1985;3:801–816.

41. Kramer ED, Cohen BH, Packer RJ. Central nervous system morbidity secondary to chemotherapy. In: Plowman PN, McElwain TJ, Meadows AT, eds. *Complications of Cancer Management.* Oxford: Butterworth; 1981:329–347.

42. Goldie JM, Coldman AJ. Quantitative model for multiple levels of drug resistance in clinical tumors. *Cancer Treat Rep.* 1982;67:923–931.

43. Packer RJ, Sutton LN, D'Angio G, et al. Management of children with primitive neuroectodermal tumors of the posterior fossa/medulloblastoma. *Pediatr Neurosci.* 1986;12: 272–282.

44. Park TS, Hoffman HJ, Hendrich EB, et al. Medulloblastoma, clinical presentation and management: Experience at the Hospital for Sick Children, Toronto 1950–1980. *J Neurosurg.* 1983;58:543–552.

45. Farwell JR, Dohrmann GJ, Flannery JT.

Medulloblastoma in childhood: an epidemiologic study. *J Neurosurg*. 1984;61:657–664.

46. Allen JC, Bloom J, Ertel LI, et al. Brain tumors in children: current cooperative and institutional chemotherapy trials in newly diagnosed and recurrent disease. *Semin Oncol*. 1985;13: 110–122.

47. Allen JC, Epstein F. Medulloblastoma and other primary malignant neuroectodermal tumors of the CNS: the effect of patients' age and extent of disease on prognosis. *J Neurosurg*. 1982;57:446–451.

48. Packer RJ, Siegel KR, Sutton LN, Littman P, Bruce DA, Schut L. Leptomeningeal dissemination of primary central nervous system tumors of childhood. *Ann Neurol*. 1985;18:217–277.

49. Gnekow AK, Bailey C, Michaelis J, Wellek S, Kleihues P. SIOP/GPO medulloblastoma II trial: sandwich chemotherapy and reduced dose radiotherapy for standard risk patients tested in a prospectively randomized international study (abstract). *Pediatr Neurosci*. 1989;15:144.

50. Laurent JP, Chang CM, Cohen ME. A classification system for primitive neuroectodermal tumors (medulloblastoma of the posterior fossa). *Cancer* 1985;56:1807–1809.

51. Diez B, Monges J, Muriel FS. Evaluation of cisplatin in children with recurrent brain tumors. *Cancer Treat Rep*. 1985;69:911–913.

52. van Eys J, Cangir A, Pack R, Baram T. Phase I trial of procarbazine as a 5-day continuous infusion in children with central nervous system tumors. *Cancer Treat Rep*. 1987;71:973–974.

53. Allen JC, Hancock C, Walker R, Tan C. PCNU and recurrent brain tumors. *J Neurooncol*. 1987;5:241–244.

54. Friedman HS, Schold SC, Mahaley MS, Calvin OM, Oakes WJ, Vick NA, Burger PC, Bigner SH, Borowitz M, Halperin EC, Djang W, Falletta JM, DeLong R, Garvin JH, DeVivo DC, Norris D, Golembe B, Winter J, Bodziner RA, Sipahi H, Bigner DD. Phase II treatment of medulloblastoma and pineoblastoma with melphalan: clinical therapy based on experimental models of human medulloblastoma. *J Clin Oncol*. 1989;7:904–911.

55. Chastagner P, Sommelet-Olive, Kalifa C, Brunat M, Zucker JM, Baranzelli MC, Tron P, Bergeron C, Demeocg F, Pein F, DeLumley L. Phase II study of ifosfamide in recurrent childhood brain tumors. *Pediatr Neurosci*. 1989; 15:147.

56. Heideman RL, Packer R, Allen J, Gillespie A,

Reaman G, Horowitz M, Ettinger L, Steinberg S, Balis F, Poplack DG. Phase II study of thiotepa (TT) in pediatric central nervous system (CNS) tumors. *Pediatr Neurosci*. 1989;15:146–147.

57. Ettinger LJ, Ru N, Krailo M, Ruccione KS, Krivit W, Hammond GD. A phase II study of diaziquone in children with recurrent or progressive primary brain tumors: A report from the Children's Cancer Study Group. *J Neurooncol*. 1990;9:69–76.

58. Kumar ARV, Renaudin J, Wilson CB, et al. Procarbazine hydrochloride in the treatment of brain tumors: Phase II study. *J Neurosurg*. 1974;40:365–371.

59. Granowetter L, Rosenstock JG, Packer RJ. Enhanced cisplatin neurotoxicity in pediatric patients with brain tumors. *J Neurooncol*. 1983;1:293–297.

60. Kovnar EH, Horowitz ME, Heidemann RL, Langston JL, Douglass EC, Kellie SJ, McHaney VA, Ogle LP, Kun LE. Cisplatin and Etoposide (VP-16) for recurrent brain tumors in childhood (abstract). *Pediatr Neurosci*. 1989;15:149.

61. Mulne AF, Kearns KM, Kamen BA, Munoz LL. Phase I/II trial of oral VP-16/Cytoxan in recurrent brain tumors (abstract). *Pediatr Neurosci*. 1989;15:154.

62. Geyer JR, Pendergrass TW, Milstein JM, Bleyer WA. Eight drugs in one day chemotherapy in children with brain tumors: A critical toxicity appraisal. *J Clin Oncol*. 1988;6:996–1000.

63. Kuhl J, Rating D, Berthold F, Riehm H, Graf N, Gnekow A, Niethammer D, Treuner J, Spaar HJ, Kaatsch P, Bamberg M, Sorenson N, Kleihues P, Neidhardt M. Intensive chemotherapy after surgery and before radiotherapy in children with malignant brain tumors: preliminary results of the West German pilot study HIT '88/89 (abstract). *Pediatr Neurosci*. 1989;15:144.

64. Packer RJ. Chemotherapy for medulloblastoma/primitive neuroectodermal tumors of the posterior fossa. *Ann Neurol*. 1990;28: 823–828.

65. Ater JL, Woo SY, vonEys J. Update on MOPP chemotherapy as primary therapy for infant brain tumors. *Pediatr Neurosci*. 1988;14:153–154.

66. Duffner P. Personal communication.

67. Cohen M, Duffner P. Ependymomas. In: *Brain Tumors of Childhood: Principles of Diagnosis and Treatment*. New York: Raven Press; 1984:136–155.

68. Ilgren EB, Stiller CA, Hughes JT, Silberman D,

Steckel N, Kaye A. Ependymomas: A clinical and pathologic study. I. Biologic features. *Clin Neuropathol.* 1984;3:113–121.

69. Dohrman GJ, Farwell JR, Flannery JT. Ependymomas and ependymoblastomas in children. *J Neurosurg.* 1976;45:273–283.

70. Lefkowitz I, Evans A, Sposto R, Wilson C, Hammond D. Adjuvant chemotherapy of childhood posterior fossa (PF) ependymoma: Craniospinal radiation with or without CCNU, vincristine (VCR), and Prednisone (P). *Proc Am Soc Clin Oncol.* 1989;8:87.

71. Walker RW, Allen JC. Treatment of recurrent primary intracranial childhood tumors with Cis-diamminoedichloroplatinum. *Ann Neurol.* 1983;14:371–372.

72. Gaynon P, Ettinger LJ, Moel D, Siegel SE, Baum ES, Krivit W, Hammond GD. Pediatric phase I trial of carboplatin: A Children's Cancer Study Group report. *Cancer Treat Rep.* 1987; 71:1039–1042.

73. Gaynon P, Ettinger L, Baum E, Siegel S, Krailo M, Hamond GD. Carboplatin (CBDCA) appears active in recurrent childhood brainstem glioma (BSG), medulloblastoma (MDB) and ependymoma (EP). *Proc Am Soc Clin Oncol.* 1988;7:81.

74. Rosenblum ML, Reynolds AF, Smith KA, Rumack BH, Walker MD. Chloroethylcyclohexylnitrosourea (CCNU) in the treatment of malignant brain tumors. *J Neurosurg.* 1973;39:306–314.

75. Ragab AH, Burger P, Badnitsky S, Krischer J, van Eys. PCNU in the treatment of recurrent medulloblastoma and ependymoma—A POG study. *J Neurooncol.* 1986;3:341–342.

76. Seiler RW. Combination chemotherapy with VM-26 and CCNU in primary malignant brain tumors of children. *Helv Paediatr Acta* 1980; 35:51–56.

77. Selansky BD, Mann-Kaplan RS, Reynolds AF Jr, Rosenblum ML, Walker MD. 4'-Demethylepipodophyllotoxin-B-D-thenylidene-glucoside (PTG) in the treatment of malignant intracranial neoplasms. *Cancer.* 19xx;33:460–467.

78. Chastagner P, Olive-Sommelet D, Kalifa C, Brunat M, Zucker JM, Barazelli MC, Tron P. Phase II trial of ifosfamide in recurrent childhood brain tumors. *J Med Pediatr Oncol.* 1989;17:355.

79. Ettinger LJ, Krailo M, Krivit W, Ruccione K, Hammond D. Phase II study of AZQ in childhood brain tumors. *Proc Am Soc Clin Oncol.* 1985;4:238.

80. Djerassi I, Kim JS, Shulman K. High-dose methotrexate-citrovorum factor rescue in the management of rain gliomas. *Cancer Treat Rep.* 19xx;61:691–694.

81. Wilson CB, Norrell HA Jr. Brain tumor chemotherapy with intrathecal methotrexate. *Cancer.* 1969;23:1038–1045.

82. Stewart DJ, Grahovac Z, Benoit B Addison D, Richard MT, Dennery J, Hugenholtz H, Russell N, Peterson E, Maroun JA, Vanderberg T, Hopkins HS. Intracarotid chemotherapy with a combination of BCNU, Cisplatin, and VM-26 in the treatment of primary and metastatic brain tumors. *Neurosurgery.* 1984;15:828–833.

83. van Eys J, Cangir A, Coody D, Smith B. MOPP regimen as primary chemotherapy for brain tumors in infants. *J Neurooncol.* 1985;3:237–244.

84. Zeltzer PM, Epport K, Nelson MD Jr, Huff K, Gaynon P. Prolonged response to carboplatin in an infant with brainstem glioma. *Cancer.* 1991;67:43–47.

85. Miser J, Krailo M, Smithson W, Belasco J, Ortega J, Hammond GD. Treatment of children with recurrent brain tumors with ifosfamide (IFOS), etoposide (VP-16) and mesna (M). Results of a phase II trial. *Proc Am Soc Clin Oncol.* 1989;8:84.

86. Rodriguez LA, Prados M, Fulton D, Edwards MSB, Silver P, Levin V. Treatment of recurrent brainstem gliomas and other central nervous system tumors with 5-fluorouracil, CCNU, hydroxyurea, and 6-mercaptopurine. *Neurosurgery.* 1988;22:691–693.

87. Levin J, Edwards M, Ward W, et al. 5-Fluorouracil and CCNU followed by hydroxyurea, mesonidazole, and irradiation for brainstem gliomas: A pilot study of the Brain Tumor Research Center and the Children's Cancer Study Group. *Neurosurgery.* 1984;14:679–681.

88. Lefkowitz IB, Packer RJ, Seigel KR, et al. Results of treatment of children with relapsed gliomas with CCNU and vincristine. *Cancer.* 1988;61:896–902.

89. Gilles F. Cerebellar tumors in children. *Clin Neurosurg.* 1983;30:181–188.

90. Gyerris F, Klinken L. Longterm prognosis in children with benign cerebellar astrocytoma. *J Neurosurg.* 1978;49:179–184.

91. Sposto R, Ertel IJ, Jenkin RDT, et al. The effectiveness of chemotherapy for treatment of high grade astrocytoma in children: Results of a randomized trial. *J Neurooncol.* 1989;7:165–177.

CHAPTER 13

New Postoperative Clinical Syndromes

John R. Ruge

Recognized postoperative neurologic changes after posterior fossa surgery include cranial nerve paresis, motor paresis, ataxia, dysmetria, and ocular nystagmus. These changes are readily understandable based on well-known neuroanatomical teachings.

This chapter addresses the recently described syndrome of cerebellar mutism after posterior fossa surgery and presents a case of transient coma. Both of these syndromes challenge our understanding of the cerebellum and cerebrocerebellar communication systems. Both of these syndromes can occur after an otherwise uneventful posterior fossa surgery.

Cerebellar Mutism

Muteness after posterior fossa surgery has only recently been reported. Rekate et al.[1] in 1985 presented six children ranging in age from 2 to 11 years who developed an onset of muteness postoperatively. Four of the children were operated on for medulloblastoma, one for cystic astrocytoma, and one for ependymoma. One 8-year-old girl not only did not speak after the gross total removal of a midline medulloblastoma, but also she had marked lateral gaze nystagmus and a mild right hemiparesis. She had normal language comprehension and full motor ability to vocalize, but she was unable to mimic the tongue movements of the examiner. Rudimentary vocalization began 6 weeks later, and by 3 months her language had fully recovered, although a mild residual cerebellar dysarthria was noted.

In another child, the onset of muteness was delayed. This 6-year-old boy underwent suboccipital craniectomy for the removal of a cystic cerebellar astrocytoma. Four days postoperatively, the child became withdrawn and whining; he could not speak. The tumor had been located in the cerebellar vermis and left cerebellar hemisphere. This child was studied closely by the speech pathology service, which noted normal motor ability for phonation and intact receptive understanding of speech, but no vocalization. The child could gesture appropriately. Three weeks after surgery, a very dysarthric speech pattern returned. At 6 months, his speech had returned to normal.

Volcan et al.[2] reported a similar case in 1986. An 8-year-old girl underwent resection of a medulloblastoma. The vermis was divided and the tumor was seen to occupy the entire fourth ventricle obstructing the aqueduct of Sylvius. Initially, the child said "Mama" in the recovery room, but on the first postoperative day was noted to be mute. In addition, the child had evidence of right cerebellar dysfunction. She was initially diagnosed as having a conversion reaction. She would cry in a "shrill, whining fashion." In 2 weeks, she could talk using monosyllables. At 1 month, the child could speak in sentences, but she was dysarthric. The author agreed with Rekate et al.'s[1] conclusion that the muteness had a cerebellar origin.

Ammirati et al.[3] reported a 14-year-old boy who had an uneventful removal of a cystic astrocytoma of the posterior fossa. The child lost the ability to talk on postoperative day 2.

He could follow commands but would only cry when asked to talk. The boy initially had right-sided dysmetria and then went on to develop a mild left-sided dysmetria. The computed tomography (CT) scan postoperatively demonstrated complete tumor removal with bilateral hypodense areas at the level of the dentate nuclei. Three weeks postoperatively, two-syllable words were uttered and at 4 months, he was only minimally dysarthric. A follow-up CT scan at 4 months revealed resolution of the hypodensities involving the dentate nuclei.

Dietze and Mickle[4] recently reported an additional two patients who had an immediate onset of muteness, lasting 3 months. One patient had a midline medulloblastoma involving the vermal and paravermal regions. The other patient had a paravermal arteriovenous malformation. Both had "mild, scanning monotonous dysarthria" at the 3-month examination.

In summary, a total of 16 patients have been reported with "cerebellar mutism" after having had a posterior fossa operation, usually for medulloblastoma.[5] In some cases, the onset of muteness was delayed for several days postoperatively. In all cases, the muteness has been transient. Improvement is noted within 4 to 6 weeks. The children are often left with a dysarthric speech of varying degrees.

The Anatomical Basis of Cerebellar Mutism

The anatomical localization of speech in the cerebellum appears to involve the vermis and paravermal cerebellar hemispheres. Holmes[6,7] first emphasized the importance of the vermis to speech. This came from his observation of World War I victims. Most of the 21 men he studied also had partial cerebellar hemispheric damage and multiple lesions. Although none of his patients had isolated vermal injury, he noted that patients with cerebellar hemispheric injury and vermal injury were most likely to develop a dysarthric speech pattern.

Lechtenberg and Gilman[8] emphasized the importance of the left cerebellar hemisphere in the control of speech. They reviewed 162 cases of patients with focal cerebellar lesions. There was no correlation between the extent of ver-

mal damage and the development of cerebellar speech. When the dissection or destruction extended into the left cerebellar hemisphere, there was a high incidence of the development of a dysarthric speech pattern. Of the 31 patients with clear cerebellar dysarthria, 22 had predominantly, or exclusively, left cerebellar hemispheric disease, whereas seven had right cerebellar hemispheric disease and two had vermal disease.

Teleologically, it may be useful for the cerebellum to lateralize function. Lateralization of cerebellar function is not without precedent. Auditory evoked potential asymmetry has been documented in cats.[9] The left cerebellar hemisphere and left paravermis project to the right cerebral cortex. In a right-handed individual, the left cerebral cortex is dominant for speech function. The right cerebral hemisphere has been shown to be important in the interpretation of melody.[10] Since it is not the meaning of speech that is interrupted with cerebellar dysarthria[11] but prosody, it may be that the interruption of the left cerebellar–right cerebral cortical connections cause the dysarthric speech patterns after some cerebellar injury.

It seems to make sense that the relatively recently acquired modality of speech should be localized in the neocerebellar cortex, not the phylogenetically older vermis. Fraioli and Guidetti[5] performed 94 stereotactic lesions of the cerebellar dentate nucleus in 50 patients for mixed dyskinetic disorders. Two patients developed the "complete absence of language." After 1 to 3 months, respectively, language returned to its preoperative state. Reviewing the coordinates used in their entire series reveals that 73 of the 94 lesions involved the entire lateral and intermediate parts of the dentate nucleus. Twenty lesions were performed again on the lateral and intermediate dentate nucleus, but, more specifically, targeted either to the dorsal or ventral side of this nucleus. In only one lesion was the medial dentate involved. So, although not clearly spelled out in their paper, it is likely that the two individuals who became mute had involvement of the lateral dentate nucleus. Coordinates to make the lesions were measured from the fastigium (or apex of the fourth ventricle). The areas between 10 and 23 mm lateral to the fastigium and between −6 and 10 mm dorsal to the fastigium were ablated using radiofrequency-generated lesions. Because not all of their patients became mute, it would seem the actual area of the cerebellum causing mutism is very near to the dentate nucleus, but not the dentate nucleus itself.

Cerebellar mutism, then, appears to be caused by the interruption of the cerebrocerebellar communication system involving language modulation. Speech is brought to a temporary halt not because there is an inability to comprehend language or formulate thought, but because the complex control of and coordination of the motor component of speech has been damaged. The anatomical locus for this appears to be just lateral to the dentate nucleus in the paravermal cortex, a distance presumed to be approximately 2 cm lateral to the midline. In right-handed individuals, there may be a left cerebellar dominance function serving the prosody of speech.

Transient Coma

Case Presentation

Kindergarten teachers recognized a change in coordination and gait in this 6-year-old boy. He was found to have bilateral papilledema, mild dysmetria on finger-nose-finger testing on the right, and a wide-based unsteady gait. CT scan demonstrated moderate hydrocephalus and a solid posterior fossa tumor. Surgery was uneventful. The surgeon states,

I was able to free completely the tumor from the vermis superiorly, from the three brachii on the right, from the floor of the fourth ventricle inferiorly, and from the restiform body on the left. I did not have satisfaction concerning the brachium pontes and brachium conjunctivum on the left. Consequently, I would say that the tumor was growing from these two brachii and minimally from the anterior medullary velum.

Postoperatively the child was comatose. He initially did not respond to painful stimuli, did not posture, and had no pyramidal or cutaneous reflexes. The cranial nerve examination, however, was normal. CT scan showed only postsurgical changes. He remained comatose for 12 days and then started to respond with hand signals. He walked 4 months postoperative. He remained mute until 6 months postoperative and then spoke with a dysarthric speech pattern that slowly improved. He returned to school 6 months postoperative. Follow-up now 11 years after surgery finds that he is an active high school honor student completing driver's education. Very vivid dreams disturb his sleep pattern at times. He has very mildly dysarthric speech made more apparent with anxiety. He otherwise has no neurologic deficits. His tumor has not recurred.

This child has remained an enigma. He became comatose after uneventful surgery for a cerebellar astrocytoma. The etiology of the coma is unclear. His brain stem was apparently spared injury as his cranial nerve examination remained normal. He has made a nearly normal recovery and 11 years later has only a subtle speech dysarthria. The prolonged cerebellar mutism (6 months) makes it attractive to speculate that the pathophysiology involved in this case is really an extension of that which is involved in cerebellar mutism.

Just as the production of speech is halted short of articulation by cerebellar injury, perhaps also all motor activity can be halted short of initiation of activity by a similar mechanism. There is neurophysiologic support for this concept.

Prior to initiating movement, the cerebellar cortex is involved in the planning and programming of that movement.[12] Kornhuber and coworkers[13,14] showed that up to 0.8 seconds before a movement is initiated a "readiness potential" can be measured over large areas of cerebral cortex. Sixty milliseconds before the movement, a sharp negative wave occurs over the appropriate motor cortex. The cerebral association cortex responsible for the planning of motor activity relays information to the cerebellar hemispheres, which in turn relay it back to the motor cortex. Movement is thus initiated. The movement is monitored by cutaneous, muscle, and joint receptors, which feed back via spinocerebellar tracts to the pars intermedia. Meanwhile, the pars intermedia

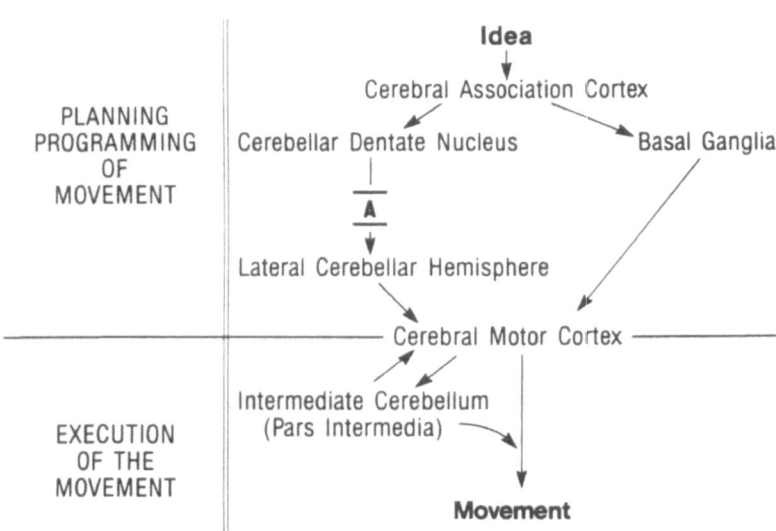

Figure 13.1. Proposed scheme of the organization of motor activity, and the cerebellar relationship tro the planning and execution of that motion. A indicates the proposed site of lesion involving cerebellar mutism and perhaps transient coma. (Modified from Allen and Tsukahara.[12])

has already received information from motor cortex for the next phase of the movement. It can use the feedback information then to modify this new information and correct movement (Fig. 13.1).

The cerebellar cortex primarily integrates information from cerebral cortical association cortex and somatosensory cortex. The cerebellar cortex feeds back to the motor area. The cerebellar cortex then participates in the planning and programming of movement. The cerebellar cortex role in movement is largely anticipatory.[12] The dentate nucleus is the major relay nucleus of the cerebellar cortex. Thach[15–17] has shown that neuronal activity of the dentate nucleus precedes that of motor cortical neurons. The activity of the interpositus neurons (globose and emboliform nuclei) tends to follow that of the motor cortical neurons.

Conclusion

Movement, whether it be the articulation of speech or the opening of one's eyelids, is first conceptualized in the cerebral cortex. The plan of action is then modulated and further organized by the cerebellar cortex and basal ganglia. The movement is then initiated. Once in progress, a spinocerebellar loop aids in the adjustment and modification of further movement.

It appears that the articulation of speech can be halted by interrupting this cerebrocerebellar system. Whether or not a comatose-like state can be produced by a similar mechanism, as perhaps occurred in the case presented, remains to be proven.

References

1. Rekate HL, Grubb RL, Aram DM, et al. Muteness of cerebellar origin. *Arch Neurol.* 1985; 42:697–698.
2. Volcan I, Cole GA, Johnston K. Letters to the editor: A case of muteness of cerebellar origin. *Arch Neurol.* 1986;43:313–314.
3. Ammirati M, Mirzai S, Samii M. Transient mutism following removal of a cerebellar tumor. A case report and review of the literature. *Childs Nerv Syst.* 1989;5:12–14.
4. Dietze DD, Mickle JP. Cerebellar mutism as a result of posterior fossa surgery (abstract). *Neurosurgery.* 1990;26:1077.
5. Fraioli B, Guidetti B. Effects of stereotactic lesions of the dentate nucleus of the cerebellum in man. *Appl Neurophysiol.* 1975;38:81–90.
6. Holmes G. The symptoms of acute cerebellar injuries due to gunshot injuries. *Brain.* 1917; 40(4):461–535.
7. Holmes G. The Croonian lectures on the clini-

cal symptoms of cerebellar disease and their interpretation. *Lancet.* 1922;2:59–65.

8. Lechtenberg R, Gilman S. Speech disorders in cerebellar disease. *Ann Neurol.* 1978;3:285–290.

9. Altman JA, Bechtereu NN, Radionova EA, et al. Electrical responses of the auditory area of the cerebellar cortex to acoustic stimulation. *Exp Brain Res.* 1976;26:285–298.

10. Shankweiler D. Effects of temporal lobe lesions on recognition of dichotically presented melodies. *J Comp Physiol Psychol.* 1966;62:115–119.

11. Zentay PJ. Motor disorders of the central nervous system and their significance in speech: Part I. Cerebral and cerebellar dysarthrias. *Laryngoscope.* 1937;3:147–156.

12. Allen GI, Tsukahara N. Cerebrocerebellar communication systems. *Physiol Rev.* 1974; 54(4):957–1006.

13. Deecke LI, Scheid P, Kornhuber H. Distribu-tion of readiness potential, pre-motion positivity, and motor potential of the human cerebral cortex preceding voluntary finger movements. *Exp Brain Res.* 1969;7:158–168.

14. Kornhuber HH. Cerebral cortex, cerebellum and basal ganglia: An introduction to their motor functions. In: Schmitt FO, Worden G, eds. *The Neurosciences: Third Study Program.* Cambridge: MIT Press; 1973: 267–280.

15. Thach WT. Discharge of cerebellar neurons related to two maintained postures and two prompt movements. I. Nuclear cell output. *J Neurophysiol.* 1970;33:527–536.

16. Thach WT. Discharge of cerebellar neurons related to two maintained postures and two prompt movements. II. Purkinje cell output and input. *J Neurophysiol.* 1970;33:537–547.

17. Thach WT. Cerebellar dentate nucleus precedes motor cortex in the initiation of a prompt volitional movement. *Abstr Soc Neurosci.* 1973; 3:155.

CHAPTER 14

Intellectual and Psychosocial Complications of Posterior Fossa Tumor Surgery and Supplemental (Radiation Therapy/Chemotherapy) Treatment

Elizabeth Hoppe-Hirsch

Some remedies are worse than the disease. It might be alluring to apply this idea to the treatment of malignant posterior fossa tumors. This would not be quite relevant since, without treatment, death is the unavoidable result of the disease. However, the problem is not only to cure the tumor, but also to assure an acceptable quality of life for the child. From this point of view, in spite of the fact that the association of surgery and radiotherapy has remarkably increased the survival of children presenting with certain malignant neoplasms of the central nervous system, the enthusiasm of the pioneers should now be somewhat reduced. The improved survival rate overshadowed for a while the late therapy-related effects: intellectual impairment, endocrine dysfunction, and secondary neoplasms.

Three main methods are now available to treat posterior fossa tumors: surgery, radiotherapy, and chemotherapy. These treatments are usually associated when the tumor is malignant. However, in the evaluation of intellectual and functional sequelae, other factors should be included such as the possible destructive effect of the lesion itself and the role of the emotional stress to the child related to multiple hospitalizations, school absence, and family reaction. As these factors are usually intermingled and perhaps even interacting, it is extremely difficult to evaluate the impact of each of them. This evaluation, however, is essential in order to improve the functional results by an eventual change in therapeutic strategy.

The sequelae observed after treatment of a posterior fossa tumor are mainly neurological deficits and/or intellectual or endocrine dysfunction. The neurological deficits are usually rapidly detected in the postoperative course; they regress more or less completely over time and are in most cases a consequence of the surgical procedure. The progress of surgical techniques that enables the neurosurgeon to respect more and more of the normal nervous tissue has considerably reduced the importance and frequency of these postoperative deficits. However, it should be pointed out that a late deafness can be the consequence of radiotherapy or that of a chemotherapy such as cis-platinum.[1] Some neurological deficits can also occur later as a consequence of radiotherapy, mainly because of its detrimental effects on cerebral blood vessels.

The neuropsychological sequelae are late-occurring and difficult to recognize, at least in the beginning. For many years, the intellectual deterioration seen in children after whole-brain irradiation and chemotherapy was for this reason underestimated. Thus in 1969, Bloom et al.[2] stated that 82% of medulloblastoma patients surviving between 5 and 17 years led active lives, with either a mild disability or no disability at all. There are two reasons for the late recognition of adverse effects on intelligence. First, the patients must be fastidiously evaluated with precise neuropsychological tests. Second, since we are dealing with a late effect essentially due to radiotherapy administered for highly malignant tumors, intellectual deterioration needs to be observed in a sufficient number of long-term survivors, a result that has only recently been achieved. This is exactly what has happened with certain tumors of the posterior fossa such as medulloblastomas and to a lesser extent ependymomas. Medulloblastomas represent one-third of the posterior fossa tumors in children. Without radiotherapy, this tumor was invariably fatal 6 to 12 months after gross removal.[3,4] The introduction of total neuraxis irradiation improved progressively the survival rate. Still, 20 years ago only one child out of three survived more than 5 years.[2,5] Today 50% to 70% of children treated for medulloblastoma are expected to be disease free 5 years after treatment.[6-8]

Therefore, as the number of survivors among children treated for a malignant posterior fossa tumor is increasing, the problem of late sequelae becomes exceedingly important since, as stated before, the problem is not only to remove the tumor but also to respect the normal nervous tissue and thus to assure a good quality of life. This problem should be discussed at several levels:

1. Is there any late intellectual deterioration after treatment of a posterior fossa tumor?
2. If there is, is it the consequence of surgery, of radiotherapy, or of chemotherapy?
3. What is its pathogenesis: cell loss, capillary damage, demyelination, alterations of dendritic arborization, or synaptogenesis?
4. What can be done to prevent or diminish this late complication of the treatment?

Posterior Fossa Surgery and Late Intellectual Deterioration

Surgery, radiotherapy, and chemotherapy are usually associated in the treatment of malignant posterior fossa tumors, and when they are it is impossible to determine what factor precisely is responsible for the late complications. The effects of surgery should be looked for in patients who are operated on but who do not receive any complementary treatment. This is the case in cerebellar astrocytomas and more generally in low-grade astrocytomas.

Cerebellar astrocytomas are especially interesting when they are developed purely in the cerebellar hemispheres and in the vermis, i.e., in nervous structures that are not supposed to be related to the development or the maintenance of intellectual function. Reviewing our series of cerebellar astrocytomas operated on before 1978, we found that most of the patients had an IQ above 90.[9,10] Some children, however, had a low IQ. These few poor results were probably related to the slowly developing preoperative hydrocephalus or to postoperative complications, such as lesion of the brain stem or postoperative infection. It has actually been shown that complications after surgery of the posterior fossa could be responsible for poor final results, especially as far as IQ is concerned.[11] At any rate, IQs in this series of cerebellar astrocytomas were by far higher than those found in a series of medulloblastomas that had been operated on and irradiated in the CNS.[9] Thus, late mental retardation does not seem to be related to surgery on the vermis or the cerebellar hemispheres.

In our series of 62 operated brain stem tumors, eight children did not receive any complementary radiotherapy after surgery. The postoperative IQ is known for seven of these children: four IQs were normal or near normal, whereas three were very low (20, 40, and 50). The number of patients is too small to draw a precise conclusion on the role of surgery per se. However, it seems clear that a brain stem tumor and the surgical procedure performed in order to remove it are responsible in some cases for mental retardation. It is reasonable to hypothesize that a surgical brain stem lesion that can lead to a postoperative coma may also cause a late intellectual deterioration.

Finally, the conclusion could be summarized as follows: when surgery is restricted to the cerebellar hemispheres or to the vermis, there is no IQ deterioration; when surgery has to deal with the brain stem, the late intellectual outcome is sometimes poor, a result that is in accordance with the knowledge of the brain stem physiology and especially with that of the reticular formation.

Radiotherapy and Late Intellectual Deterioration

The problem of the late effects of radiotherapy delivered to the central nervous system has to be studied in malignant tumors of the posterior fossa in which radiotherapy is precisely the mandatory complementary treatment. The first question to answer is the following: Is there any late intellectual deterioration in children treated for malignant posterior fossa tumors?

To answer this question, we have reviewed in 1978 our series of 57 medulloblastomas.[9] This tumor had been chosen because of the relatively large number of long-term survivors. This study showed that survival rates were very high, whereas functional results were very poor. Only 12% of the children had an IQ above 90; 70% were between 70 and 90; emotional and behavioral disorders were observed in 93% of the patients, and specific types of retardation (spatial orientation, speech, writing, reading) in 82%. Academic failure was the consequence in 75% of the cases. On the one hand, these results were in complete contrast with the optimistic papers published previously.[2] On the other hand, we felt that these poor results were related to radiotherapy, since they were by far worse than those observed in cerebellar astrocytomas that were operated on but did not receive any radiotherapy. However, our children had received a total central nervous system irradiation and in most cases a chemotherapy so that two questions could not be answered: What were the respective effects of the irradiation on the hemispheres and on the posterior fossa? Was chemotherapy partly or totally responsible for this intellectual deterioration?

Raimondi and Tomita[12] reported in 1979 that, in their series, only 3 out of 15 children surviving medulloblastomas had an IQ above 80. These patients had been irradiated on the whole central nervous system, but had not received any chemotherapy. Thus it was clear that radiotherapy, without chemotherapy, could be responsible for the poor functional late results.

This study was confirmed by the report of Danoff et al.[13] who assessed the long-term effects of radiotherapy without chemotherapy for various brain tumors in children and found that 50% of their patients had an IQ below 90. Moreover, they pointed out that the younger the patient, the higher the risk of late mental retardation.

The conclusions were similar in the study of Kun et al.,[14] in which 53% of the patients who had received a supra- and infratentorial irradiation had an IQ below 80, and 63% of the patients attended a specialized school. Radiotherapy was delivered to the posterior fossa alone in six patients. Only one of these patients exhibited an intellectual disability. Therefore, it seems that the main danger is at the level of the supratentorial irradiation.

However, the functional results reported by Packer et al.(11) were slightly better since the mean IQ 4 years after treatment was 97, even though the children, in most cases, showed significant learning difficulties. Therefore we decided to review again, 10 years after the initial study, our series of medulloblastomas to see if a larger number of patients and a longer follow-up would confirm our first conclusions. This study[8] showed that, 5 years after treatment, only 58% of the patients had an IQ above 80. More important was the demonstration that the intellectual degradation was progressive over the years. At the 10-year evaluation, only 15% of the patients maintained an IQ above 80 (Table 14.1) and 46% had an IQ

Table 14.1. IQs 5 and 10 years after treatment.

IQ	5 years	10 years
<60	18%	46%
60–80	24%	38%
>80	58%	15%

Table 14.2. Scholastic integration 5 and 10 years after treatment.

Scholastic integration	5 years	10 years
Special	26%	62%
>2 years late	34%	31%
Normal	39%	7%

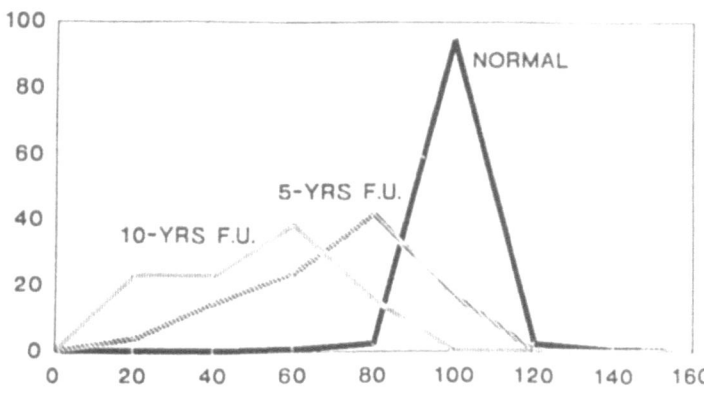

Figure 14.1. Comparison of IQ distributions in a normal population (normal), in medulloblastomas 5 years after treatment (5-yrs F.U.), and in medulloblastomas 10 years after treatment (10-yrs F.U.). The displacement of the peak toward the left demonstrates the progressive intellectual degradation over the years.

below 60. Five years after treatment, 39% of the children attended a normal school, whereas 5 years later this percentage had dropped to 7% (Table 14.2). No patient had normal employment, whereas 64% worked in a protected environment. This progressive decline in IQ was also demonstrated in the study of Packer et al.,[15] which also showed that the decline started very early, in the first 2 years after treatment.

This progressive worsening over the years is probably related to a serious impairment of the learning abilities of the child. Performances do not improve with time, so that the result is a more and more important divergence with the performances required for a normal IQ.

All in all, the different studies lead to the same conclusion: children treated by surgery and radiotherapy for a posterior fossa tumor show a poor intellectual outcome. The degradation is progressive over the years (Fig. 14.1) and more important in very young patients (Table 14.3). The far better results of surgery alone, as far as IQs are concerned,

point to the role of radiotherapy in this degradation.

Another demonstration of the deleterious effects of radiotherapy on the developing brain of a child results from the study of series of children with leukemia who receive prophylactic radiotherapy to the central nervous system without any associated surgical treatment. The studies of Moss et al.[16] and Meadows et al.[17] showed that a 2,400-rad cranial irradiation resulted in a significant intellectual deficiency that was more important in very young children. Although the results of McIntosh et al.[18] and those of Ivnik et al.[19] are less conclusive, it can be accepted that a dose of 2,400 rad has a significant effect on the brain of a child. It should be pointed out that deficiencies are mild. The majority of treated children still perform within the low average range at most tasks. However, this performance probably represents a significant reduction from their previous level of ability. Therefore, the detrimental effect of radiotherapy on the brain is certainly dose related. It is of utmost impor-

Table 14.3. Influence of the age of the child at the time of treatment on the IQ.

Age (years)	5 years				10 years			
	Nb	<60	60–80	>80	Nb	<60	60–80	>80
<3	11	18%	36%	45%	4	50%	50%	0%
3–6	18	28%	22%	50%	6	33%	50%	17%
6–10	16	12.5%	25%	62.5%	3	67%	0%	33%
>10	10	10%	10%	80%				

Nb,

tance to know that the intellectual outcome is by far worse with 3,500 rad on the cerebral hemispheres than with 2,400 rad.

Various neuropathologic changes can be seen after central nervous system irradiation. It has been assumed[20] that the primary site of damage was the capillary endothelial cell or the glial and oligodendroglial cells. Antigens released from damaged glial cells have also been thought to be responsible for an allergic reaction. A spectrum of clinical syndromes may occur, including radionecrosis, necrotizing leukoencephalopathy, mineralizing microangiopathy with dystrophic calcification, cerebellar sclerosis, and spinal cord dysfunction.[21]

However, the clinical features related to necrosis or to leukoencephalopathy are very different from the sequelae on cognitive function that are seen after posterior fossa surgery associated with central nervous system irradiation. Alterations of dendritic arborization and synaptogenesis have been related to mental retardation.[21] It is conceivable that radiotherapy could damage dendrites and synapses and be responsible for the intellectual sequelae, but this hypothesis remains to be demonstrated.

Chemotherapy

The degree of responsibility of chemotherapeutic agents in central nervous system lesions and in sequelae is extremely difficult to assess accurately, for various reasons. Chemotherapy is practically always used in association with surgery and radiotherapy in the treatment of central nervous system tumors, so that it is often hazardous to assess the respective role of these three treatments in the determination of sequelae. However, some facts are well documented. As already stated, radiotherapy without any chemotherapy can be responsible for the late sequelae. In contrast, if methotrexate is excepted, late intellectual impairment has not been described in those tumors developed outside of the central nervous system that are treated by chemotherapy alone. Finally, it is well documented that some chemotherapeutic agents like methotrexate may have a deleterious effect on the central nervous system. Given through the ventricular route when there is a blockade of the CSF circulation[22,23] or intravenously in large doses,[24] methotrexate has been reported to cause a leukoencephalopathy.

Less dramatic changes in functioning may result from various combinations of radiotherapy and chemotherapy.[25] Several studies[26–29] tend to demonstrate a synergic, adverse effect of the association of methotrexate and radiotherapy. The mechanism of this interaction is not well understood, but it has been postulated on the one hand that a radiation-induced disruption of the blood-brain barrier might increase the concentration of the methotrexate in the nervous tissue and thus its toxicity. On the other hand, several experimental and clinical studies have shown that methotrexate reduces cerebral glucose metabolism and induces an alteration in blood-brain barrier function.[30–32]

Besides methotrexate, there are many other chemotherapeutic agents. Some agents cross the blood-brain barrier and are thus able to reach the isolated tumoral cells that spread in the normal nervous tissue; others do not and are therefore less toxic, since they reach only the tumor, where the barrier is disrupted. There are now at least four main classes of anticancer agents with four different mechanisms of action: DNA-lytics, antimetabolites, alkylating agents, and antimitotics. These anticancer agents can produce CNS clinical symptoms such as ataxia, blindness, paresis, hallucinations, cranial nerve palsies, slurred speech, seizures, inappropriate antidiuretic hormone (ADH), and orthostatic hypotension.[33] In most cases, several of these agents are used in association. But the precise role of these different chemotherapeutic agents, if any, in the late functional outcome of children treated for malignant posterior fossa tumors will be very difficult to assess accurately because of the usual association of different therapeutics. However, it seems that chemotherapy alone is less deleterious than radiotherapy. It might therefore be a candidate to replace radiotherapy if, in the future, it becomes as efficient.

The severity of the late intellectual deterioration after treatment of a malignant posterior fossa tumor raises the last question: What can be done to avoid or at least reduce this complication? Assuming that it was the consequence of the large x-ray dose delivered to the hemispheres, we have checked in the second SIOP trial whether a reduction of this dose would lower the survival rate or not. For the time being, the survival rates of the children who received the standard dosage (35 Gy) and that of the patients who had only 25 Gy are not statistically different. However, it is too early to form a conclusion, and the possible advantages of the reduced dosage have not yet been assessed.

Another problem is raised by those patients under 2 years of age who present with a malignant posterior fossa tumor. The late sequelae after radiotherapy are in these cases so heavy that new strategies have to be tried. In the pediatric neurosurgery service of *Les Enfants Malades* in Paris, we try to give chemotherapy after surgery and to postpone radiotherapy as much as possible. Again, it is too early to know if this new strategy is of any interest.

In conclusion, consideration of this late intellectual deterioration is essential. However, we should not forget that 30 years ago all the children presenting with a medulloblastoma were dying, whereas 60% now survive. Some remedies are worse than the disease, but we should remember that death is the worst disease. Therefore, when we decide to change our treatments or our strategies, we should do it step by step, slowly, and very carefully.

References

1. Granowetter L, Rosenstock J, Packer RJ. Potentiating effects of CNS radiation on cisplatinum neurotoxicity with brain tumors. *J Neurooncol.* 1983;1:293–297.
2. Bloom HJG, Wallace ENK, Henk MB. The treatment and prognosis of medulloblastoma in children. *Am J Roentgenol.* 1969;105:43–62.
3. Cushing H. *Intracranial Tumors.* Springfield, IL: Charles C. Thomas; 1932.
4. Matson DD. *Neurosurgery of Infancy and Childhood.* 2nd ed. Springfield, IL: Charles C. Thomas; 1969.
5. Hoffman HJ, Hendrick EB, Humphreys RP. Metastasis via ventriculoperitoneal shunt in patients with medulloblastoma. *J Neurosurg.* 1976;44:562–566.
6. Berry MP, Jenkin RDT, Kun CW, Mair BD, Simpson WY. Radiation treatment for medulloblastoma. A 21 year review. *J Neurosurg.* 1981;55:43–51.
7. Park TS, Hoffman HJ, Hendrick EB, Humphreys RP, Becker LE. Medulloblastoma: clinical presentation and management. *J Neurosurg.* 1983;58:543–552.
8. Hoppe-Hirsch E, Renier D, Lellouch-Tubiana A, Sainte-Rose C, Pierre-Kahn A, and Hirsch JF. Medulloblastoma in childhood: progressive intellectual deterioration. *Childs Nerv Syst.* 1990;6:60–65.
9. Hirsch JF, Renier D, Pierre-Kahn A, Benveniste L, George B. Les medulloblastomes de l'enfant. "Survie et résultats fonctionnels." *Neurochirurgie.* 1978;34:391–397.
10. Hirsch JF, Renier D, Czernichow P, Benveniste L, Pierre-Kahn A. Medulloblastoma in childhood. Survival and functional results. *Acta Neurochir.* 1979;48:1–15.
11. Packer RJ, Sposto R, Atkins TE, Sutton LN, Bruce DA, Siegel KR, Rorke LB, Littman PA, Schut L. Quality of life in children with primitive neuroectodermal tumors (medulloblastoma) of the posterior fossa. *Pediatr Neurosci.* 1987;13:169–175.
12. Raimondi AJ, Tomita T. The disadvantages of prophylactic whole CNS postoperative radiation therapy for medulloblastoma. In: Paoletti P, Walker MD, Butti G, et al., eds. *Multidisciplinary Aspects of Brain Tumor Therapy.* Amsterdam: North-Holland; 1979:209–218.
13. Danoff BF, Cowchock FS, Marquette C, Mulgrew L, Kramer S. Assessment of the long term effects of primary radiation therapy for brain tumors in children. *Cancer.* 1982;49:1580–1586.
14. Kun LE, Mulhern RK, Crisco J. Quality of life in children treated for brain tumors: Intellectual, emotional, and academic function. *J Neurosurg.* 1983;58:1–6.
15. Packer RJ, Sutton LN, Atkins TE, Radcliffe J, Bunin GR, D'Angio G, Siegel KR, Schut L. A prospective study of cognitive function in children receiving whole-brain radiotherapy and chemotherapy: 2-year results. *J Neurosurg.* 1989;70:707–713.
16. Moss HA, Nannis ED, Poplack DG. The effects of prophylactic treatment of the central nervous system on the intellectual functioning of children with acute lymphocytic leukemia. *Am. J. Med.* 1981;71:47–52.

17. Meadows AT, Gordon J, Massari DJ, Littman P, Fergusson J, Moss K. Declines in IQ scores and cognitive dysfunctions in children with acute lymphocytic leukaemia treated with cranial irradiation. *Lancet.* 1981;2:1015–1018.

18. McIntosh S, Klatskin EH, O'Brien RT, Aspnes GT, Kammerer BL, Snead C, Kalavsky SM, Pearson HA. Chronic neurologic disturbance in childhood leukemia. *Cancer.* 1976;37:853–857.

19. Ivnik RJ, Colligan RC, Obetz SW, Smithson WA. Neuropsychologic performance among children in remission from acute lymphocytic leukemia. *J. Dev. Behav. Pediatr.* 1981;2:29–34.

20. Rottenberg DA, Chernik NL, Deck F. Cerebral necrosis following radiotherapy of extracranial neoplasms. *Ann Neurol.* 1977;1:339–357.

21. Packer RJ, Meadows AT, Rorke LB, Goldwein JL, D'Angio G. Long-term sequelae of cancer treatment on the central nervous system in childhood. *Med Pediatr Oncol.* 1987;15:241–253.

22. Duffner PK, Cohen ME, Brecker ML, Berger P, Parthasarathy KL, Suraj Bakshi, Ettinger LJ, Freeman A. CT abnormalities and altered methotrexate clearance in children with CNS leukemia. *Neurology.* 1984;34:229–233.

23. Packer RJ, Zimmerman R, Rosenstock J, Rorke LB, Norris D, Rosenstock J. Focal encephalopathy following the administration of methotrexate via misplaced intraventricular catheter. *Arch Neurol.* 1981;38:450–452.

24. Allen JC, Rosen G, Mehta BM. Leukoencephalopathy following high-dose IV methotrexate with leucovorin rescue. *Cancer Treat Rap.* 1980;64:1261–1273.

25. Meadows AF, Evans AE. Effects of chemotherapy on the central nervous system. *Cancer.* 1976;37:1079–1085.

26. Duffner PK, Cohen ME, Thomas P. Late effects of treatment on the intelligence of children with posterior fossa tumors. *Cancer.* 1983;51:233–237.

27. Bleyer WA, Griffin TW. White matter necrosis, microangiopathy, and intellectual abilities in survivors of childhood leukemia, association with central nervous system irradiation and methotrexate therapy in radiation damage to the nervous system. In: Gilbert HA, Kagan AR, eds. New York: Raven Press; 1980:155–174.

28. Eiser C. Intellectual abilities among survivors of childhood leukaemia as a function of CNS irradiation. *Arch Dis Child.* 1978;53:391–395.

29. Pratt RA, DeChiro G, Weed JC. Cerebral necrosis following irradiation and chemotherapy for metastatic choriocarcinoma. *Surg Neurol.* 1977;7:117–120.

30. Phillips PC, Thaler HT, Allen JC, Rottenberg DA. High-dose leucovorin reverses acute high-dose methotrexate neurotoxicity in the rat. *Ann Neurol.* 1989;25:365–372.

31. Phillips PC, Dhawan V, Strother SC, Sidtis JJ, Evans AC, Allen JC, Rottenberg DA. Reduced cerebral glucose metabolism and increased brain capillary permeablity following high-dose methotrexate chemotherapy: a positron emission tomographic study. *Ann Neurol.* 1987; 21:59–63.

32. Phillips PC, Thaler HT, Berger CA, Fleisher M, Wellner D, Allen JC, Rottenberg DA. Acute high-dose methotrexate neurotoxicity in the rat. *Ann Neurol.* 1986;20:583–589.

33. Byfield JE. Central nervous system toxicities from combined therapies. In: Vaeth JM, ed. *Combined Effects of Chemotherapy and Radiotherapy on Normal Tissue Tolerance.* Basel: Karger; 1979:228–234.

CHAPTER 15

Family and the Child with a Posterior Fossa Tumor

Yoon Sun Hahn and Erica Ciro

Introduction

Children with brain tumors are living longer now with improved methods of treatment. This generates a concern for their quality of life. Chronic illness has been shown to impact not only the child, but parents and siblings as well. The child with a brain tumor will experience a number of effects from the tumor and its treatment, and, in fact, more than 50% of children, whether radiated or not, experience major problems in cognitive, emotional, academic, physical, and psychosocial functions.[1] Undoubtedly, the family will also be affected during the course of the child's illness.

Pain Reaction and Suffering of Children

Children with posterior fossa tumors experience a number of physical effects from the tumor itself, as well as from the treatments they receive. Bloom[2] in 1971 reported that 82% of children who underwent posterior fossa surgery for medulloblastoma presented with various neurological impairments including nystagmus, learning disability, tremor, and ataxia. LeBaron et al.[1] in 1988 found that the neurological and neuropsychological deficits include higher cortical function, although the affected site was the posterior fossa. Children with posterior fossa tumors often present with headache due to the mass effect of the tumor, as well as increased intracranial pressure re-

sulting from obstructive hydrocephalus.[3] Most of the children experience headache that is worse in the morning, followed by vomiting. Others experience lethargy, anorexia, personality changes, and irritability.[3]

Most children with posterior fossa tumors will undergo surgery and its associated discomforts. The pain response varies with each child and is influenced by several factors. Katz et al.[4] in 1980 examined the pain response in children of varying ages, undergoing a bone marrow aspiration. The younger children ages 2 to 6 displayed the greatest range of distressed behaviors as compared to children in the 7 to 12 or 13 to 20 age groups. Further, girls tended to cry, cling, and request emotional support, and boys tended to utilize stalling tactics. The ability to understand and respond to pain is related to the child's level of development.

Infants have a generalized response to painful stimuli.[5] They will usually cry loudly, and as the infant grows older, will withdraw or physically resist. The toddler is aware of where the pain stimulus originates and tends to respond by resisting. Toddlers often will seek their parents as a means of comfort. The preschooler has a limited ability to understand causation, often engaging in "magical thinking." The child may attempt to postpone a painful procedure. The school-aged child is able to characterize his or her pain and rate the severity. Distraction and relaxation techniques are often helpful in this age group to control pain.

Adolescents are able to use abstract thought and problem-solving in response to pain. Though they often experience anxiety as well as the pain, the adolescent's response tends to be more positive than younger adults.[6] In addition to the child's developmental level, several other factors influence the child's response to pain. The child's personality and temperament, past experience with pain, and gender influence pain perception.[5]

Unfortunately, pain management in pediatric patients has been less than ideal. Several studies have examined this issue with startling results. A study done in 1983 by Schechter et al.[7] utilized 90 adults and 90 children matched for sex and diagnosis. The results revealed that adults received between $1\frac{1}{2}$ and 3 times the number of narcotics as children.

In 1984, Beyer et al.[8] performed a similar study in which 50 adults and 50 children who had undergone open heart surgery were compared. Twelve of the 50 children received no analgesics within the first 3 postoperative days. Of those children who did receive pain medication, only one or two doses per day were given. On the other hand, the adults received 70% of all analgesics given, whereas children received 30%. Analgesis for children are often withheld for several reasons: (a) the fear of addiction, (b) the fear of respiratory depression, (c) the child may not display overt signs of pain, and (d) the child may not ask for pain medication.[9] However, pain management is a necessary part of the child's care and must be carefully assessed, diagnosed, and treated.

Children with posterior fossa tumors will also undergo painful procedures as a component of their treatment plan, including staging myelograms beginning within the first month of surgery, bone marrow aspiration, venipuncture for labs, intravenous needle insertion for multiple computer tomograms, and magnetic resonance imaging with contrast enhancement. Therefore, proper emotional preparation, is necessary for these invasive procedures. The scope and timing of the preparation is based on the cognitive level of the child. For very young children, preparation immediately prior to the event is best because of limited attention span and memory. The older child, depending on level of development, can be prepared for a procedure in advance to allow time for the

child to develop a coping response. Preparation can involve a simple verbal explanation, or include charts, pictures, video, or demonstration. It is important to assess the child's previous experience with similar procedures, and parents' perceptions of the child's ability to tolerate or not tolerate advanced preparation. Further, if the child is experiencing anxiety the parents may have anxiety of their own. Therefore, it is very important to include parents in the preparation of the child, lest they convey their own fears and anxiety reactions to their child. A number of techniques can be utilized to help the child through painful procedures related to the tumor. Distraction imaging, rhythmic breathing, and encouragement may be helpful. These techniques must be chosen based upon the child's level of development.

Body Image

The child with a posterior fossa tumor will experience some changes in appearance that can negatively impact the body image. Surgical intervention results in shaving all or a portion of the child's hair, leaving a large scar, with additional incisions if a shunt is necessary for hydrocephalus. This alone can be very traumatic, but the fear of being teased by peers is equally distressing. The child may also receive chemotherapy and radiation treatment, which will increase the hair loss. Wigs and hats can help to ease the child's anxiety about his/her appearance. Steroids such as Decadron are frequently used to control cerebral edema perioperatively and for the duration of radiation therapy. Side effects can include cushingoid appearance and increased appetite, which may contribute to weight gain. The child with a posterior fossa tumor and on Decadron will have a very different appearance, one that can alter the body image and further increase the child' anxiety. Therefore, it is extremely important to prepare the child and parents in advance for these temporary changes.

If chemotherapy is selected as a means of treatment, a central venous access device may be surgically placed. Though central lines are easily hidden under clothing, for some children this line may be embarrassing or threatening. Such children need support and reinforcement that they are still the same child as before, but with a slightly different appearance.

Emotional Reactions of Children

Depending on their age, children diagnosed with a life-threatening illness have some basic fears and concerns. It is imperative that health care providers are aware of these concerns so that fears can be identified, addressed, and allayed. Depending on the age of the child, each age group has some specific stressors and coping strategies to deal with these fears. The infant's primary stressor is separation from the family. The infant will respond by crying, temper tantrums, and possibly withdrawal.

In early childhood, separation continues to be a stressor, as well as the fear of bodily harm and mutilation. Because of the inability to discern reality from fantasy, "magical thinking" may persist. Coping behaviors include protest, ritualism, fantasy, and regression. Infants and toddlers cannot appreciate the concept that people and objects that are out of sight continue to exist. Similarly, young school-aged children fear abandonment. Therefore, it is essential that when the child is hospitalized, parents are encouraged to visit. When the parents must leave, the health care team must reinforce that the parents will be back. Also, leaving pictures of family members and/or a cassette tape with messages from the family or a favorite story or songs can provide a sense of security for the child.

Middle childhood is characterized by a fear of loss of control, fear of the unknown, and separation from family. Possible coping behaviors include denial, projection, identification, and randomization. In late childhood, fear of separation persists and includes family as well as peers. Coping mechanisms include displacement and withdrawal. Adolescence is characterized by a need for independence; therefore, fear of loss of control and dependence are common. Coping responses include rebellion, denial, rationalization, fantasy, daydreaming, and identification.[10]

Many children associate the cause of illness with wrongdoing and therefore perceive illness as punishment. The child may feel he/she did something to cause the tumor to occur. Such children need support and must be reminded that the tumor is not their fault.

In middle and late childhood, as well as adolescence, the loss of control is a major stressor. For the child with a posterior fossa tumor, hospitalizations are inevitable. Normal routines for eating, sleeping, bathing, and playing are altered. An ill child, possibly with neurological deficits may be unable to perform activities of daily living. This loss of control and dependency upon others can be upsetting to the child. To alleviate some of this stress, the child should be allowed to make as many choices as possible, and an attempt must be made to maintain a daily routine.

Surgery, chemotherapy, radiation therapy, and other invasive procedures performed on children with posterior fossa tumors can evoke the fear of bodily mutilation. This is especially true because of their cognitive inability to discern fantasy from reality. Young children require simple but honest explanations about their illness and procedures they will undergo. When information is not provided, children tend to fill in the gaps with their own explanation, which is often comprised of fact as well as fantasy. These children also need to be reminded that surgery and other procedures are being done to help them get better, not to punish them for being sick.

Because of the strides being made in medicine, children with posterior fossa tumors are living longer lives, with death extending over a period of months or years. This places a responsibility on health care workers to assure the child the maximum quality of life, as well as death.

The child's perception of the concept of death is dependent on their level of cognitive development. Nagy[11] identified three developmental stages in the child's response to the meaning of death. In the first stage, children ages 3 to 5, see death as a form of sleep. They are unable to grasp the finality of death. In the second stage, ages 5 to 8, children are able to appreciate that death is final. Death may be personified at this stage, possibly as a means of making death seem less frightening. In the third stage, death is seen in a mature sense as final, inevitable and universal.

Bluebond-Langer[12-14] has further added to the understanding of children's perception of death. Her study of terminally ill children and their perceptions of death led her to describe five different stages that are applicable to children of all ages beyond infancy and are overtly expressed as fears, concerns, and anxieties.

It is not uncommon for parents and health care providers to feel the need to shield the child with a posterior fossa tumor from the negative prognosis. However, studies have shown that children are able to detect the anxiety of others and infer the severity of their situation. Currently, it is believed to be most beneficial for everyone involved to acknowledge the child's fears and proceed in an open and honest manner. Discussions about death must be age-appropriate and follow the cues of the child. Information should be simple and direct and only the questions asked should be answered. Additional counseling may be necessary depending on the individual.

At our institution, upon diagnosis, a discussion between the parent(s) and staff is conducted. A frequent concern of parents is, What do we tell our child? We encourage parents to use their child's own language to explain the tumor and seriousness of the condition. Our staff supplements the parents' explanation using diagrams, a model of the brain, and other methods to clarify the diagnosis for the child. We also remind the child that we will always be honest about treatments and prognosis. All discussions are tailored to the individual child and his level of development.

The importance of play and its benefits are well documented in the literature.[15-19] Play is an activity of learning that infants and children engage in spontaneously. Play can involve physical exercise or quiet activity, but is an active process with several important functions. Play is a means of communication, a way of exploring the environment, a means of practicing and refining fine and gross motor skills, a way of practicing roles and behaviors, a means of

socialization in a particular group, an outlet for stress and negative feelings, a means of coping with unpleasant situations, a means of expressing creativity, and most importantly, it is an activity that is fun. Play opportunities for the child with a posterior fossa tumor must be included in the plan of care. Toys and games from home help to provide a sense of familiarity and stability for a child upset by hospital routines and procedures. The manipulation of equipment such as syringes (without the needles), stethescopes, bandages, etc. can assist the child to work through fears about them.

We have also found it helpful for school-aged children and adolescents to see an actual shunt catheters for hydrocephalus. Often they are quite surprised to see that the shunt is much smaller than they had expected. Allowing the child to see the shunt seems helpful in reducing fears about it. It is also helpful to encourage children of the same age to engage in group activities. This fosters socialization and may help to distract the child.

For the child in the terminal phase of illness, play can be altered to meet his/her needs. Quiet activities such as reading a book to the child, watching a movie specifically for children, or singing favorite songs can provide enormous benefit. Such activities prevent total isolation, may provide distraction from discomfort or fear, and simply make the child feel better. The involvement of a play therapist is essential in caring for children who are hospitalized.

Radiation

Brain growth occurs rapidly within the first 3 years of age. Myelinization of the central nervous system is pretty well developed by the age of 2 but not complete until puberty. Radiation therapy in the early years, therefore, is expected to have serious effects on the child's brain. Radiation treatment can cause demyelination, white matter cavitation, and leukoencephalopathy months to years following therapy. The actual incidence and extent of cognitive dysfunction among children treated with irradiation are difficult to determine. A number of variables complicate the data including the underlying disease and its associated pathology (hydrocephalus or increased intracranial pressure), other therapies (chemotherapy and surgery), and the impact of the illness on body image, as well as school attendance. Psychomotor retardation may alter intellectual development as a result of radiation treatment.[20] Furthermore, alterations in intellectual,[20] emotional,[21] and academic functions, and problems of visual-motor integration, spatial placement, mild to moderate global loss in ability including decreased attention span and learning disability are not uncommonly observed.

Fifty percent of the children were found to have emotional disturbances including reactive depression, oppositional behavior, anxiety reactions, and schizoid disturbance.

LeBaron et al.,[1] in 1988, identified a number of deficits in the 15 children entered in their study. Ages ranged from 6 to 19 years. Nine patients had medulloblastoma, one had ependymoma, and five had astrocytoma. Radiation therapy was given to all of the children with medulloblastoma and ependymoma, and one of the children with astrocytoma. Results demonstrated that 50% of children experienced serious problems including motor, sensory, cognitive, academic, and emotional difficulties.

All of the above studies demonstrate the need for careful assessment of children prior to the initiation of therapy, as well as regular follow-up. Children with posterior fossa tumors are at risk for neuropsychological impairment in relation to their treatment.

At our institution, children undergo neuropsychological evaluation prior to onset of therapy. Reevaluation is done after completion of therapy. Children with deficits are identified and referred for appropriate therapies and special education as needed. To facilitate the child's return, a staff meeting is held at the child's school. Included are the principal, classroom teacher, school nurse, and any other teachers involved with the child, as well as our Neurosurgery nurse clinician, Pediatric Hematology/Oncology nurse clinician, and Oncology social worker. Information about the child's diagnosis and treatment are provided, as well as the results of the neuropsychological

evaluation. Efforts then are made as a team to provide the most appropriate education program for the child as needed. Overall, we have had a very favorable response to this approach.

Cerebellar Mutism

At our institution, the family receives advanced preparation about a peculiar phenomenon that may occur following posterior fossa craniotomy: cerebellar mutism. Disturbances in speech following resection of posterior fossa tumors have been reported in the literature. The term "cerebellar mutism" has been used to refer to the complete absence of speech in a conscious person, without lesions of the neuraxis or, more rarely, with such lesions.[22]

Six forms of mutism have been identified, depending on the area of the nervous system affected: (a) lesions in Broca's area, (b) lesions in the supplementary motor area of the dominant hemisphere, (c) lesions in the mesencephalic reticular formation, (d) bilateral thalamotomy, (e) pseudobulbar palsy, and (f) bilateral pharyngeal or vocal cord paralysis.[23]

Since 1985, a number of cases have been published that would fall under the category of "cerebellar mutism." These children, who ranged in age from 2 to 11 years, underwent removal of a large midline posterior fossa tumor; preoperative symptoms were primarily cerebellar deficits and intracranial hypertension. In addition, the mutism usually began 18 to 72 hours postoperatively with no change in level of consciousness, no deficits of the lower cranial nerves, and no disturbance of the phonatory organs. The duration of the mutism was usually 3 to 16 weeks, with speech recovery after a period of dysarthria in a number of the children.[24]

Ammirati et al.,[25] in 1988, reported a case of a 14-year-old boy who underwent a suboccipital craniotomy for resection of an astrocytoma. On the second postoperative day, the child was unable to speak. He was able to follow commands but could only cry when asked to speak. In the third postoperative week he was able to speak two-syllables words; by 5 weeks he was dysarthric but able to speak in two- to three-word sentences. At 4 months postoperatively, the dysarthria was minimal.

Recently, we had a $3\frac{1}{2}$-year-old girl who was diagnosed with an ependymoma of the posterior fossa at the age of 21 months. The tumor was completely resected and a ventriculoperitoneal shunt was inserted at that time. Thirteen months later, she was found to have a 2-cm lesion in the left cerebellar peduncle. She underwent a suboccipital craniotomy for total removal followed by 30 fractions of radiation therapy. Seven months later, a lesion was noted in the fourth ventricle and 3 months later, the patient again underwent a suboccipital craniotomy for debulking of the tumor. Prior to this surgical intervention, the patient was talking without difficulty. Postoperatively, she was unable to speak, and could only whine or cry. She was able to follow commands and gesture for what she wanted but was emotionally regressed. Within 4 weeks, the mutism had almost completely resolved. The child continues to have dysarthric speech but is improving.

The exact mechanism involved with cerebellar mutism is uncertain at this time. However, a combination of functional and organic factors may be involved.[24] We believe this is a complex phenomenon of emotional regression. Because recovery has been noted to occur once the child is discharged home, negative feelings on the part of the child who may feel betrayed by parents and medical staff are a possibility. Substantiating this viewpoint are the following: the absence of cranial nerve deficits, integrity of the supratentorial speech centers, and the ability to understand spoken language and to communicate by gesturing.[24,26]

The functional theory, however, does not explain either why this only occurs with children who have posterior fossa tumors, or the dysarthria that follows the mutism. Possible organic factors may include extensive damage to the cerebellar parenchyma, vascular disturbances—either ischemia or edema, disturbances in cerebraspinal fluid (CSF) circulation, and postoperative meningitis.[24] Further investigation of this phenomenon is warranted.

The occurrence of cerebellar mutism can be quite upsetting to children and their families.

Because these children are alert, the sudden inability to speak can be frightening as well as frustrating. If appropriate, parents and their children should be prepared for its possibility when discussion and consent for surgery are undertaken. If mutism occurs, the child and family need further information regarding the phenomenon and assurance of its self-limiting nature. Also, the child needs assistance in communicating his/her needs and feelings. The speech therapist is invaluable in assisting with this process.

Effects of Posterior Fossa Tumors on Parents

The family is a dynamic, interdependent unit that can weaken in the face of disequilibrium. When a child is diagnosed with a posterior fossa tumor, the illness touches every member of the family. The impact can be felt in the relationships of family members, in job performance, in social relationships, and in financial concerns.

When a child is diagnosed with a brain tumor in the posterior fossa, the parents are confronted with a number of challenges. The ability of the family to respond to these challenges can influence the manner in which the child will cope with the tumor. After receiving the news that their child has a brain tumor, the parents may experience a number of emotions including disbelief, shock, anger, fear, guilt, and confusion. How the information is presented to them can influence their emotional responses. It is important when giving the diagnosis to avoid overwhelming the parents with excessive medical jargon, prolonged explanations of pathophysiology, and specific details of the treatment process. In most instances, this amount of information will be beyond their comprehension. The parents will need to hear the information repeatedly before they are able to understand it.

It is extremely important for parents and the child to understand the illness. The child's symptoms are complicated first by the presence of the tumor in the posterior fossa, which can cause ataxia, titubation, incoordination, and difficulty with speech (disarticulation). The presence of obstructive hydrocephalus can further complicate the situation. Because of the associated signs and symptoms of increased intracranial pressure, the hydrocephalus may be more problematic for the child than the tumor itself.

After the initial shock of the diagnosis, some parents, in an effort to find answers to their multitude of questions, will go on a search for information. It is at this time that more details can be given to the family about the tumor and treatment plan. Pamphlets and other literature may be helpful for parents. In our experience, a number of families have requested to meet other families of children with the same diagnosis. Advice and support are shared between them and friendships often develop in the process. The entire family can benefit from such a relationship.

The child with a posterior fossa tumor can absorb much of the parent's time and energy. It is often difficult for the parents to find time to care for themselves. Outings with friends or even a "date" for the parents may be nearly impossible. Lack of child care coupled with guilt on the part of the parents may prevent them from spending much needed time away from their child. Heffron et al.,[27] in a group discussion of parents with leukemic children, reported some problems with friends. Many friends were found to be well meaning but unable to talk with the parents about the severity of the illness. In addition, friends slowly began leaving the parents out of activities until finally they were completely isolated. Others reported that they were fortunate enough to have several close friends who maintained their support while other friends faded away.

The failure to maintain a balance between competing needs in a family may be expressed in marital difficulties. Review of the literature on divorce noted that divorce is no more likely in families with a chronically ill child than in families with healthy children.[28-30] However, the degree of tension and stress in such families runs higher than in families without a child who is chronically ill. Marital integration, harmony, distress, agreement, and friction have been assessed and, overall, parents of chronically ill children appeared more distressed than those with healthy children. Parents of children with posterior fossa tumors will require much support and assistance in working through their problems. They must be encouraged to maintain communication between themselves and to seek support and counseling as needed.

Having a child with a posterior fossa tumor can greatly impact on the parents' ability to effectively perform at work. Today, many families require both parents to work to meet financial demands. However, this is not always possible. Frequent hospitalizations, clinic visits, and diagnostic tests mean taking time from work to be with the child.

Employers may be sympathetic, initially, but as the requests for time off continue, they may be less willing to allow the parents to be away from the job. Further, preoccupation with their child's illness may prevent the parents from putting forth their full effort at work. As the child's condition deteriorates, more time is needed for care and one or both parents may have to leave work indefinitely. This can further add to the stress of an already difficult situation.

Though it is not the primary concern of most families, financial matters are a major and constant burden. Regardless of the type of insurance coverage, it is often insufficient. The specific financial burdens arise from a number of sources. Surgery, hospitalizations, clinic visits, diagnostic tests, medications, and nursing care can slowly drain the family of its resources. In addition to these major expenses, smaller costs related to the daily care of the child are incurred. Fees for transportation and parking for hospital and clinic visits, the cost of babysitters for other siblings, and the cost of equipment add to the cost of care.

The combined costs of medical care for the child with a posterior fossa tumor can lead to financial hardship for the family. Parents and siblings may be deprived of basic needs as well as luxuries such as a family vacation because of the expenses of the child.

The impact of chronic illness on the patient and parents is well identified in the literature. The effects of the illness on healthy siblings has received far less attention. Groundwork began in the 1960s, looking at the effects of a child's death on the siblings. Since the late 1970s, the focus of research was on the perceptions of siblings and parents about what living with a child with chronic or catastrophic illness means for the sibling(s).[31] A number of studies looked at the parents' perceptions of the siblings' response to the illness, with fewer studies focused on the siblings' perceptions of the illness.

Binger et al.,[32] in 1969, found that in approximately 50% of the families of leukemic children, one or more previously well siblings showed behavior patterns that indicated coping difficulties. Problems described by the parents included headaches, enuresis, abdominal pain, depression, separation anxiety, and school phobia. In addition, siblings felt guilty and feared they too might suffer a fatal illness.

Cairns et al.,[33] in 1979, studed 71 families of children with cancer. Results revealed that siblings of children with cancer have significant anxiety, fear for their own health, and social isolation from both family and friends. Iles,[34] in 1979, also investigated siblings' perceptions during the illness experience of the child with cancer. A number of losses were identified including disrupted relationships, physical changes in the ill sibling, and disturbed family routines.

Because of the nature of the illness, siblings of children with posterior fossa tumors face a number of stressors. Frequent hospitalizations result in separation of the healthy sibling from the parents as well as the ill sibling. The healthy child may be shuffled between family members and babysitters. The financial strain caused by the illness may result in the loss of vacations and other leisure activities with the family. Also, the healthy child may have to sacrifice some personal items to enable the family to meet medical expenses.

Further, the healthy sibling may lose the relationship once had with the ill sibling. Playing together, sharing secrets, and teasing each other may no longer be possible because of the illness. The sibling has to look elsewhere for children to share these activities with and may or may not be successful in doing so. The experience of having a sibling with cancer, however, cannot be assumed to be totally negative. Iles[34] found in interviewing siblings

of children with cancer that the illness provided an opportunity for growth and increased knowledge of the disease and its treatment; the development of respect for the ill sibling also identified the healthy children's perceptions of what has helped or would help them through the experience. Having a best friend, knowing what to expect, being there, feeling special, and having others think the child is someone special were mentioned by healthy siblings to be helpful.

It is important, therefore, to remember the siblings when we deal with the child with a posterior fossa tumor. They are often overlooked in the process of caring for the sick child. The parents must be reminded to provide support for the siblings and include them in the treatment plan as much as possible. Though the siblings may not verbalize their feelings, they undoubtedly are affected.

Summary

Caring for children with posterior fossa tumors is a challenge. An aggressive approach must be taken to meet the many needs of the child and family. Education of the patient and family are essential to the plan of care and preparation is needed for treatments and tests. Neuropsychological testing should be performed to identify problems and evaluate long-term progress. Based on the results, an individualized educational plan must be devised in collaboration with the school system. Parents and teachers must be educated about the effects of the tumor, hydrocephalus, and radiation treatment on cognitive function. Psychomotor retardation will make new learning for the child more difficult. Patience on the part of the parents and teachers is essenital to prevent frustration. Cerebellar symptoms such as ataxia and titubation can place the child at risk of injury. Parents and teachers must be prepared for the child's safety in the home and school. The early initiation of rehabilitation medicine is also important to promote function. Preparation of the child's peers for the return to school is also helpful for everyone. By educating the classmates, they may be less frightened by the child's altered appearance. This may prevent or minimize teasing of the child and make the transition back into school less traumatic. There is a need for additional studies that focus specifically on posterior fossa tumors. Much of the present literature has been on brain tumors in general. Retrospective as well as prospective studies are needed with larger sample sizes to examine the long-term effects of the tumor on the child as well as on the family. Further, the role of hydrocephalus and cognitive disturbances must be identified.

References

1. LeBaron S, Zeltzer PM, Zelter LK, Scott SE, Marlin AE. Assessment of quality of survival in children with medulloblastoma and cerebellar astrocytoma. *Cancer.* 1988;62:1215–1222.
2. Bloom HJG. Concepts in the natural history and treatment of medulloblastoma in children. *CRC Crit Rev Radiol Sci.* 1971;2:89–143.
3. Bonner K, Siegel K. Pathology, treatment and management of posterior fossa brain tumors in childhood. *J Neurosci Nurs* 1988;20(2):84–93.
4. Katz SR, Kellerinan J, Siegel SE. Behavioral distress in children with cancer undergoing medical procedures: Developmental considerations. *J Consult Clin Psychol.* 1980;48:356.
5. Posnanski E. Children's reaction to pain: A psychiatrist's perspective. *Clin Pediatr.* 1976; 12:1114–1119.
6. Broome E. The child in pain: A model for assessment and intervention. *Crit Care Q.* 1985;8(1):47–55.
7. Schechter NL, Allen DA, Hansen K. Status of pediatric pain control: A comparison of hospital analgesic usage in children and adults. *Pediatrics.* 1986;77(1):34–35.
8. Beyer JE, Ashley LC, Russell GA, DeGood DE. Pediatric pain after cardiac surgery: pharamacological management. *Dimens Crit Care Nurs.* 1984;3:326–334.
9. Eland JM. Pharamacologic management of acute and chronic pediatric pain. *Issues Comprehens Pediatr Nurs.* 1988;11:93–111.
10. Mott SR, Fazekas NF, James SR. *Nursing Care of Children and Families.* Menlo Park: Addision-Wesley; 1985.
11. Nagy M. The child's view of death. In: Feifel H, *The Meaning of Death.* New York: McGraw-Hill; 1959:3–27.
12. Bluebond-Langer M. Field Research on Children's and Adult's Views of Death. Field Notes, 1975.
13. Bluebond-Langer M. Field Research on Children's and Adult's Views of Death. Field Notes, 1976.
14. Bluebond-Langer M: Meanings of death to children. In: Feifel H, ed. *New Meanings of Death.* New York: McGaw-Hill; 1977.
15. Bruner JS, Jolly A, Sylva K, eds. *Play.* New York: Basic Books; 1976.
16. Cass J. *Helping Children Grow Through Play.* New York: Shocken Books; 1973.
17. Chance P. *Learning Through Play.* New York: Gardner-Press; 1979.
18. Ellis MJ. *Why People Play.* Englewood Cliffs, NJ: Prentice-Hall; 1973.
19. Millar S. *The Psychology of Play.* London: Cox & Wyman; 1968.
20. Spunberg JJ, Chang CH, Goldman M, Auricchio E, Bell JJ. Quality of long-term survival following irradiation for intracranial tumors in children under the age of two. *Radiat Oncol Biol Phys.* 1981;7(6):727–736.
21. Kun LE, Mulhern RK, Crisco JJ. Quality of life in children treated for brain tumors. *J Neurosurg.* 1983;58:1–6.
22. Brain WR. *Speech Disorders: Aphasia, Apraxia and Agnosia.* 2nd ed. London: Butterworths; 1965:1–121.
23. Benson DF. *Aphasia, Alexia and Agraphia.* New York: Churchill Livingston; 1979:163–164.
24. Ferrante L, Mastronardi L, Acqui M, Fortuna A. Mutism after posterior fossa surgery in children. *J Neurosurg.* 1990;72:959–963.
25. Ammirati M, Mirzai S, Samii M. Transient mutism following removal of a cerebellar tumor. *Childs Nerv Syst.* 1988(5):12–14.
26. Rekate HL, Grubb RL, Aram DM, Hahn JF, Ratcheson RA. Muteness of cerebellar origin. *Arch Neurol.* 1985;42:697–698.
27. Heffron WA, Bommelaere K, Masters R. Groups discussions with the parents of leukemic children. *Pediatrics.* 1973;52(6):831–840.
28. Kalnins I. Cross-illness comparisons of separation and divorce among parents having a child with a life-threatening illness. *Child Health Care.* 1983;12:72–77.
29. Lansky SB, Cairns NU, Hassanein R, Wehr J, Lowman JT. Childhood cancer: Parental discord and divorce. *Pediatrics.* 1978;62(2):184–188.
30. Lansky SB, Cairns NU, Lansky LL, Cairns GF, Stephenson L, Garin G. Central nervous

system prophylaxis studies showing impairment in verbal skills and academic achievement. *Am J Pediatr Hematol Oncol*. 1984;6(2):183–190.

31. Lynn MR. Siblings' responses in illness situations. *J Pediatr Nurs*. 1989;4(2):127–129.

32. Binger CM, Ablin AR, Feuerstein RC, Kushner, JH, Zoger S, Mikkelsen C. Childhood leukemia, emotional impact on patient and family. *N Engl J Med*. 1969;280:414–418.

33. Cairns NU, Clark GM, Smith SD, Lansky SB. Adaptation of siblings to childhood malignancy. *J Pediatr*. 1979;95(3):484–487.

34. Iles JP. Children with cancer: healthy siblings' perceptions during the illness experience. *Cancer Nurs*. 1979(2):371–377.

35. Bluebond-Langer M. *Awareness and Communication in Terminally Ill Children: Pattern, Process, and Pretense*. Unpublished doctoral dissertation, University of Illinois, 1975.

36. Duffner PK, Cohen ME, Thomas P. Late effects of treatment on the intelligence of children with posterior fossa tumors. *Cancer*. 1983;51:233–237.

37. Mulhern RK, Kun LE. Neuropsychologic function in children with brain tumors: III. Interval changes in the six months following treatment. *Med Pediat Oncol*. 1985;13:318–324.

38. Rowland JH, Glidewell OJ, Sibley RF, Holland JC, Tull R, Berman A, Brecher ML, Harris M, Glicksman AS, Forman E, Jones B, Cohen ME, Duffner PK, Freeman AI. Effects of different forms of central nervous system prophylaxis on neuropsychological function in childhood leukemia. *J Clin Oncol*. 1984;2(12):1327–1335.

39. Sabbeth B, Leventhal J. Marital adjustment to chronic childhood illness: A critique of the literature. *Pediatrics*. 1984;73:763–768.

40. Spinetta JJ, Rigler D, Karon M. Anxiety in the dying child. *Pediatrics*. 1973;52:841–845.

Index